WHE[illegible] WOODHAM FERRIS?

by

Les A. Holden

Illustrated by John Frankland

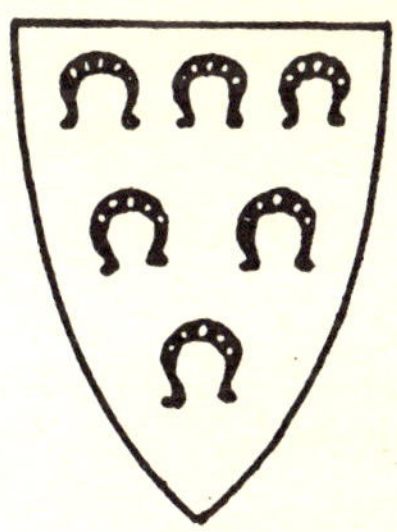

The Shield of Henry de Ferrers
who was given
The Manor of Woodham
for his part in
The Battle of Hastings, 1066

Printed in England
by
Simmons Printers, Chelmsford 266005

Preface

It was not easy for a small village like South Woodham Ferrers to absorb the large housing estates which were built there in the 1960s. To be then told that it is to be a mini-new town, with a population rise of from 950 to 18,000, was most disturbing for the residents. Particularly so for Les Holden, who had lived in this quiet rural haven for fifty years. However, Les is a craftsman, and as he worked with his wood, he quickly reverted to his old habit of thinking out ways in which he could help the growing community.
For seven years, I was the project manager for the new town, and I had many quiet talks with Les. We agreed that new residents in the town needed to know something of its roots, of the history of the area in which they now lived. The result is this book: his gentle tale of rural Essex, which I commend to all who love this land of ours.

Paul S Chester
April, 1986

Foreword

I first visited South Woodham Ferrers inadvertently in 1977, when I got lost late at night between Maldon and Rettendon. The road I was driving on petered out in a sea of mud surrounded by new buildings on all sides, and I slowly realised that what I saw in my headlights was a new town being born. New, that is, to me - Les Holden had lived there for years - and when, as the local Member of Parliament, I got to know the town better, I soon realised that he was the local historian.

Appropriately then, his book describes life a hundred years ago, and is the story of a ship's boy, whose first journey by sailing barge is from Wapping to Woodham, via Canvey and Leigh, on the Thames, and past Burnham, Fambridge and Hullbridge, on the Crouch.

As time passes, and the lad becomes a sea captain hardened by war, he makes further journeys into Essex and describes our homes and villages of yester-year. The generous use of dialogue, masterly illustrations, and the fascination of familiar place names linked together in an historical novel, make for easy reading.

Truly, a local book by a local man, enshrining the past for us all.

Michael Clark, MP
House of Commons, June, 1986

Acknowledgements

It is not easy for one with limited qualifications, such as myself, to write a book and its outcome is the result of people's encouragement and conation. 'Where's Woodham Ferris' would never have been written had it not been for the initiative of Mr Paul Chester, the then project manager for the new town of South Woodham Ferrers, whose sincere persuasion convinced me that my memories were worthy to record.

To Kathleen Peyton, whose literary works are so well known, saying the right word at the right time - in fact, just when I had decided to cast my waning effort overboard.

To John Frankland, my illustrator, whose skill and insistence for perfection can only enhance any production.

To the many senior citizens of South Woodham and Woodham Ferrers who suffered my questioning and cross-questions in persuit of information.

To Alf Pinner, and others of the bargeing fraternity.

To all who feel that they may have helped, please accept my thanks.

To Audrey, my wife, and Hazel, my daughter, who endured me living in a trance while 'Where's Woodham Ferris' was being conceived in my mind.

Not forgetting Avril, my daughter, who deciphered and typed my script.

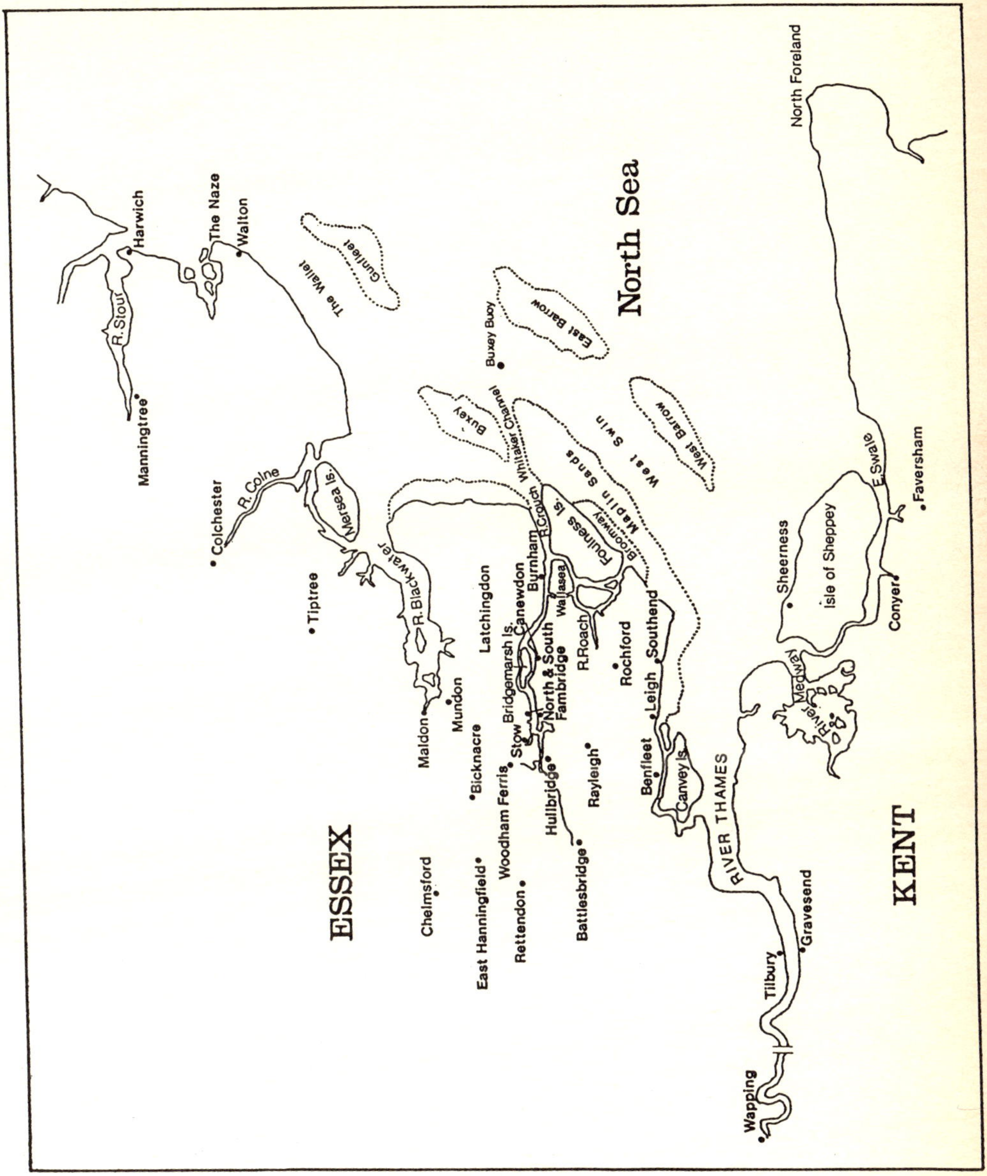

JIMMIE'S INITIAL SAILING AREA

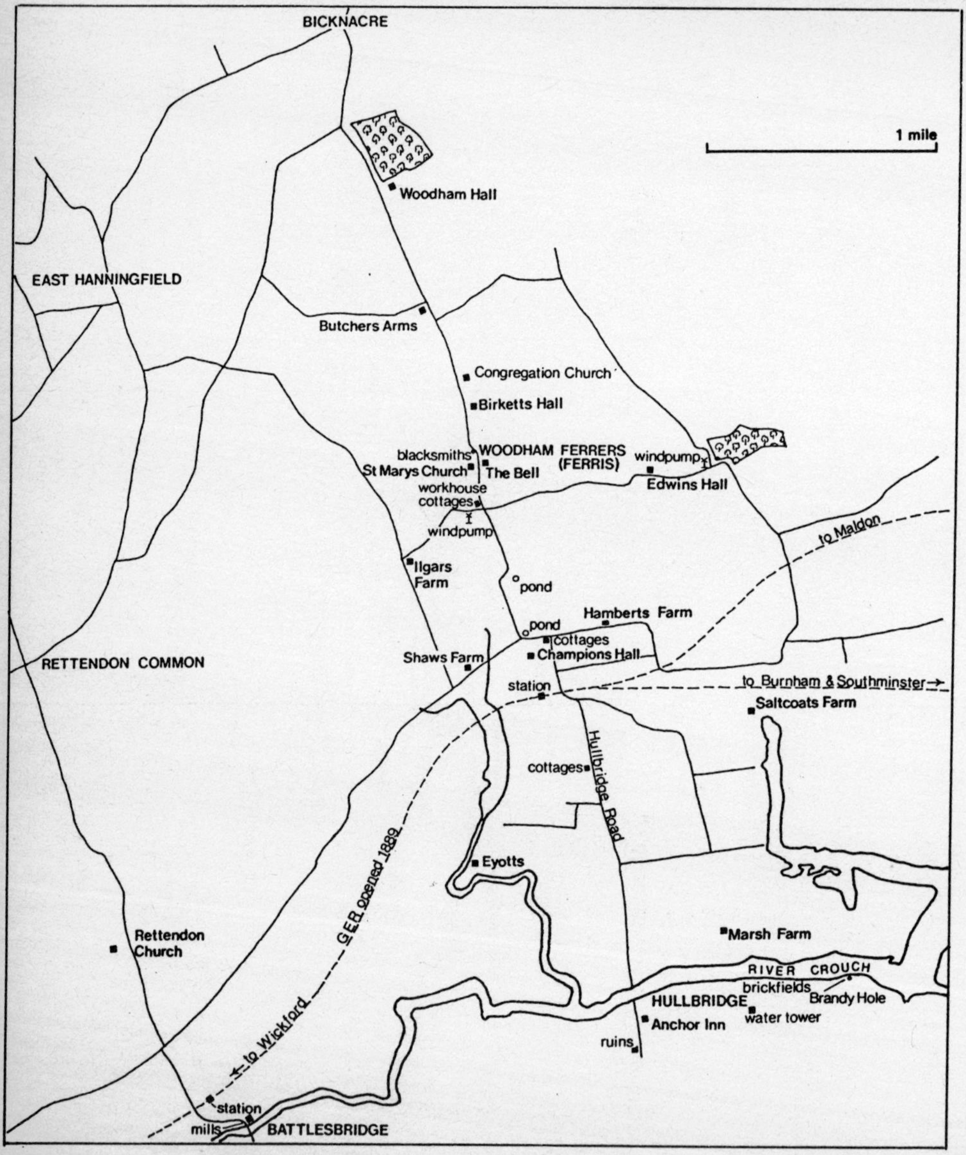

JIMMIE'S INITIAL AREA OF DISCOVERY INTO ESSEX

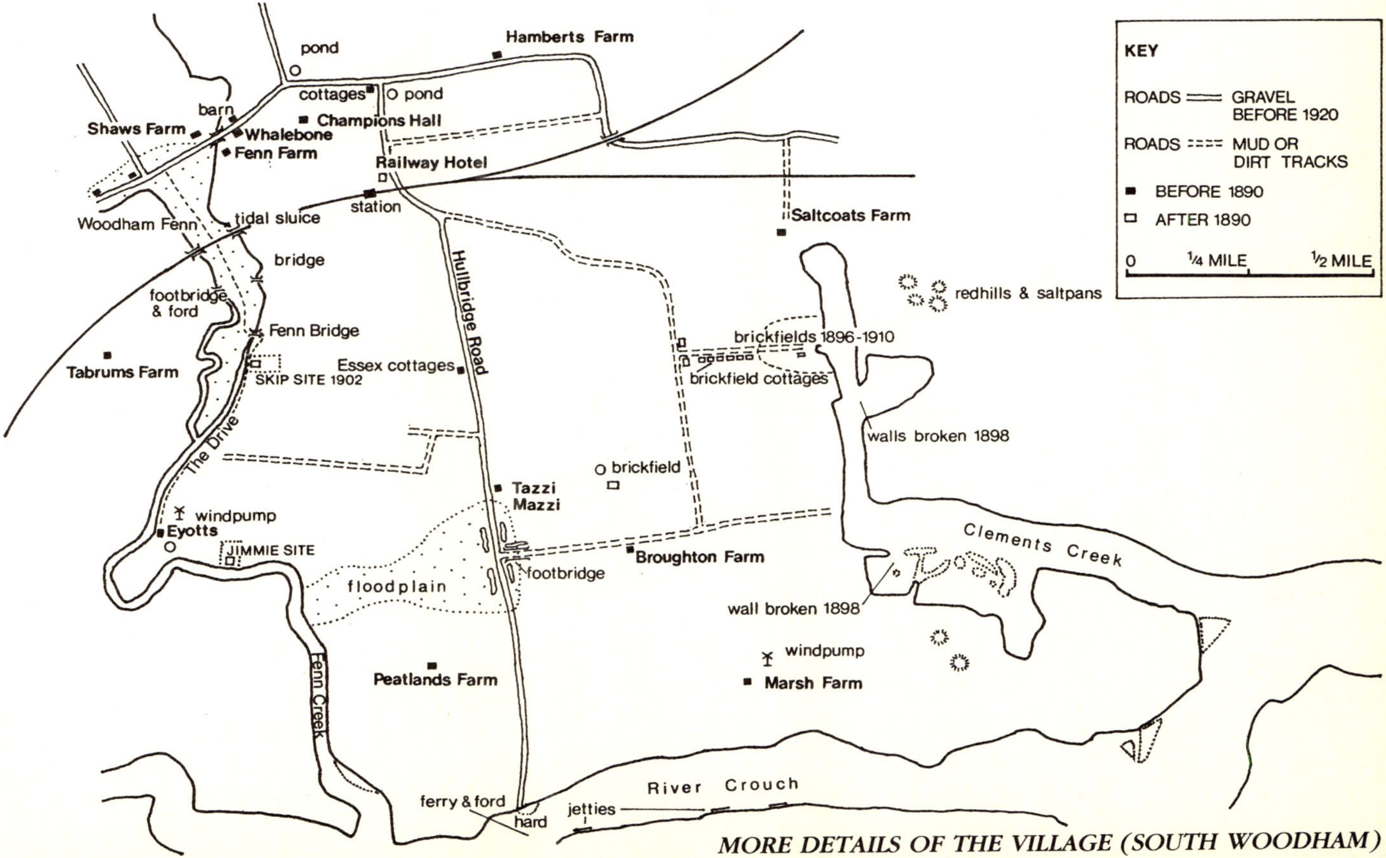

MORE DETAILS OF THE VILLAGE (SOUTH WOODHAM)

CONTENTS

MAPS AND ILLUSTRATIONS

MAPS

ILLUSTRATIONS

Introduction

Two men, strangers, stood admiring the stately form of Tower Bridge which spans the River Thames.

"From what I can see of it, it certainly is a most wonderful example of man's ingenuity, but I'm darned if I can fathom out how it works."

"It's what you cannot see that makes it work, sir," said another man standing close by. He was the engineer responsible for the construction of the bridge.

The villages of the British Isles are often lonely, rugged, fascinating and quaint. Some are really wonderful. We drive through them, we park our cars and walk their cobbled streets, we take a drink in their old pubs and visit their ancient churches. We walk around their country manors and while away our time in little museums, but like the man looking at Tower Bridge, we call them wonderful and walk away not really knowing how they work. Villages, like bridges, have beginnings and some, sad to say, have drastic endings.

The south ward of the village of Woodham Ferris (Ferrers), alias South Woodham in the county of Essex, has, during the last hundred years, been conceived, born, matured and died.

No, not quite.

In the process, it has itself given birth to a New Town, now called South Woodham Ferrers, which has left the parent village of Woodham Ferrers to retain its own identity.

This has happened, not by the wish or desire of its locals, but by progressive man, raping the Old to create the New: and it has happened not once, but twice, since 1889.

This book is dedicated to those people who resided in the area from 1840 onwards, and to those who came from all parts of the world, between 1889 and 1939, to create not a medieval village, not even an olde worlde English village, but to establish a cosmopolitan community that would, unknowingly, bridge the eras of sail, steam and the combustion engine and on into the space age. The first birth occurred because of the steam era, when the Great Eastern Railway Company introduced the wonders of the steam engine to the Dengie Hundred in 1889.

I knew personally some of the characters who lived before that happened, who worked on the building of the Wickford to Southminster and Maldon lines; others who sailed their barges from London to serve the villages and transported the materials to build the railways; and others who settled here in order to start a new life.

Although young, I listened intently as they related their experiences, I tried to understand their problems and heartaches. From an abundance of stories I learned to laugh when they laughed and felt like crying when they cried.

With that background of information, I have endeavoured to condense the many characters into just a few, and the many stories into one, hopefully that you, my readers, may get to know some of the deep emotional feelings that lie hidden deep down in a growing village community.

"It's what you cannot see that makes a village work."

Look at the old man trudging wearily away from the local river. You may think he is just a village yokel, with little to contribute to society. He touches his cap in respect and passes on. In fact, you could be in any village in our country. Read "Where's Woodham Ferris?" and you may discover that you have misjudged him.

PART ONE

Chapter One

Jimmie Meets Skip

Wapping, Friday 13th June, 1879

The old boarded door of number twelve, Riverview Cottages, crashed against its rickety frame, the impact reverberating through the equally rickety building. An old scraggy mongrel dog, lying on the worn brick floor, opened one eye and looked in the direction of the interruption of his siesta. He had heard it all so many times before, so he tucked his nose down again.

"Where's Wudum Ferrus?" The shout echoed through the cottage like the crash of the door. This time, the old mongrel really came to life, jumped up and raced round the table, barking furiously. From a door at the rear of the room, a rather voluminous woman in a tattered frock appeared. Her sleeves were rolled up above her elbows, and round her waist was tied a large hessian apron, from which the water from the washing tub dripped. Shaking her fist, she enquired as to the cause of all the commotion.

"Jimmie Brown," she shouted, "You'll do that once too often, an' the 'ole damn place will fall on our 'eads. Ain't you got any savvy at all?"

"I'm sorry, Mum. I never fort."

"You never do, do yer? Wotever yer told goes in one ear an' out t'uther. 'Eaven knows wot sort of a man you'll grow up ter be. Wot's it all about this time?"

"I only wanna know where Wudum Ferrus is, Mum."

"Is that all! The way yer came in I thort the River Thames 'ad cort fire. Wot yer wanna know for, anyhow?"

"'Cos I'm goin' there termorrer."

Jimmie's mother shook the copper-stick in his face. "Not till after yer've mucked the stables out, my boy. Yer not gettin' away wiv it two days!"

"But I've got anuver job, Mum."

"Oh ye'. An' wot's it this time? A sentry outside Buckin'am Palace? 'Cos I can't imagine 'er Majesty would want you struttin'up an' down outside 'er 'ouse wiv a gun!"

"No, Mum. I'm goin' to be a sea Cap'n."

"Good Gawd! Wapping's answer to Nelson! Any'ow, it makes a change from an ingin driver. I've no idea w'ere this Wudum Ferrus is, but I've a good idea yer father wants 'is dinner, so yer 'ad better come down to earth an' go an' tell 'im it's ready."

Jimmie turned and left the house, followed by the scraggy dog, with much of his enthusiasm for sailing dampened. Meanwhile, his Mum had forgotten all about the crashing door, and was feeling somewhat anxious about her eldest son, thirteen years old that day. He could hardly read or write, yet had a vivid sense of imagination and was full of hopes for a future at sea, but had little chance of fulfilling those dreams.

Turning suddenly in the alley outside the cottage, Jimmie grabbed the dog by its collar and dragged it up onto its hind legs. Then, looking straight into its eyes, he said, "Bingo, one of these days I'll show 'em all that Jimmie

Brown is not as daft as 'e looks." He then let go of his collar and kicked a stone along the alleyway for the dog to retrieve.

Dad was a stable-man for a large firm of carriers who collected the freight from the docks by the riverside and delivered to warehouses all over London. Keeping the stables clean for some two hundred horses was a major operation. A team of men and stable-boys would toil from early morning until late afternoon to keep pace with the task. The muck removed from the stables was taken to the nearby quayside, and stacked. Week after week, red-sailed barges would tie up, unload hay or straw, then sail off into the unknown, laden with horse manure.

It was the mystery of where it all went that intrigued Jimmie. He had questioned his father, but received only negative replies. "Dunno son, as long as it's out of my way I don' care wot they do wiv it."

That reply, as well as others, did not satisfy Jimmie. He wanted a positive answer. So it was, when his father had called him to go to work that morning, that he had pretended to have stomach-ache. After all, he was thirteen today, and a day away from the stables would not come amiss, though he was still surprised when Dad told him to come along later.

By eight o'clock Jimmie was up and making his way to the river. On the quayside, men with long forks were throwing the dung into the moored barges. Having spent so many of his boyhood days playing around the dockyards, and on the boats, he knew where to find the crew. He jumped the eighteen inches down onto the deck and quickly made his way to the crew's quarters. He timidly knocked on the cabin door.

He waited with a certain amount of apprehension, and wondered whether he had done the right thing. A rather gruff voice told him to come in. Slowly opening the door, Jimmie stepped inside.

Lying on a bunk bed, fully dressed even to a black bowler perched on his head, was the skipper. His long black beard flowed down, covering his hands folded on his chest. What could be seen of his face was as red as the sails of the barge. Both man and boy stared at each other. Jimmie felt his legs getting weaker, and quickly looked around the cabin to escape the glare of the man before him. In the forced silence, he noticed that everything was trim and perfect. The brasses shone, even the little cast-iron stove was polished black.

"And who told you to come aboard my ship?" the skipper shouted.

This quickly brought Jimmie to face again the man he thought to be very old and fierce.

"N n n no one, sir," he stuttered.

"Then what are you doing here?" was the curt reply.

Jimmie began to wish that he had not set out on his investigation, then mustered up sufficient courage to say, "I only came ter find out where yer take the 'orse dung to, sir."

"Stop on board, then you'll find out," was the quick answer.

These words caused Jimmie to gasp for breath. He had heard many stories of boys and men being forced to serve on boats under terrible conditions. And now he had walked into a trap. He turned towards the open door, but his suspected captor was ahead of him.

"Close the door, boy," he shouted, "or I'll set the dog on you!"

With a trembling hand, Jimmie did as he was told.
"Now, sit on that stool! No one comes aboard my ship asking impertinent questions and leaves until I give my permission. Do you understand that, boy?"
"Y y yes, sir," Jimmie feebly murmured.
The old man turned on the bunk, swung his legs round, and sat up straight. It was then that the lad saw the skipper's right hand. It made him feel sick! It had a knarled thumb, but the rest was just a ghastly, gory mess of torn, red flesh. He turned away in horror, closing his eyes and catching his breath. He wished that he had gone to work.
"How old are you, boy?" was the skipper's next question. This time, Jimmie sensed a more civil approach.
"I'm firteen today, sir."
There was another period of silence, broken only by the thud of the dung being loaded on board. Jimmie watched as the old man buried his face in his hands. The sight of the gory one, pressed against the skipper's eyes, made Jimmie wince. Perhaps this would be his last chance to get away. He raised himself quietly from the stool, but at the same time a growl and a scuffle came from under the bunk. A brown and white terrier bared its teeth at the terrified boy, and he sat down at once.
"You can start tomorrow." This time the man's voice was subdued.
"Start wot?" asked Jimmie.
"Work, boy. Work. If you know what that is."
"Yes, sir. Wot'll I 'ave to do, sir?"
"Keep an eye on that stuff in the hold."
Jimmie detected a slight grin on the skipper's face. It would seem he was not now a prisoner, or maybe it was still a trap.
"Be here at seven o'clock sharp. We'll be sailing on the morning ebb."
"Where to?" chipped in Jimmie.
"Woodham Ferris. Now off you go. Bring along a change of clothes, if you have one, and tell your parents, if you have any, that we'll be back in ten days. And call me Skip in future."
In a rather bewildered state of mind, Jimmie got up from the stool and lifted the latch on the cabin door.
"Before you go, what is your name?" asked Skip.
Jimmie stopped. Looking back, he thought the skipper seemed a different man from when he had entered the cabin. Somehow, he felt a strange affection towards him.
"Aw, call me Jimmie. That's wot me muvver calls me, sir. Skip, I mean."
Suddenly the skipper's head dropped forward. Once more he covered his face with his hands. Jimmie turned and went down on his knees in front of the older man.
"Is there suffink wrong, sir? Can I go an' get some 'elp?"
Putting his good hand on the boy's shoulder, Skip mumbled, "No lad, all I need is a good sleep. So off you go, and don't be late in the morning."
Jimmie left the cabin, then made his way onto the quayside. He wandered along the dockside to find a quiet spot where he could sit down, and have a think. Some bales of straw made a suitable place for him to sit and collect his thoughts. With his head resting in his cupped hands, he watched the

ever coming and going of men busy with their boats. While he had spent his life beside the river and docks, and had many dreams of sailing off one day, Jimmie had never before seriously thought he might really go to sea. The events of the morning had set new ambitions afire in his thinking. Unfortunately there was a large 'but'. Could he really work on a barge with that old man and that dreadful-looking hand?

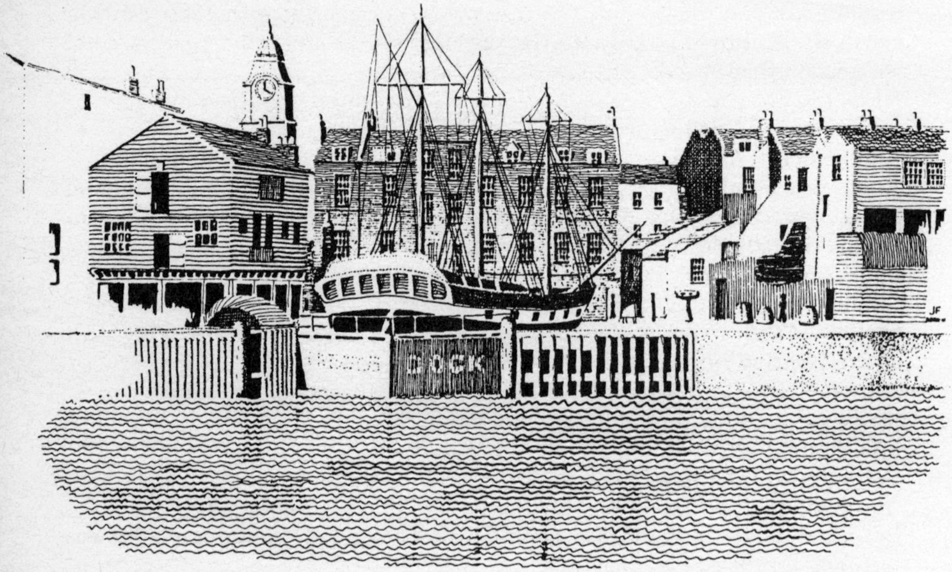

RIVERSIDE AT WAPPING

In his mind, Jimmie went through the scene again. He realised that he had surprised the skipper; then he had thought him a cruel and cunning man who had trapped him. It also occurred to him that the old man had spoken like a gentleman in the Big House where he took the washing: so different from the other barge men. Despite all the peculiarities of the skipper, Jimmie still felt he would like to sail with that boat on the morning tide. He then tried to picture where this place called Woodham Ferris might be.
He knew that big ships sailed all over the world. His schoolmaster had shown him the routes they took, by pointing out the dotted lines on the globe of the world. India, America, China, all sorts of places. Yet he could not remember any dotted lines going to Woodham Ferris.
The sun shone down and gave every indication of another sweltering day. Jimmie lay back on the straw, and pictured himself on the mighty sea, giving the crew their orders, as new lands came into view. Gradually sleep overtook him.
Some time later, a shout from one of the stablemen to shift his body brought Jimmie to his feet, his morning of dreaming over. He then decided he could not face this predicament alone and must now seek his Mum and Dad's advice.

But so far his Mum had been no help, and at her bidding he made his way to the stable block that his father was responsible for, and found him spreading clean straw over the floor.

"A clean bed them 'orses get every night. We're lucky if we get one once a month!"

Jimmie had been working with his father for nearly twelve months and had heard the same quip every day, so it seemed.

"'Ave you come to work, or just look?" shouted his father.

"No, Dad. To tell you your dinner's ready."

"I can do wiv it, 'avin' dun two men's work this mornin'."

"If you count me as a man, I should get a man's pay," retorted Jimmie.

"Orl right, me boy. Enuff ov the back chat. Let's get 'ome to dinner."

Dad took off his leather apron while Jimmie collected the tea-can from its hook. Then he gave Bingo, busy sniffing out a rat, a call. The three set off for number twelve. This time, the boy decided to use a more casual approach in finding out where his intended boat trip would take him.

"Ave you ever bin to Wudum Ferrus, Dad?"

"Where the 'ells that?"

"I dunno. I fort, you 'avin' gorn to so many places, you would 'ave known."

"Well, it's nowhere rawnd 'ere, Jimmie."

"I know that, Dad, 'cos you 'ave to go on a boat ter get there."

"Then why ask me? I've only ever bin on a 'orse, an' it's never taken me to Wudum Ferrus. Wot you wanna know for anyway?"

"'Cos I'm goin' there termorrer."

"Like 'ell you are! You're 'elping me muck out them stables, an' that's that."

Jimmie was flabbergasted. It did not matter what else happened, any thought or suggestion he made, if it upset the mucking out of the stables, then Mum and Dad did not want to know.

His hard thinking slowed his pace and his Dad was now some ten feet ahead of him. Suddenly he stopped and turned round to face his son.

"An' just 'ow were you goin' ter this Wudum Ferrus place, me boy?"

"On the 'Maywell', Dad."

"Oh, that stinkin' crate. 'Ave you bin talking to the skipper?"

"Yes, Dad, 'e's given me a job."

Jimmie saw his father thrust his thumbs into the thick leather belt round his waist. The sign was ominous to him. He turned to run. He did not want a strapping in the roadway.

"Come back 'ere you clot. I only want to talk."

Jimmie, holding Bingo's collar, walked nervously back and faced his father.

"Now look 'ere son. I reckon the smell of that 'orse dung as gorn to old Todd Summers' 'ead to arsk a gormless hulk like you ter work wiv 'im."

"I'm not that daft, Dad. I'll prove it to you one day."

"Let's 'ope you do, boy, but for the present you can forget abawt Todd Summers and the 'Maywell', an' learn ter be a decent 'orseman. I don't reckon 'e's ever sailed past Gravesend, let alone to Wudum Ferrus. 'E don't even talk like a bargeman! All 'e's fit for is to be a schoolmaster. So, forgit it naw, let's go an' 'ave our dinner, or your Mum'll be slinging it out the back door for the seagulls."

Jimmie knew it would be senseless to pursue the issue. Dad's word was final. The remainder of the journey home was made in silence.

Mealtimes at the Brown's were not of the highest standard. Around a rough boarded table sat Jimmie's two younger brothers, two younger sisters, Mum, Dad, then himself, Bingo and the two cats. In the middle of the table stood a large cast-iron saucepan, thickly coated with soot, and from which issued a rather fatty smell. The contents Mum ladled out into basins and then a lump of bread was given to each of the children. This was immediately submerged in the stew and, despite the unpleasant smell, the whole lot was devoured in minutes. The only remark passed was that Dad thought the scrag-end stew was a little short of scrag-end.

Jimmie was relieved that no remarks had been made about the morning's episode, so he proudly reminded the family that it was his thirteenth birthday. Mum confirmed that he was correct; Dad said it could be possible, as you have one each year, but he preferred to forget such occasions because it made him feel older.

"Now I know why you didn't come to work, young man, and seein' I've dun your share already, yer may as well 'ave the rest of the day orf."

"Thanks, Dad, now I can go and see Grandad."

"And you can also take the washin' back to Mrs Marshall on the way," said his mother.

Jimmie knew this would make a longer walk, but he would be sure of a penny when he got there, so it would be well worthwhile.

Grandad was held in high esteem by Jimmie. He could not only listen for hours on end to the stories the old man could tell, but Grandad always had time to listen to him. Today he had a problem. Should he ignore the advice of his father and mother, and leave home against their wish? Should he join the 'Maywell', or stay put and be a stable-boy?

He knew of other boys who had done just that. Fortunately, his parents were not cruel to him, as were some other boys' parents, but life was not at all easy. He worked a full day at the stables, then was general dogsbody for all the errands and jobs at home. For this he got little praise and lots of grumbles.

Whilst he was a big boy for his age, he objected to being called an awkward gawk and daft. He was certain Grandad would listen and give him good advice.

Grandad had been born in 1791 and was now the ripe old age of eighty-four, and still alert in his mind. He had been a sailor all his working life. Jimmie was always proud of the fact that his Grandad had served under Lord Nelson as a powder-boy at the Battle of Trafalgar.

The washing delivered, and the penny for doing so received, Jimmie made his way through the hot, dusty back-streets, stopping only to buy six large mint humbugs from the lady at the corner of the High Street. With a halfpenny change in his pocket, he headed for the river, hoping there would be a cool breeze blowing.

Within five minutes he arrived outside the cottage, which was almost on the river's edge. Grandad had chosen to retire there so that he could follow the activities of the river and sea-going ships. The afternoon being hot, he had made himself comfortable in a hammock in the garden, positioned so that he could see downstream. On noticing Jimmie, he removed the clay

pipe from his mouth and greeted him.
"Hallo, Jimmie-boy. And why are you looking so sad on a lovely day like this?"
"I wanna be a sailor, but Mum and Dad won' 'ear of it."
"Oh dear, that sounds serious. I had the same problem some seventy or more years ago, and my Dad said that I wasn't strong enough."
"What did you do, Grandad?"
"I ran away from home and joined the Navy, and stayed there for nearly fifty years."
"Did you ever sail to Wudum Ferrus, Grandad?"
The old man scratched his head. "Do you know, Jimmie, I have sailed to all different parts of the world many times, but I cannot recall ever going to Woodham Ferris. Perhaps you can tell me where it is?"
"I don't know neiver, Grandad, but I was 'opin' to go there termorrer."
"How were you going there if you don't know where it is, young man?"
"The skipper on the 'Maywell' told me I could start work on 'is barge, and we would be sailin' to Wudum Ferrus."
Grandad coughed. "Now I begin to see what it's all about. You have come for advice."
"Yes, please."
Jimmie had to wait for a while before the old man spoke again.
"Now, I happen to know the skipper of the 'Maywell'. He talks to me from time-to-time, when he walks into town. Todd Summers is his name. He's rather different from most bargemen. I'm sure he must be the son of a gentleman, and why he is satisfied sailing a dung barge puzzles me, but I expect he has a good reason. I am sure he is a most capable young man. I find him most interesting. He has a great knowledge of all the rivers along the east coast. He can talk about wildlife and birds and the history of ships, but he never talks about himself."
Then, giving Jimmie a wink, "You listen carefully to what he says, and do what he tells you, and I'm sure you'll be as clever as him one day."
"Fank you, Grandad," was Jimmie's immediate response, "but wot's wrong wiv 'is 'and?"
"I'm not sure, Jimmie. He always has a glove on it."
The boy was relieved to hear that.
"Now tell me, what else has happened since I saw you last?"
Jimmie thought for a while. "Not much, Grandad, but it's me birfday today. I'm firteen naw."
"Well, I must say you're a big lad for thirteen, and I'm sure you're strong."
That remark helped Jimmie to make up his mind. "Me Dad says it's the 'orse dung gittin' fru me boots wot's made me grow so tall, but he reckons it ain't done no good to me brains."
"You mustn't take that remark to heart, Jimmie. Your Dad has always been one for pulling people's legs. Now, will you go into the parlour and fetch me my Diddi box?"
Jimmie knew exactly where to go, and returned a few seconds later. From his watch chain Grandad chose a key and unlocked the box. It was about fifteen inches square and six inches deep, made from rich red rosewood and inlaid with mother of pearl: a souvenir from his travels around the world. From its contents, Grandad picked out a sailor's clasp knife. It was

beautiful.

"If you're going to be a sailor, Jimmie, you will need one of these. It is yours, on one condition: that you do not sell it, or give it away, until like me you have no practical use for it."

"I promise, Grandad."

"Keep it tied round your waist and inside your trousers, otherwise you'll soon have someone take it from you."

After a cup of tea and a slice of cake from the lady next door, it was time for Jimmie to return home. Grandad took Jimmie's hand.

"If you decide to join Todd Summers tomorrow, you will be starting on a journey that will take you into a world which will be totally different from what you have experienced so far. You will come into contact with good men, bad men and cruel men, and that goes for women as well. You will see beautiful places and, if you think that this part of London is bad enough, you will find places that reek with sin and iniquity. You will have to decide, as you grow older, the way you will conduct your life. I do hope that you choose to be honest and upright, and win the respect of your fellow men. And a word of warning – be prepared for disappointments and learn to surmount them. Goodbye, Jimmie. I'm confident in you, and may God bless you."

Jimmie gave his Grandad a hug and ran from the garden. He made his way along the riverside until he came in view of the 'Maywell', then sat down on a crate, popped one of the humbugs into his mouth, and began to think out how he could be on that barge at seven o'clock without raising the suspicions of his Mum and Dad. The problem was that Dad started work at six-thirty, and he had to start at seven o'clock. If he left home too early, Mum would wonder why. She always called out to remind him when it was time to go to work. If he was not at work at seven, Dad would be making his way to the 'Maywell' and dragging him back to the stables.

It would be necessary for him to take a longer route to the quay because he dare not pass the stables. He decided that he would leave home at the usual time and run like mad. Providing the barge sailed on time, he would be away and safe. If it had sailed before seven o'clock, he would return to the stables and hope Dad would excuse him for being late.

He gave another glance at the 'Maywell' before setting off home. The men were still throwing on the dung. What caught his eye was the sight of the skipper making his way back to the boat. On his shoulder he carried a sailcloth bag and, just as Grandad had told him, he was wearing a glove on his hand. This made Jimmie feel much easier.

On arriving home, he discovered that his family were all out, which suited him. He found a small sack, then went upstairs and there rummaged through a heap of clothes lying on the floor of a cupboard. To his surprise, the clothes he considered to be his best were missing, and he realised that he could not ask his mother their whereabouts. So he took the next best, and hid them under the straw mattress.

Going into the garden, he untied Bingo and, in his own way, explained to the dog what he would be doing on the morrow.

"Yer the only one 'oo knows, 'sides Grandad. Don't fret about me, an' I'll bring yer back suffink nice."

Later, a call from one of his younger sisters announced tea, and he went indoors expecting bread and dripping, which never excited him. What he saw on the table came as a complete surprise: Chelsea buns, jam tarts, bread and margarine.
"Cor blimey! Where's all this come from?"
"Never you mind, Jimmie. It's your birthday, ain't it?" was his mother's quick reply. "You'd better git eatin', but save some for yer Dad."
While Jimmie enjoyed the feast, he could not help thinking that Mum had pawned his clothes to buy the cakes. Even at thirteen, he already understood that it was a way of life for them. The evening passed as any other evening. He helped his Dad in the garden and, after a cup of cocoa, made his way to bed. To his great relief, nothing was mentioned about going to Woodham Ferris.
"No guts-ache tomorrow morning and be there sharp at seven," shouted his father, as Jimmie scrambled up the rickety staircase to bed. The bedroom was as sparse as the rest of the house. On the floor lay three straw mattresses and a collection of rough blankets: here Jimmie and his two brothers slept. He decided not to undress; just take off his boots, in case he overslept in the morning. The excitement of the day robbed him of any chance of getting to sleep early, and he heard the church clock strike eleven, twelve and then one o'clock.

Chapter Two

On Board the 'Maywell'

The shout of "It's nearly 'arf past six" from his father brought Jimmie to his feet, but before his father could open the door of the bedroom he was back under the blankets again, pretending to be asleep. Everything must appear normal, he told himself.

Dad put his head round the door. "You awake, Jimmie?"

"Yes, Dad."

"Then get up. You're to be there by seven."

"Alright. I'll be there, Dad," Jimmie groaned.

"Right. Make sure you are then. Goodbye for now."

As soon as his Dad had shut the front door, Jimmie was downstairs. He ate a slice of bread, the remaining Chelsea bun and then took a long swig of milk straight from the jug.

"Funny, Dad should say goodbye," he thought to himself, "I suppose 'e's tryin' to make a fuss of me. 'E's got a bee in 'is bonnet about bein' on time."

He heard the church clock strike a quarter to seven. Any minute Mum would shout "Time you were off". He had another swig of milk, woke Bingo to say goodbye, then picked up his sack of belongings. His mother's voice rang down the stairs, "Time you were off, Jimmie."

"Alright, Mum, I'm going."

Usually that meant another few minutes, but this morning he was away. He just heard his mother shout, "Goodbye, Jimmie. Try and do your best."

While that remark seemed strange, he had no time to meditate upon it. It was now a race against time. As he arrived at the quayside, a man was slipping the rope from the bollards which moored the barge.

Jimmie jumped onto the deck and there he stood, panting for breath and feeling rather embarrassed, as the skipper came over to him.

"So, you have decided to join the 'Maywell', Jimmie. Welcome aboard. I will give you your orders."

Jimmie stood as smartly as he could.

"Firstly, do what you are told at once. Secondly, always be on the lookout and be prepared for whatever happens. Thirdly, try to remember what you see and hear. If you train yourself to do these three things, they will help you to become a good seaman, and we shall get along together. Have you understood?"

"Yes, Skip."

"Now, take that bucket of coal into the galley, make up the fire and put the kettle back on top. Then you can come up on deck and watch us set sail, but keep well out of the way. And by the way, the dog's name is Trip. Now off you go."

In the distance, Jimmie could just hear the church clock striking seven. He was off like a shot and into the galley, afraid of his father arriving on the quayside and demanding his return. He knew his Dad would not hesitate to use his belt. He felt like asking Skip to please get going. In a few minutes, the fire was stoked and kettle returned to its rightful place. It was then he felt that the boat was in motion. He turned to ascend the gangway, but a scuffle and a growl brought him to a swift standstill. In his excitement, Jimmie had forgotten the dog. It was now holding his trousers in his teeth and growling. Jimmie, without fear, put his hand on the dog's head.

"Now, Trip. You an' me 'ave got ter learn ter be friends. So, let's start now."

He gave the dog a pat, at which Trip let go of the trousers and wagged his short tail.

"That's better. I'll tell you about Bingo later."

Then, in a few strides, he was on the deck. The 'Maywell' had already turned into the tide. Skip was standing at the tiller, and giving orders to the short fat man busy working at the rigging. As the topsail picked up the wind, Jimmie felt the boat gather up speed. The quay was now some hundred feet away and, as there was still no sign of Dad, he breathed a sigh of relief.

"I bet 'e'll be down 'ere in a few minutes, shoutin' 'is 'ead orf, but I'll be gorn then," he thought.

It was not long before Jimmie realised that it was not only the 'Maywell' making its way downstream. Ships of all shapes and sizes seemed to be on the move, each jockeying for a position to get a clear way. The abuse and banter between the seamen and river pilots was, for Jimmie, a new experience. The swear words he knew quite well, but the river terminology was completely baffling.

He watched, with fascination, the buildings on each side of the river. They looked so different from off-shore. All the time, the little fat man seemed busy running up and down, untying ropes, pulling ropes and then tying them up again. Gradually more and more sail began to be unfurled, and the speed of the 'Maywell' increased. It gave Jimmie a sense of exhilaration. He was getting away from those smelly stables and, for the first time in his life, he felt free. He felt like shouting, "Hurrah" - when he heard another shout, "Stand by!"

He felt his head hit the hatch boards, his neck seemed to be on fire. The little fat man picked him up, shook him by the shoulders, and looking into his eyes told him, "You'll live me boy, be bejabbers, your neck will be sore for a day or two. You sure need two pairs of eyes on a barge."

"What 'appened?" blurted out Jimmie.

"A free line from the rigging twisted round your neck. It happens to all seamen from time to time. That's why you must always keep a watch when we are hoisting. You had better sit down on the covers for a while."

Skip, from the tiller, had seen the incident. Although he considered himself to be a hard-hearted man, he found himself being unusually sympathetic towards the lad. Strangely, he could not rid his mind of the thought that he had acted on impulse in taking the lad on. Could this be a bad omen? He shouted to Paddy and was relieved to get a fair report. Jimmie sat rubbing his head. He could feel a large bruise rising and his neck was still burning. He could easily have cried, but he told himself he was a man now, and choked back his feelings.

"A few minutes ago I was so 'appy," he said to himself.

Closing his eyes, Jimmie found comfort in the movement of the ship and the wind rustling through the sails. A cold, damp pressure on the back of his hand suddenly alerted him. Looking down, he found Trip making a friendly acquaintance. He pulled the dog closer to him and realised he had made another friend. Sitting there, nursing his wounds and Trip at the same time, he watched the countless ships. Smokey steamers pulling lines of small barges, large full-riggers, their sails collecting every available movement of air to head out to sea and foreign parts. The fact that he was now a part of this huge armada helped him to forget his wounds. Skip's shout brought him to his feet, and Trip scuttling along the deck to his master. He walked back to the stern, where Skip and the fat man were drinking. Skip, putting his hand on Jimmie's shoulder said, "I can now introduce you to Patrick Donovan, partner of the 'Maywell'."

Jimmie thrust out his hand, to the surprise of Skip and Paddy, and shook hands with them both.

"That's a very fine gesture, Jimmie. Who told you to do that?"

"Me Grandad. 'E said, shake 'ands wiv ya superiors, an' yer less likely ter get yer ears boxed."

"You have a wise grandfather," said Skip. "Do you think we can knock Jimmie into a seaman, Paddy?"

"I'm sure of that, Skip. He's made of the right stuff. That bump on his head shows he can take a knock or two."

"Yes, I'm sorry about that, Jimmie. Now you know why I said always have your eyes about you. Help yourself to bread and drink and then, after that, I'll show you round the ship."

With the excitement of the morning, Jimmie had forgotten he was hungry. Now he readily made his way into the bread and cheese, his first meal on board.

Paddy took over the tiller whilst Jimmie followed Skip around the deck. The wind freshened, filling the sails and speeding the 'Maywell' on its way down to the sea.

As Jimmie walked the narrow gangway between hold and gunwhale, he realised the speed they were travelling, and was ready to clutch on to every available rope. Pointing to the top-sail, Skip asked him how he fancied climbing to the top. The boy, holding tight, gazed above.

"I don't fink I could do it while your movin'. It makes me feel funny just lookin', Skip."

"Well, you've no need to get anxious. We will not be asking you today, but by the time you have been aboard a few months, you will be able to scramble along any of those spars. You will also have to know the names of each line and pulley, and carry out orders at once. Do you still fancy being a seaman?"

"Yes, Skip. I want to try."

The river now began to widen. Fields and marshland bordered the banks, so different from the inner London river that Jimmie had grown up to know.

"What's that place over there, Skip?"

"That's Tilbury. It's quite an important place along the river. In fact, it's where the largest ships berth. Queen Elizabeth came from London to visit her army there in 1588. They massed on those fields there, ready to protect the city from the Spanish Armada. Do you like learning about the past, Jimmie?"

"Yes, Skip. Me Grandad has told me all 'bawt the Armardar, but 'e reckons Lord Nelson would 'ave got rid of 'em in next ter no time. Me Grandad, 'e served wiv Lord Nelson, so 'e no's a lot abawt those sort ov fings."
"I'm very pleased to know that, Jimmie. I hope to hear more about your grandfather, when I have time. That's Gravesend on the starboard side, and a very busy place that is too. You have got to learn the names of all these places, and in which order they come when we are sailing."
"Are we nearly there?" asked Jimmie.
"Not for a long while. What made you ask that?"
"Well, me Dad said yesterday that 'e reckoned that you never sailed past Gravesend."
"Well, you will be able to enlighten him when we return. I expect he was pulling your leg."
"Oh! 'e's good at that," said Jimmie.

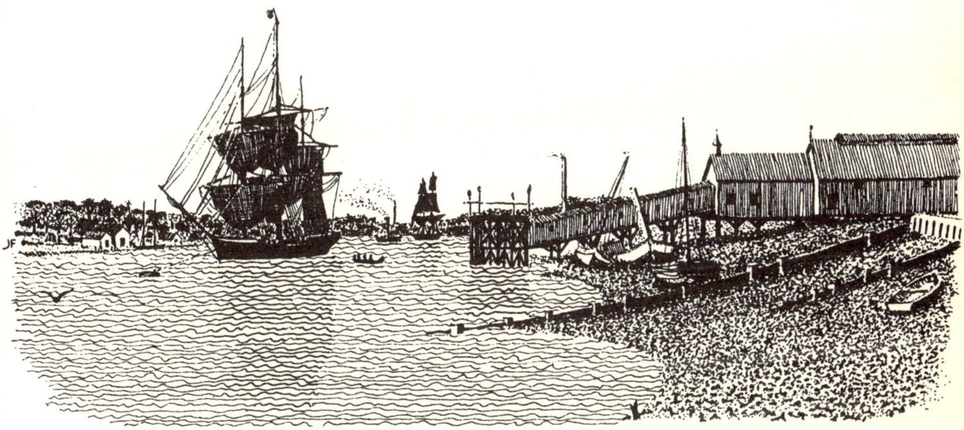

TILBURY

For a while the lad was left on his own, so he made himself comfortable in the bows and watched the water part into two cascades as the prow cut its way through. Every now and again, a wave would clip the bows and send a spray into his face. The taste of salt surprised him. It was so different from the murky, foul water that gurgled round the docks at home.
On one bank, he noticed the high ground coming down to the water, and on the other, the low, flat marshland stretching for miles. Jimmie enquired of Skip, when he next came by, "Why's all that land so flat over there? It looks lower than the water."
"You're quite right, Jimmie. It is lower than the water at Spring tides. I will explain to you how it happens another day. It's all marshland. That, over there, is called Canvey Island. The wall surrounding it was built by a Dutchman called Coppenburgh, in 1621. It enables farmers to graze sheep

and cattle at all times, though when its stormy, the sea will break over the top and flood the land."

Jimmie was quiet.

"Must 'ave taken 'im a long while to build a wall round an island on 'is own, Skip."

Skip laughed. "Not quite on his own. I should imagine there would have been a few hundred men working at once. Coppenburgh was the engineer, or man responsible for the work."

"My schoolteacher told us about that Dutchman 'oo built that wall. It all comes back to me now."

Skip listened with interest. "That boy's brain never stops," he thought to himself.

"'E told us that Coppenburgh's boy was walkin' 'ome from school one day when 'e noticed a little spurt of water comin' out of the wall. At first, 'e fort 'e'd run and tell 'is Dad. Then 'e fort it would get bigger and flood the 'ouse where 'e lived, so 'e stuck 'is finger in the 'ole and waited for 'is Dad to come along when 'e knocked orf work. But the 'ole kept gettin' bigger, so 'e put 'is 'and in, and then bofe 'ands'. Then it got dark, an' the poor kid got colder an' colder. 'Is father didn't find 'm till ever so late, an' by then 'e were dead. But the people on the island reckon 'e saved them all from drowning, an' made 'im there 'ero. I don't remember me teacher sayin' wevver it were Canvey Island or not."

"I've heard similar stories, Jimmie. They are attributed to Holland, where most people live below sea level, and everyone is taught to keep watch on the sea walls for their own protection. Now, you can follow me to the galley, then I will show you how to make the tea and prepare a simple meal."

Once there, Jimmie was interested to see where things were to be found, where things were to be put, and most important, how everything must be kept spotlessly clean.

"I will insist on that at all times," said Skip.

"Yes, Skip. I will do my best," was Jimmie's reply. At the same time he thought to himself, "It's a good job Skip 'as never bin in our 'ouse or 'e wouldn't 'ave taken me on."

By four o'clock the 'Maywell' was heading for the estuary. The open sea was a sight Jimmie's vivid imagination had never been able to conceive. He stood in the bows, holding Trip with one hand, and the rigging with the other. Although it was a hot day, he could feel the cool wind blowing through his threadbare clothes.

"Cor, lummy, I never fort there was so much water." For the first time, a sense of fear came over him. The barge seemed so small on such a mighty expanse of sea.

The appearance of Paddy to the fo'c'sle brought some reassurance to him.

"Where abouts is Wudum Ferrus?" he asked.

"Now, you may not believe it, Jimmie, but we are heading in the opposite doirection to where it is, yet we finish op there in a copole o' days. But don't you worry, me boy, the skipper knows his way orl round the world. You're quoite safe."

"Thank you, Paddy. I were gettin' a bit frightened."

"Yes, I could see it in your face as I walked along. Now, take a tip from me, and you will get along with the skipper quite well. He's taken a liken to you already, which rather sorproises me. Do what he tells you at once. You can ask him as many questions as you loike about boats and the sea and the places we go. He is a very educated man, not loike an ordinary seaman. But, never ask him questions about himself or you will soon get shrugged off."

"Thank you, Paddy. I'll remember wot you've said."

By early evening, Skip had the long arm of Southend Pier clearly in view. With a slackening breeze and the fast-flowing flood, the 'Maywell' was making slow progress.

"We'll bring up in the 'Ray'," shouted Skip to Paddy, who was enjoying a pipe on the hatch covers. "I presume you will be going ashore."

The 'Maywell' turned to port and came in near to shore. Jimmie became fascinated as Paddy began to take in the large red sails. The flapping and cracking as they lost the wind was quite frightening to the young newcomer to the sea.

The call by Skip to assist in dropping anchor brought Jimmie to the foc's'le. He listened carefully as Skip emphasized the things not to be done.

"Now watch me. Do as I tell you and soon the whole procedure will become second nature to you."

Later, after they had enjoyed a bowl of the stew that had been simmering on the stove for most of the day, and a large chunk of bread, Paddy rowed the dinghy ashore. The fact, as Skip explained, that the place was Leigh-on-Sea, and that Paddy would be meeting his mates on shore, was of little interest to Jimmie. The sleepless night plus the excitement of the day had expended the boy's strength. Skip noticed his physical condition.

"Right, young man, get your boots off, and your head down."

Pointing to a boarded platform above the dining quarters, he said, "That's your bunk for tonight."

Jimmie scrambled into the niche, pulled a rough blanket over himself and, with a "Goodnight Skip", fell straight asleep. Within an hour though his sleep was disurbed and he thrashed his arm. At home, rats were not uncommon visitors to the bedroom, but now the cold nose of Trip reassured him of his new surroundings, and he slept on. It was another two hours before Skip rolled onto his bunk. The fact that he had this lad, now soundly sleeping, in his care, came as quite a challenge to him.

Chapter Three

From the Thames to Burnham

Sunlight poured down through the gangway hatch. Jimmie could see Skip preparing to light the stove. He jumped from his shelf almost straight into his boots.

"I'll do that. I'm good at lightin' fires."

"That may be so, Jimmie, but you can light fires in one place only on a barge and that's in the fire box. So I will watch you carry out the task."

With a couple of minor corrections, he was satisfied with his assistant's ability. "Very good. From now on that will be your first task of the day. But remember, I want it kept perfectly clean."

The morning was hot, showing the first signs of another true flaming-June day, but to Jimmie's surprise it did not please Skip or Paddy. Without a whisper of breeze to fill the 'Maywell's' sails, she was becalmed.

"It's proof the Lord does not want us working on a Sunday," said Paddy over their breakfast meal.

"I'll take the boy ashore and show him the cockle sheds and let you have a quoite day, Skip."

"Take Trip with you. He will keep Jimmie occupied when you are supping beer," was the older man's reply.

The day in Leigh passed very quickly. Paddy was good company and showed

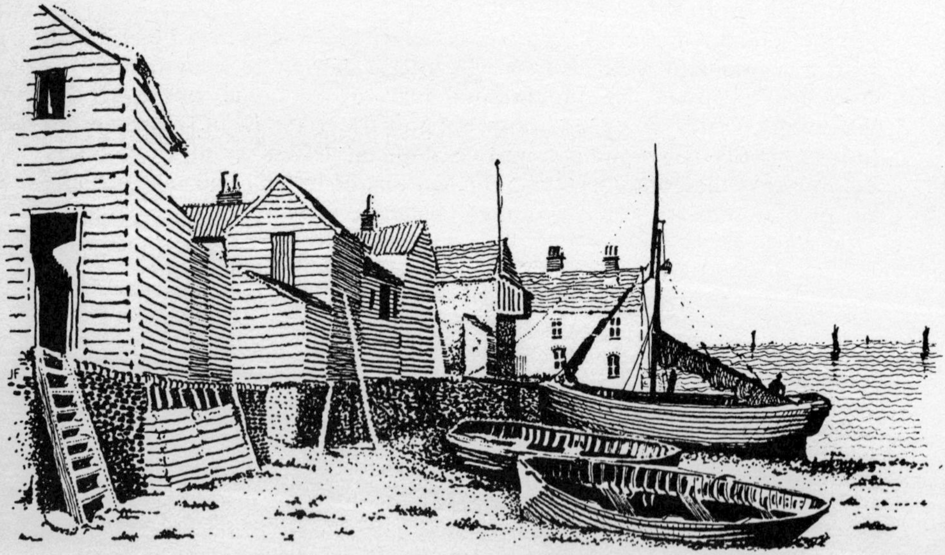

LEIGH-ON-SEA

Jimmie all his favourite haunts, treating him to plenty of food and drink. When they returned to the 'Maywell', the boy was happy to climb into his cupboard to sleep.

Monday morning was kind to them, so it was a quick breakfast, sails up and away, and around Southend Pier. Jimmie watched the coastline to starboard gradually disappear, and the ships and barges take on different routes.

"I'm blowed if I knows 'ow they know where they're goin'," he thought to himself.

The 'Maywell', following in line with other barges, seemed to him to be making its way along the coast. To portside, there seemed to be miles and miles of marshland. Skip came and explained to him the route they were taking.

"We are now sailing the North Sea, Jimmie. Those ships making their way south are on the way to France, in fact, any part of the world. That is the way to the English Channel. We are heading north. That land there," he said, pointing to port, "is known as the East Coast."

"Do you get to the Norf Pole this way?" piped in Jimmie.

"If you sail far enough, but I have no intention of doing that. We are making for the River Crouch and Burnham, and to do that we must skirt this waste area known as the Maplin Sands. When the tide is high there is a temptation to make a short cut, but it is a risky thing to do, very risky. That land is Foulness Island. The whole area you see before you is made up of islands. Can you see all those poles? That is known as the Broom Way. Horses and carts make their way from island to island at low tide along that route. The wind has been very favourable today, and we should turn the Buxey buoy in another hour, into the Crouch, and take the tide up to Burnham where we shall be staying the night."

"When do we get to Wudum Ferrus, then?"

"Not for another two days, Jimmie."

"Cor blimey! It's a long way, ain't it?" exclaimed the boy.

The journey up the Crouch to Burnham was no less exciting than the rest of the day. Jimmie was fascinated by the cluster of houses near the quay, and the barges moored in straight lines along the waterway. Paddy was busy furling the sails, and Skip showed him again the procedure of dropping anchor.

"You say we're stoppin' 'ere for the night?" asked Jimmie.

"Yes. After we have tidied up and had a wash, we shall be going ashore."

From somewhere, Skip produced a tin bath, gave Jimmie a bucket on a short line, and told him to fill the bath. After a short while, Skip returned with a lump of red soap and a large rough towel.

"There we are. You can get washed first."

Jimmie rolled up his sleeves, splashed the water over his face, and was about to dry himself when Skip's voice rang from the bows. "Not so fast, boy! Off with your clothes and into the water. I want to see you a mass of soap suds from head to foot." The order came as a shock to Jimmie. Skip suddenly became the dreadful man he had seen that recent morning, and he hesitated. Paddy arrived on the scene.

"Get his clothes off and scrub him down," shouted Skip, "I want him perfectly clean."

Jimmie winced as Paddy pulled the shirt over his head.
"Do as you're told, Jimmie. No harm will come to you."
The rest of his clothes were off and he stood in the bath. Paddy gave him a scrubbing brush, "Use plenty of soap. You'll feel lovely afterwards."
With no possible chance of getting out of the task, Jimmie turned his back to any onlookers and gradually worked a lather over his body. He felt somewhat ashamed as the soapy water made pink patches appear on his body and legs.
"I s'pose I must be dirty," he thought to himself, "It's ages since I 'ad a barf."
He rinsed away the suds and turned to see Skip throwing his clothes into the river. In fury he jumped from the bath.
"Me 'nife, me 'nife. You thrown away me Grandad's 'nife. I hate you," he shouted, as he rushed headlong at Skip.
"Calm down, calm down, Jimmie. Here is your knife, and a very nice one at that. Get yourself dried, I have a nice surprise for you."
The feel of the knife in his hand made Jimmie feel better. With the back of his hand he wiped away the tears, and walked slowly back to the towel and began to dry himself. He was now uncertain what to do. It was too far to swim ashore and they would soon catch him.
In a few minutes Skip returned, "Here, Jimmie, your first seaman's uniform. I hope everything fits. Get yourself dressed, we want you looking really smart when we get ashore." Jimmie looked starry-eyed. The garments were all brand new. He had never in all his life put on new clothes. "So that was why Skip made me scrub meself," he thought.
He slipped the blue shirt on. It felt lovely and clean. There followed dark serge trousers, navy jersey, long socks, white spotted handkerchief, kneb cap and a comb. He suddenly forgave the man he had so recently attacked. Fully dressed, with a little help from Paddy, he was ready to report for duty again.
"Go and tell Skip you are ready for inspection. He will have forgotten your fit of temper."
Feeling rather self-conscious in his new rigout, Jimmie presented himself meekly to Skip.
"Not bad, Jimmie, but you're standing as though your clothes don't belong to you. Are you pleased with them?"
"Oh yes, sir."
"Right then. Stand up to your full height, throw out your chest, and be proud of what you own. Now, go and help Paddy lower the dinghy."
In a few minutes, the two men and Jimmie, with Trip, were seated in the little boat, and Paddy was pulling to the shore. They were greeted, as they neared the quay, by a group of seamen.
"What's on board this time, Todd?" shouted the Harbour Master.
"Equine excreta, bound for Eyotts Farm, Woodham Ferrers."
"Why don't you call it by it's common name? It would save me explaining to this lot here. Anyway, we're pleased you have moored in mid-stream and spared us the smell."
Paddy tied up the dinghy. Jimmie followed Skip up the steps and stood to one side while his employer was engaged with the Harbour Master.
"Who have we here?" shouted one bystander. "He looks like a paying guest!"

At the same time he was feeling the quality of Jimmie's jersey. This made the lad feel nervous, then remembering Skip's advice, he pulled himself to his full height. "I'm Jimmie Brown, and Skip is training me to be a seaman."
The men gathered round and gave a hearty laugh.
"You've a bright one there, Todd. Where'd you pick him up?"
"That, gentlemen, is my business. I do have my connections in the right circles."
Picking up his bag, he told Jimmie to follow, and wished the seamen 'Goodnight'.
Jimmie trailed Skip and Paddy between a few buildings into what seemed like the town centre. Then the two older men stopped, and had a few words together. Paddy turned to make his way up the street. He wished Jimmie all the best, "I'll see you next week," he said, and was gone.
Skip and Jimmie crossed the road, then made their way down a side turning and stopped outside a cottage named 'Plovers'. Passing through the gateway and following the garden path, Jimmie was attracted by the flowers on either side of him.
"I like them," he called to Skip.
"Good, then you will have to tell my sister, Nell."
A knock on the door brought Todd's sister to greet them. Jimmie's mouth opened in surprise. What a lovely woman she looked, dressed in beautiful clothes, and such a lovely smile.
"Hello Todd, and who have you brought with you?"
"This is Jimmie Brown, my new second mate."
Jimmie stretched out his hand. "Pleased to meet you, ma'am."
Skip secretly noted the lad's courtesy.
"I'm pleased to meet you, Jimmie. Come indoors. You must both be ready for a meal."
Skip made his way upstairs, and Jimmie was ushered into a small room.
"Make yourself comfortable, Jimmie. Here are some books you can look at whilst I prepare dinner."
"Thank you, ma'am," said Jimmie, sitting down rather awkwardly on a chair.
As she left the room she turned, "I think it will be easier if you call me Aunt Nell. Will you do that?"
"Yes, ma'am."
Both laughed. It broke the ice, and somehow Jimmie knew they were going to be friends. He looked around the room. Hanging on the walls were paintings of the river and boats. In the corner stood a tall bookcase filled with books. On the floor was a large rug with a most wonderful pattern, and near the window stood a lovely bowl of flowers. Everywhere was so clean and smelt so fresh. Jimmie was quite satisfied to just sit, and look.
"Now I know why Skip dressed me up like this. He could never 'ave brought me 'ere, all mucky an' rough."
For some thirty minutes the boy just sat and stared. "If only I could read, I could understand the books."
The door opened and Skip beckoned him to follow. "I'm sure you're ready to eat."
Around a small table were four chairs. On one sat a ginger-haired lad, and Jimmy quickly decided that he was younger than himself.

Aunt Nell told him, "Stand up, William. This young man, who your Uncle Todd has brought along, is called Jimmie Brown. I want you to shake hands and entertain him in a gentlemanly fashion."
Both lads reached out their hands.
"Pleased to meet you," said Jimmie.
"Pleased to meet you," replied William. Both eyed each other with a degree of suspicion. Having sat down, there was a silence while Aunt Nell filled the plates with steaming meat and vegetables. The savoury smell made Jimmie's mouth water.
"Before you start, I will say Grace."
William put his hands together and closed his eyes. Skip just nodded his head. Jimmie followed Skip, hoping that he was doing the right thing. "For what we are about to receive, Lord, make us truly thankful. Amen."
The food, to Jimmie, was just wonderful. He soon realised that he must slow up eating or he would finish first. Skip and his sister were busy talking, while Jimmie listened. When all the first course was eaten, a dish of apple tart was brought in to finish off the meal.
The rest of the evening was spent with William showing Jimmie his rabbits, and a quick walk to the waterfront and back. Both boys had now overcome their shyness and were fast becoming friends. After a drink of cocoa, William was sent off to bed, and Jimmie was shown to his room. It was tucked away in the crutch of the roof rafters.
"It's rather small, Jimmie, but I'm sure you'll be comfortable. Goodnight and God bless you."
Jimmie said, "Goodnight, and thank you, Aunt Nell, for 'avin' me."
The door closed and Jimmie inspected his surroundings. On one side, rucked against the wall, was a bed with a pretty patterned quilt on top. He put his hands on the pillows, and they were so soft. By the bed was a chair and a large box stood against the opposite wall. Jimmie expected it was for storing things in. On the floor was a large rug made with lots of little pieces of cloth. By standing on the chair he could see the river through the window high in the roof. A candle and tinderbox stood on a little shelf above the long box. On one of the walls, which were clean and white, was a painting of a tiger and the jungle.
It was now getting dark, and he sat on the rug to remove his boots. For the first time he realised he was tired. He felt the bed once more. It was inviting, but he had never slept in a proper bed. Dare he chance it? The rug was also soft to the touch, so removing his jersey, he rolled it in a ball, laid his head on it and was asleep.
A knock on the door startled him. "Are you awake, Jimmie?"
It was Skip.
"Yes, I'm awake." He jumped up, wondering what was the matter.
Skip entered the room. "Lay down, Jimmie. I'll light the candle."
Skip's eyes went quickly round the room. It was obvious to him that Jimmie had not been in bed, and that he had been asleep on the rug.
"Why are you sleeping down there, young man?"
"I was takin' off me boots and I just dropped orf, Skip."
The answer seemed plausible enough, but Skip had his suspicions.
"Right, off with your trousers and into bed." Jimmie knew he must obey at

once, and was between the sheets in seconds. Skip pulled the chair up towards him and sat down.

"I know you have had a busy day, but I want to know if you are pleased with your decision to come with me."

"Yes, Skip. I'm glad I came wiv you, but I'm worried wot me Mum an' Dad will be finking ov me. I don't really wanna 'urt them."

"That is why I have come up here, to tell you that, after you left me the other morning, I called at the stables to see your father. Then we went to your house to discuss the matter with your mother. Your mother reckoned that if you were like your grandfather, and you were, then nothing on earth would stop you being on the 'Maywell' in the morning. Your Dad reckoned you would have changed your mind before you went to bed. So we left it for you to decide. I have a few things which your mother gave me. You can sort them out in the morning."

Skip nipped out the light. "I'll see you in the morning. Sleep well."

As he closed the door, Jimmie called out, "I'm sorry I said I 'ated you. I'll never say that again."

"That's quite alright. You're forgiven."

Jimmie lay there, his mind in a whirl. He suddenly realised that the room was getting lighter. Looking up he could see the moon shining on the white walls.

So Mum and Dad knew, and they never let on. That accounted for their odd remarks, and explained why Dad had not come to the dock, "I never fort they cared abawt me." His mind quickly relived the last two days: the kindness of Aunt Nell, the new clothes from Skip, the lovely food, the feel of the clean sheets and the beautiful smell of lavender.

For the tough awkward kid from London dockyard slums, it was more than he could take. He knew he was going to cry. Looking up, he thought, "There's only the man in the moon to see me, an' I don't suppose 'e'll bovver." Laying his head deep on the pillow, he sobbed freely. He could feel the tears running down his face and smarting on the red wheal on his neck. But he was the happiest boy ever to leave London.

For Skip, reflecting on the day was quite different. Because of circumstances, he had committed himself to employ and train a young lad to be a seaman. It was going to alter his way of life. The first two days had revealed certain facets of this teenager's character that he had not appreciated before. Was he capable of training this urchin to be a man of responsibility in a future society?

Chapter Four

On to Hullbridge

The shout of "Breakfast's ready" from William awoke Jimmie. He was dressed and down the stairs in a few minutes.

"Good morning, Jimmie. Go into the washroom. You will find water, soap and a towel. Then come in for your breakfast," said Aunt Nell.

On a long slate slab stood the bowl. Jimmie went through the ritual of washing, though he could not understand why, after sleeping in a clean bed, it was necessary. In any case, he had a bath only yesterday. However, the smell of breakfast cooking hastened his task. He returned to the kitchen, where William was waiting.

"Where's Skip?" asked Jimmie.

"He has gone to the 'Maywell'. You're to follow after breakfast."

Some half-an-hour later, their stomachs full, William and Jimmie stood by the quay.

"Uncle Todd will be stowing-up this morning, and we are to help. He is teaching me to row. I expect you can row already."

Jimmie avoided the answer. While he had played in boats at the docks, he wasn't sure whether he could row well enough to please Skip.

The morning was spent taking on coal, water, food, various pieces of rope, tubs of grease, and all manner of bits and pieces, which they collected from the boatyard. All were stowed in special places aboard.

Their next job was to clean all the brasses, scrub the galley floor and generally tidy up. When all was done to Skip's satisfaction, William was given his rowing lesson and they returned to shore for a midday meal.

Skip had explained to Jimmie how Paddy would not be rejoining the 'Maywell' until after they had returned from Woodham Ferrers, and that from now on he would be required to carry out duties. They would be sailing to Hullbridge on the afternoon tide. After another fine meal, they said goodbye to Nell and made their way along the quay. This time Jimmie was told to row the dinghy. Having watched and listened to the instructions given to William earlier, he felt more confident and applied his arms to the oars to the best of his ability. With a few corrections from Skip, and advice from other bargemen, he pulled alongside the 'Maywell'.

Skip told Jimmie that he could now take off his new clothes and sort out the best from his bag for working in, and that this would be the order from now on, "Always put your best clothes on when you go ashore."

Then he explained to Jimmie each operation in detail for getting underway and taking up anchor.

Having lashed the tiller to allow minimum freeway, Skip explained what 'to port' and 'to starboard' meant, how to hold the tiller and what to do when he gave the orders. After a few practice orders, and Skip being satisfied with Jimmie's reactions, the anchor was raised. This tested the boy's strength as he helped turn the windlass.

Slowly, the 'Maywell' moved with the tide. Jimmie took his position by the tiller as Skip attended the setting of the sails. The feeling of movement, and the resistance of the tiller to water as Jimmie held it tight, was for him a new and proud experience. "If only me Grandad could see me now," he thought to himself. But a sharp order from Skip soon stopped his mind from wandering.

Once satisfied with the sails, Skip took up position by Jimmie. The wind was light and favourable, and he knew there would be little to worry about. The tide alone was quite enough to get them to Hullbridge.

"Have you ever heard about the River Crouch before, Jimmie?"

"No, Skip. I only knows the Thames, an' I never knew that was so big 'till yesterday."

"Well, it's a tidal river, about fourteen miles long, and it gets narrower as we make our way upstream. That means you have to pay special attention to positioning your boat for all the twists and turns. You have to watch out for the mud bars, and not take risks. You will see for yourself tomorrow."

Skip pointed, "That place over to starboard is Creeksea. We may see the ferry as we pass. They have a special boat for taking animals over. The church on that high ground to port is Canewdon. That's a very special place: the Saxons and the Danes fought it out there many years ago. Do you know anything about the history of England, Jimmie?"

"I do remember some bits. It comes to me from time to time. Whether 'e were a Saxon or Dane I don't know, but our teacher told us 'e lost 'is 'orse, and was walkin' 'ome and lorst 'is way, and busted 'is leg in the dark. 'E stopped at an 'ouse, where an old woman said she would get some 'elp if 'e would look after some cakes she were bakin' on the grate. Anyway, while she were away, 'e went to sleep. I fink 'e were a king."

"Alfred," said Skip.

"That's 'im, Alfred the Grate. They called 'im that because 'e burnt the cakes on it. Anyway, the old woman knocked 'im about when she got back, 'cos of the cakes. When 'e told 'er 'e was a king, she just laughed, and they put 'er in the Bloody Tower."

Skip laughed, "You're talking about the Saxon king, Alfred, who fought the Danes on those hills. The story about the cakes is just make-believe."

"My Grandad's told me a story about 'istory, cos 'e's bin to the place where it 'appened."

"And where was that, Jimmie?"

"I can't fink of the name of the place now, but 'e says there were all these chaps 'oo 'ad 'orns growin' out of their 'eads, like cows, an' they come in fousands of boats, and landed on some beach, an' they were s'posed to come to London, but lorst their way. They orl got out the boats and found they couldn't get up the cliff, 'cos the people up the top kept rollin' stones on their 'eads. Then these chaps wiv the 'orns on their 'eads started to ping away wiv their bows an' arrows, but they couldn't do any good, 'cos they couldn't ping 'em high enough. An' the fellers firin' from above were knockin' 'em orf like flies. 'Astins it was, I just remembered. Do you know where 'astins is, Skip?"

"Yes, I know where Hastings is, but go on. I'm interested to hear the end of the story."

"Well, these chaps wiv the 'orns run out of arrows, and they orl got back in their boats and the people on the top of the cliffs were roarin' their 'eads orf. Then one of the chaps wiv 'orns found 'e got an arrow left, an' 'e didn't fink it were worf takin' back, so 'e stood up and stretched 'is bow until it nearly busted, and let go, and the arrow came down, an' it 'it this chap right between the eyes an' killed 'im. And 'e were a king. 'Arold, I fink. Me Grandad said it were rough luck, because he were just thankin' God, 'cos 'e fort 'e 'ad won the battle, an' after that, these fellows all got out their boats and found a way up the cliffs and fought the English with their choppers, and won. Me Grandad reckons that's why you should always look down when you say your prayers."
"Well, I must say, you fascinate me with your stories, Jimmie. The men you referred to were the Normans, and they came from France. I'm not so sure that they actually wore horns, and the battle took place some four or five miles inland from Hastings.
The rivers of the East Coast were ideal inlets for the raiders of that day. They ransacked the villages and farms, then made off to do the same further along the coast. Sailing these rivers has increased my interest in local history and I spend many hours reading up about it. Perhaps you would like to read some of my books."
Jimmie looked down on the deck.
"Aunt Nell told me I could look at 'er books yesterday, and I didn't like to tell 'er I couldn't read."
"Would you like to be able to read, Jimmie? I'm prepared to teach you, providing you work hard."
"Thank you, Skip. I promise to work hard. Can you teach me to write as well?"
"In due course, Jimmie. Take hold of the tiller while I slack off the sail. I can see we have a visitor."
Ahead, Jimmie could see a boat being rowed out to meet them. As the 'Maywell' lost speed, the dinghy pulled alongside.
"Be you stopping at Hullbridge, Todd?" shouted the man.
"Yes, for tonight," replied Skip.
"Would you oblige me by taking this sack to the 'Anchor'?"
"Put it in the dinghy, Bill, and I will deliver it tonight. Am I supposed to know what it is?"
"No, Todd. Just leave it."
The sack was transferred from the dinghy. Bill gave a loud cheerio. Skip adjusted the sails and they headed upstream.
"We are now at Fambridge, North Fambridge to starboard and South to port. That was the ferryman wanting another mystery package delivered. It pays to keep on the right side of these rivermen, and not to ask too many questions. They are a law unto themselves."
For the next ten minutes, Skip was busy checking the rigging. Jimmie, holding tight the tiller, noticed that the river ahead was divided. In fact, water seemed to flow in all directions.
"Which way do we go now?" he shouted.
"Remember what I told you earlier about the river. This is where the river changes its mind. Over to starboard is Stow Creek, we go there at times. Straight ahead is Clements Green Creek. That takes you to Saltcotes Farm,

another of our stopping places. Today, we shall turn to port and follow the main stream, so you must pay special attention to what I tell you, because we have to negotiate two bends. So, stand by for orders!"

Having successfully carried out the instructions and been complimented by Skip, Jimmie felt proud of himself. The river ahead again appeared straight and Skip once more took over.

"This part of the river is known as Brandy Hole and is accredited as being a hideout for smugglers. I don't have any hard and fast facts, but I'm well aware that much goes on under the cover of dark, and the least questions asked is better for you."

"Me Grandad reckons they were always after smugglers. He says that for every one you caught two would pop up, and they were a bloodthirsty lot. He would rather fight the French than smugglers!"

"I'm sure he was right, it's a very old profession and very difficult to eliminate. Now, can you tell me what is different on this part of the river from that which we have already passed?"

Jimmie looked around. "No, Skip. It all looks the same to me."

"What did I tell you the other morning when you came aboard, Jimmie? Keep a good look about you, and take a note of what you see. It is important that you should now see a change about you. Have another good look."

For a while the boy looked up and down.

Then, suddenly, he shouted, "There's no sea wall on that side."

"And what side do you call that?"

"The port side."

"Good, now remember that. It can help you to tell where you are in foggy weather. In fact, it is about the only stretch of the Crouch which has a natural bank, and it is known as Hullbridge. Where you can see those wooden cottages by the waterside is the village, and that is where we shall stop tonight, alongside the bank, there, where two other barges are, with men working on them."

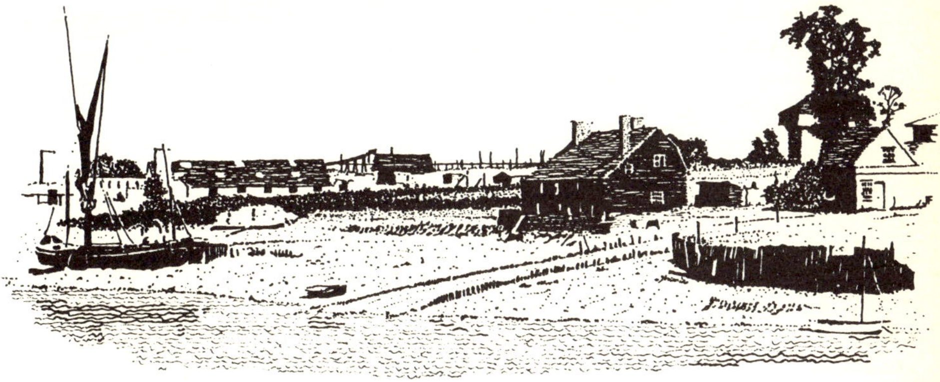

HULLBRIDGE

Large elm trees grew almost to the water's edge, creating a different picture from what Jimmie had been looking at all the afternoon.
"Why don't trees grow on the other side?" asked the boy.
"That is a very good question. It is because all the flat land beyond the river wall is really marsh land and, before the walls were built, it was covered by the Spring tides. The land is too salty for trees to grow. The trees on that bank collect their water from the high ground."
The 'Maywell' brought up, and Jimmie helped Skip with the slipping of the anchor and the reefing-in of the sails. Except for a few children sitting on the water's edge, watching the 'Maywell', all seemed quiet. The odd seagull circled overhead, waiting for a titbit to be thrown overboard. A moored barge, with its sails reefed, had an unusual effect on Jimmie. Like a live creature requiring your full control, it lay there, almost still and robbed of its glory. Jimmie walked from stem to stern, feeling that he had lost something - from the busy London dockside, with its swarming bustle of men, horses, boats and noise, to this. Tonight he would be sleeping on the 'Maywell' again.
"I 'ope its goin' to be better than this when I get there," he said to himself.
On the other bank, his eye followed rows of wooden piles protruding from the water and leading to a gap in the sea wall. Beyond were fields, and further away, low hills. He turned back, "Ain't much to look at there".
"What's that place?" called Jimmie, pointing to the gap in the wall.
"That's Woodham Ferris, Jimmie."
The answer came as an anti-climax and Jimmie's heart sank. The pictures of the place he had imagined were obliterated from his mind. Whatever could he tell his mates at home? Whatever could he tell his Grandad? He was sure they would laugh at him. He just stood staring, his mind now blank. Skip looked across and read the boy's mind. "Somehow, I must put that right," he thought.
A shout brought Jimmie to the galley. Tea was made, and the beef sandwiches that had been made by Aunt Nell were soon eaten. Jimmie was quiet and uneasy.
"Now, don't get over-anxious, Jimmie. We do not get to our destination until tomorrow. For the present, we will have a wash, go ashore and deliver the mystery parcel."
"Does that mean I've got to 'ave anover barf?"
Skip laughed, "I don't think that will be necessary, but it will do no harm to freshen yourself up."
"Do I put me uvver clothes on?"
"Why not? Let those youngsters over there know you are proud of your ship."
Half-an-hour later, Jimmie rowed the dinghy ashore and tied up on the wharfside. They carried the sack and its contents to the Old Anchor Inn. Skip suggested that Jimmie could take a look round the village with Trip, while he made arrangments for help tomorrow.
The little cottages nestled between high trees. Red and white roses rambled over the black tarred boards, reflecting the setting sun. The little gardens, all a mass of colour, seemed to lift Jimmie out of the doldrums. Talking aloud to Trip, who seemed to be enjoying his walk with his new master, he said, "Those 'ouses look really nice; suffink diff'rent to our street. I'll 'ave to tell me Dad to grow some flowers like them up our wall."

For a while he inspected some ruins which looked like an old church, then retraced his steps to the river, turned right and made his way along a footpath between the high elm trees skirting the river bank. Suddenly, three lads came into view and quickly disappeared into the bushes. Somehow, he suspected they were watching him. He called Trip to heel, and passed them sitting on a tree branch.
"Where do you come from, Smarty?" they shouted.
"Lundun," replied Jimmie.
"Then be off back. We don't want you round here."
Jimmie walked on. He was not turning back for them. His assailants sat back, surprised that their threats should be ignored. Some hundred yards on, Jimmie stood and inspected a barge tied alongside the wharf. It was obvious that they too were unloading dung. Then, looking at the name on the bow, he realised it had been loaded at Wapping the week before the 'Maywell'. Calling Trip to heel, he began the walk back to the ship. No sign of the lads was apparent. Trip trotted proudly along, when suddenly, a tree branch crashed onto the path, catching the dog squarely across the back. With a yelp the dog jumped, then fell to the ground. Jimmie ran to its aid, picked Trip up and comforted him. From behind a tree one lad appeared.
"Why don't you clear off, Smarty, to your hoity-toity skipper?" he laughed.
Jimmie, holding Trip, went to walk past, but from behind he felt a clump to his head and he fell to the ground. In the next five minutes Jimmie expended more energy than he had for a very long while. His thirteen years in the rough and tumble of the docks had hardened him to attack and self-defence, and it was obvious that his three assailants had expected the smartly dressed lad to be a London softie.
Each boy gave of his best: shouts and threats; punches and kicks; and Trip barked and growled. The noise attracted Skip's attention, waiting on the causeway, and he quickly headed in the direction of the affray.
It was Trip, who had recovered from his blow, who settled the fight. As each lad in turn retreated from Jimmie's onslaught, they felt the dog's teeth in their buttocks. This brought them to a state of final surrender. The arrival of Skip ended the matter. Exhausted, the four stood before him. Trip lay panting at his master's feet.
"Don't move, any of you, before I say, or the dog will get you." Having already felt his teeth once, the lads waited.
Grabbing a ginger-haired lad, Skip shouted, "You are from the 'Acacia'. Go and get back on board, or I'll sling you in the river."
With a shove of the boot he was gone.
"You're from the 'Swale'," he roared at a tubby, red-faced lad with blood pouring from his nose. "You can tell your skipper who hit you when you get aboard, and you will most probably get his belt across your arse! Now be off!"
"And who are you?" Skip shouted at a lanky lad standing sheepishly before him.
"Oi live 'ere." Blood poured from his mouth as he spoke.
"In that case, you can inform your local lads in the morning that Jimmie Brown of the 'Maywell' spoilt that pretty face of yours, and in future don't regard us as a couple of spoufs. Now, get off home and do something about

your bloody face." With one eye on the dog, the boy turned and was gone.
Skip then addressed Jimmie, "Pick up your cap, and let's get back to the boat. I'll deal with you then."

The message only just registered. Jimmie's brain was in turmoil. He saw Skip and Trip heading their way along the path. He leaned forward to recover the cap, then everything went black. Trip heard the fall and scampered back, quickly followed by Skip. Gently, he lifted the boy to his feet, then, putting his shoulders onto Jimmie's stomach, raised him over his back. By the time they had reached the ferry hard, Jimmie had regained consciousness. With assistance, he settled down in the dinghy while Skip skulled the short distance to the 'Maywell'. He was then lifted on deck and given instructions to make his way to the cabin. As Jimmie waited for Skip to tie up, he could feel the results of his melee - aching arms, sore mouth and shins, and still more to come when his employer came down. While he had not been afraid of the three lads, he trembled at the thought of facing Skip.

Meanwhile, Skip was contemplating how he would deal with the situation. The last thing he wanted was a lad who threw his arms around on the slightest provocation. He was pleased that Paddy was not aboard. His judgement would have been short and sweet: "Boys are a bloody nuisance, get rid of him!"

It was obvious that the lad was in pain. He must attend to his wounds first, and then sort out the cause of the trouble afterwards. Calling Trip to follow him, he then realised the dog too was walking with difficulty. Picking him up, the animal cried out with pain. Skip's mind worked fast. "I reckon the lad was defending the dog." He cursed himself for his previous thought. Carefully, he laid Trip in his sleeping box, then turned to Jimmie sitting doubled up on a stool.

"Right, get yourself laid on my bunk, then I can look and see what has happened to you."

Slowly Jimmie transferred himself from the stool and was pleased to lay his weary limbs on the bunk. Skip looked at the pathetic scene: Trip whimpering in his box, and his new helpmate shivering with fear and pain. Any hardness over from the past was suddenly removed. His heart went out to the boy. "Have you ever drunk rum before?"

"No, Skip," came the feeble reply.

"Well, I am going to give you some now, but drink it slowly. It will relieve your pain and help you sleep." The tone of Skip's voice at that precise moment gave greater solace to Jimmie than the thought of the pending drink. He sipped, and coughed, and then sipped again. Skip looked at the boy's face. It was puffed and red. Blood dripped from the side of his mouth and one eye was quickly closing up. The knuckles of both hands were raw.

"Why, oh why?" he quietly said to himself. "I'm sorry, Jimmie. It was my fault. You keep drinking the rum and I will tidy you up."

With hot water and flannel, Skip carefully washed the wounds. The rum, meanwhile, had its effect. Jimmie lay sleeping. Skip bandaged the boy's hands with a piece of linen, and looked sadly at his own right hand. He removed Jimmie's boots and then found his shins were bruised and clotted with blood where he had been kicked. Carefully, he undressed the lad, bathing each wounded part and finally covering him with a blanket.

For him, tonight, it would be sitting, watching and thinking. Exhausted from the day and the evening's ordeal, Jimmie slept soundly.

Making himself as comfortable as he could, with a large drink beside him, Skip began to re-assess the day. Paddy now gone, he was on his own with a boy who was already showing capabilities. What could he expect from him? What could he teach him, because teach him he must? Already the lad had proved himself. Despite coming from the slums, he was polite, he had a heart of gold, he showed affection and was determined. While Skip did not know the facts of what had really happened on the river bank, he was certain that Jimmie had been defending Trip and himself. He was well aware of the nicknames the bargeing fraternity had for him. "I was a fool to let him off on his own, with those lads knocking around."

In spite of his discomfort, Skip slept. Morning broke with heavy rain. It would be three hours before Joe Hymas arrived. He lit the fire, made some tea, and toasted some of the sandwiches that Nell had packed.

The movement at last woke Jimmie, who found it hard to come to grips with where he was. He tried to turn, but every bone in his body ached.

"Wot's 'appened, Skip? Me 'ands are all wrapped up."

"You stay where you are, Jimmie. I have some tea for you to drink."

Skip helped him to sit up, and Jimmie drank.

"Cor, me jaw don't 'arf 'urt. I don't fink I did very well against that lot last night. Me Dad don't like me fightin'. 'E would say, serve you right, if 'e could see me this mornin'. But they 'it Trip wiv a lump of wood, and called you Hoity-Toity. But I didn't start the fight, Skip, really I didn't. Someone clobbered me from the back and I fell to the ground, then I just went mad."

Jimmie had said enough to tell Skip that his suspicions were correct, but he was surprised that they should take it out on the dog as well. Holding Jimmie's battered hands, Skip explained how he was not liked by all the seamen, and he was sorry that Jimmie should suffer on his behalf. On the other hand, he was proud of the way Jimmie had defended Trip and himself.

"I can assure you, Jimmie, that your three assailants are also nursing their wounds this morning. Now, we must get you better."

By soaking the bread, Jimmie managed to get some food down. Then he lay back on the bed and fell asleep.

Chapter Five

Eyotts Farm

By eight o'clock the rain had cleared and the sun shone brightly. Joe, the huffler, came on board. Jimmie could hear the talking, and called out. When Skip arrived, he asked to be helped up the ladder. "I wanna see where we're goin'."

Skip admired the lad's courage, and made him comfortable on deck on some sailcloth.

"Can you see with one eye, Jimmie?"

"Yes, Skip. I won't miss a fing."

Jimmie watched the two men. Only the topsail was unfurled, and they moved off slowly. The river branched to starboard, the direction the 'Maywell' took. Jimmie realised how narrow the river was getting. Skip seemed busy with a long pole, moving from side to side, preventing the bows from touching the saltings. Slowly, the 'Maywell' negotiated the sharp bends. The mile trip from Hullbridge to Eyotts Farm was nearly completed. The barge slowly made its way round the last large bend. Jimmie, lying on his makeshift couch, could see the farmhouse and buildings close to the river's edge. On the bank stood men and children awaiting their arrival. The 'Maywell' came almost to a standstill. Lines were thrown ashore, fore and aft, and were passed through pulley blocks. The barge was slowly pulled sideways onto the bank. Likewise, the gangplank was pulled across the gap. Skip paid Joe for his assistance, and Joe then untied his dinghy from the stern and began the row back to Hullbridge.

Quickly, the waiting men began the task of laying a platform from the sides of the 'Maywell' to the bank. A tumbril was drawn up to the board and unloading proceeded. Onto the ship walked a large, portly man and shook hands with Skip. After talking business, he turned towards Jimmie, "Hello, young man. It would appear that you must have run into pirates on the way. I hope you gave a good account of yourself."

"I can assure you he did, Harry, but three against one tells a story."

Harry, turning to one of the men unloading, told him to nip to the house. "Get my cane fireside chair, and tell the wife we have a special guest."

That done, the workmen soon lifted Jimmie into the armchair. With one holding the front legs, and the other the back of the chair, they carried him over the gangplank and into the farmhouse, followed by Skip and the man called Harry. The procession into the house was greeted by tones of anquish from the womenfolk as they gathered around Jimmie.

"Oh, you poor boy, whatever happened?"

"Make the lad comfortable, Mary, we can have the details later," said Harry.

Above the fireplace was a large mirror, and for the first time Jimmie saw himself. The sight took him back. "No wonder the ladies screamed," he thought.

Raising his voice the best he could with his stiff jaw, he murmured, "I'm

sorry I frightened you, ma'am, wiv me funny face, but me Mum reckons I'm pretty!"
"Of course you have a pretty face," came the motherly voice of Mrs Millard, "but for the time being it needs a little make do and mend."
Quickly, a makeshift bed was prepared in the farmhouse parlour, then Jimmie was transferred from the uncomfortable whicker chair to a soft mattress and clean sheets. With loving care, Mary and Rosy the housemaid, began to assess the extent of Jimmie's wounds. Arms, legs and even his back had bruises and large wheals, caused by the thrashing of a stick. Carefully they bathed and bandaged his battered frame. Frequently he cringed as they carried out their task.
"You poor boy!" cried Mary. "How can you smile at us when you are obviously in so much pain?"
"You're all so luv'ly to me, Ma'am," was his weak reply.
For the next three days Jimmie had neither the strength nor the inclination to leave his bed. His only request was that he should be moved nearer to the window, so that he could see the river and watch the tide come in and go out again.
The incident caused a problem for Skip. It would delay his return to Burnham and Paddy. Taking the dinghy, he rowed back to Hullbridge to contact a passing barge, to pass on a message to Paddy and Nell.

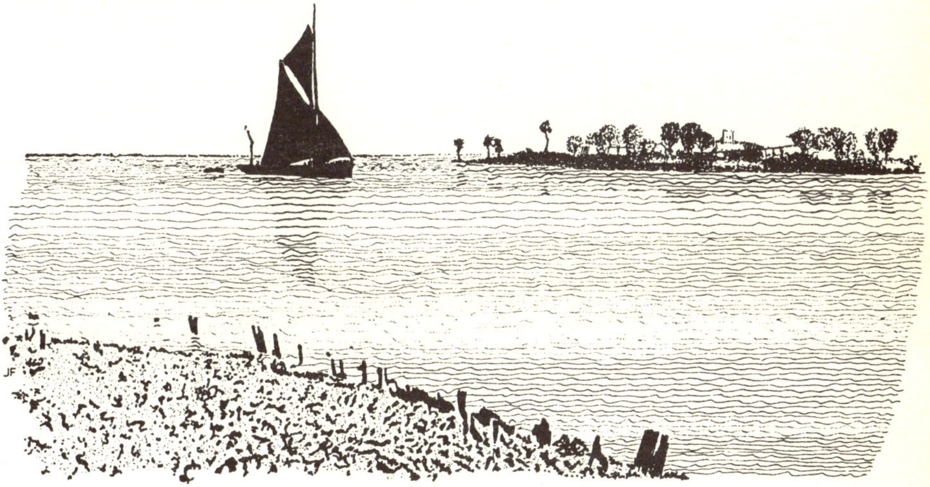

SAILING BARGE NEAR HULLBRIDGE

Twice a day Skip visited his patient and, throughout the day, when conditions permitted, Mary's children brought in their pets, even a jackdaw, to entertain Jimmie.
The care and attention paid by Mary and Rose embarassed him. His insistance that he was alright, lying there, seemed to make them fuss over him the more. On the fourth evening, when Skip came to see his charge, Jimmie was sitting dressed, looking at a book.

"I'm gettin' better nar, Skip. I wanna start work termorrer!"
"I'm very pleased to hear you say that, Jimmie, but I think a couple of days convalescence would be more appropriate. The children are anxious to show you around the farm, and the exercise will get your limbs in trim again."
The expression on the lad's face was one of disappointment. "Can I sleep on the 'Maywell' tonight, Skip?"
"Whatever for, Jimmie? Aren't conditions good enough for you here?"
"No, Skip. They're too good. I'm not used to it. I don't deserve it."
Skip took the point and realised that the boy was really out of his depth. Hard boards and straw were his ideal.
"Right then, we will compromise."
"Wot's that mean?" Jimmie asked, inquisitively.
"It means, I will go part-way with your request, and you will obey my instructions. Tonight you will sleep here, and tomorrow night you can sleep on the 'Maywell', but for the next two days you will spend your time on the farm with the children."
"Ta, Skip," was the doleful reply.
To his surprise, he found the two days being escorted around the farm more than interesting. Other than horses, it was his first experience of animals such as cows, goats and poultry. The art of building haystacks intrigued him: he had only ever seen hay eaten by horses, he had never imagined the way in which it was prepared.
The workmen on the farm likewise became interested in the lad they thought to be a bargeman's son, yet who had a great knowledge of horses. Meals were still provided from the house and, with his jawbone and gums healing, Jimmie could now enjoy the wholesome food.
Meanwhile, all the dung had been removed from the 'Maywell'. Jimmie began to realise that it was a far more odorous task to unload than to load. He watched with interest as men with buckets of disinfectant and brooms scrubbed out the hold, overseen by Skip. Cleanliness of the ship was a fact of life he was to learn over the next few years. With Skip, cleanliness came before godliness, and was exercised at all times. Six days after arriving at Eyotts Farm, Jimmie was officially returned to duty. Workmen were busy now loading hay bales into the hold for the return journey.
"I expect your father will be feeding his horses with that fodder in a few days time."
Mr Millard's voice made Jimmie jump. He was absorbed by the way the men were stacking the trusses.
"Yes, sir. 'E's fussy wot 'e gives 'em. I'll be able to tell 'im 'ow it's made and where it cum from. That should please 'im."
Jimmie's duties were light that morning, cleaning the cabin and preparing a meal. Then Skip showed him how to whip a frayed line, and gave him a few ends to practise on, with instructions to bring them to the cabin when completed.
It was an hour before Jimmie ventured back with his effort.
"That's not the way I showed you, Jimmie. Do I suspect your grandfather has been giving you instructions?"
"Yes, Skip. 'E said it would cum in useful one day."
"He was quite right, but it will not come amiss to learn my way as well.

Now, you can make a cup of tea for us, and a jug for the workmen. After that I want you to come and sit down. I want to have a talk with you."

The look on Skip's face suggested to Jimmie that this talk would be of a serious nature. He quickly brewed the tea, thinking all the time that he would be scolded for fighting and missing out on work. Man and boy drank their tea in silence.

"Any minute 'e's goin' to explode," thought Jimmie, but what he did not know was that his employer was also fighting a mental battle. One week with this young urchin had completely disrupted his mode of life. Every decision seemed to revolve around him and he had asked himself, time and time again, whether he had acted on impulse, ignoring the consequences. Now he must decide whether or not he was man enough to carry out his original plan. Jimmie washed the two mugs and prepared himself inwardly for the sharp edge of his employer's tongue.

"Sit down, Jimmie, and make yourself comfortable. We shall be talking for a long while. I will light my pipe and you can eat some of Nell's toffee."

The permission to dip into the toffee tin relaxed the boy at once.

"Unless I am mistaken, did I suspect a hint of disillusionment on your face when we brought up at Hullbridge last week?"

Jimmie looked somewhat puzzled.

"I don't 'no wot yer really mean, but I were right upset wen yer told me it were Wudum Ferrus over that wall."

"Well, Jimmie, you have answered the question correctly and confirmed my assumption, and that is now the question for immediate discussion. Would you like to describe to me what you were expecting to see on your arrival at Woodham Ferris?"

For a few seconds Jimmie strove to separate his teeth from the toffee, then he answered sheepishly, "Weel, Skip, I fort it were gonna be suffink like Lundun, but orl luvly an' clean, an' lots ov sand instead ov mud, an' lots ov them trees wiv dirty great long leaves, like yer see on the tea chests at the docks. An' orl I could see was nuffink but grass and a few trees."

There was quite a pause in the conversation as Skip assessed Jimmie's reply. He cleared his throat, "Whilst I apologise for not describing our destination, the experience of discovering for oneself should not be denied, Jimmie. It is now my intention to prove to you that Woodham Ferris is not as you described: grass, a few trees, and nothing else. I have always found it a place of great interest, so I am proposing that we go on a tour of discovery this afternoon, hopefully to whet your appetite for the Essex countryside."

"Fank you, Skip, I shall enjoy that. I fort you were gonna tell me orf for 'avin' that dust up wiv them kids."

"On that matter, I am well aware that you did what you considered right and honourable, and I appreciate your action. The outcome was that everyone suffered because of my lack of foresight. From now on that matter is closed."

Chapter Six

Woodham Ferris

One hour later, Skip and Jimmie, followed by Trip, left the 'Maywell' and headed in a northerly direction along a rugged cart track which led to the fenland and rolling countryside beyond. Jimmie was dressed in his best rig and Skip carried a canvas bag roped over his shoulder. He had a five-foot staff in his hand.

The first stop was but a matter of five hundred yards. Here the river parted its way to encircle the fifty or more acres of fenland. They stopped to watch the rising tide rush up the two creeks, each in an effort to outstrip the other in its penetration inland. Between the two arms of water, moving gently in the breeze, lay acre upon acre of pink and mauve thrift. With the reflection of the sunlight and clouds it looked like a vast shimmering lake.

"Cor, look at that! There must be fousands and fousands of them flowers. 'Oo the 'ell planted that lot?"

The sudden outburst rather startled Skip. The boy's description of the scene showed deep appreciation, but his vocabulary lacked the beauty of the flowers.

"How come you have not seen them before? You have been running about here for two days."

"I dunno, Skip. I expect we 'ave always gorn the uver way."

"Those flowers you are looking at are known as thrift, and the plant thrives on the land partly covered by the sea water. We shall be crossing over the area shortly.

"Good," said Jimmie. "When I go 'ome I'd like to take some for me Mum. She loves flowers."

They continued their journey, but within a short while Skip had brought the trio to a halt. Then, pointing with his staff into the sky, asked Jimmie, "What sort of bird is that?"

The boy's eyes scanned the sky. At last they rested on what appeared to be a stationary dot above him.

"Blimie, I've never seen a sparra' standin' still in the sky before. Owed they do it, Skip?"

"That sparra', as you call it, is a skylark, and it is hovering. In fact, if you listen you can hear it singing, but what it really is doing is keeping a watch on us, or any predators who could destroy its nest and young. It will hopefully frighten them away."

He told Trip to sit and Jimmie to stand still and watch. Quickly the bird dropped from the sky and landed in the grass nearby.

"Follow me," said Skip, then pointed to a tuft of green grass with his staff, "Have you seen anything like that before?"

Jimmie went down on his knees quickly. Nestled together in their home of moss and feathers were five little fledglings, their mouths wide open for food.

"Blimie, the poor little buggers! They ain't got no fevvers, and fancy 'avin'

them on the ground w'ere someone's gonna tread on them!"
Once more, Skip flinched at the boy's manner of expression and felt a word of reproof was necessary. Looking sternly at the lad he said,
"Jimmie, while I agree that your style of expression and dialect has a charm of its own, and is a natural part of you, I do not like to hear you swear. It does nothing for your character and quickly becomes a nauseating habit."
Jimmie got the message. "Sorry, Skip. I do that when I get excited. You'll 'ave to tell me if I do it again, 'cos I soon forgets."
"Have no fear, young man, your memory will definitely improve if you remain in my employ."
Their next stop was to open the gate of a very old rustic bridge which spanned the creek. "It was re-built by the prisoners of the Napoleonic wars," explained Skip.

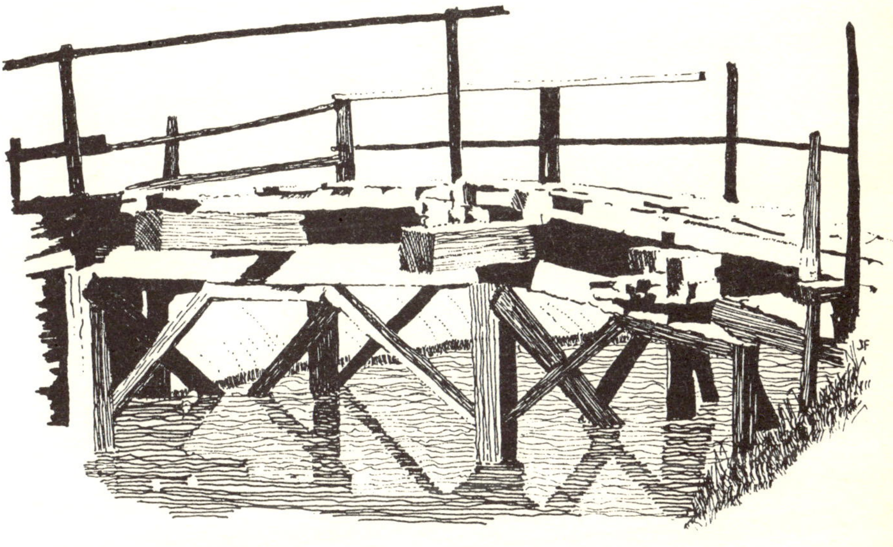

BRIDGE OVER FENN CREEK

They made their way onto the bridge and rested their arms on the protection rails. "Wot's it got two gates for?" enquired Jimmie.
"To prevent animals getting on it from both sides. You must always remember to close gates when you are in the country, to prevent animals roaming away."
"It was on me Grandad's ship they took that fella to some island. Me Grandad reckoned 'e chucked 'is orders around like nobody on earf, instead of be'avin' like a prisoner."
"I presume you are now talking about Napoleon. You are correct when saying they took him to an island. It was St Helena in the South Atlantic. That man caused a tremendous lot of misery to countless thousands. A few years in that lonely place must have given him time to reflect on his misdeeds. I am certain your grandfather was right. Napoleon had been throwing his orders around all his life and would have found it difficult to curb his tongue, even as a prisoner. Right. Fasten the gates and lets get going."

Trip proudly led them along the raised track which formed the roadway across the fenland.
"This track on which we are now walking must be one of the oldest, and often one of the busiest in the area," said Skip. "For centuries, seamen have rowed or sailed their craft to the head of the river, loaded or unloaded their freight of corn, lime, timber, stone and coal. Men with horses and carts have pulled their merchandise backwards and forwards over this very road to the hinterland, and yet now it is all so peaceful and quiet, with birds, flowers and bees to cheer us on our way."
Jimmie took little notice of what Skip was saying, for he had a burning desire to jump the shallow ditch bordering the track and go scuttling through the sea of flowers.
His wish was soon granted. "We turn left here and follow the footpath. Its the way the farmworkers take to get to Tabrums Farm, on the far side of the creek."
The feel of the springy turf under foot and the constant tap of flower heads on Jimmie's boots gave him a peculiar sensation. Without warning, he gave a loud "Whoopee!", threw his arms skywards, did three somersaults and lay flat on his back. Trip raced around him, barking furiously.
This latest intrusion into Skip's methodical and reserved way of life was not readily accepted. His reaction was immediate. "Get up from the ground at once, and conduct yourself like the man you are to be, not like a seven-year-old child!"
Skip's tone of voice quickly made Jimmie realise that there was no time to delay. He jumped to his feet immediately.
"I'm sorry, Skip. I don't know wot came over me. It felt so nice, walkin' fru them flawrs, it made me wanna do summit 'cos I was so 'appy."
"I suppose it's understandable. I was romancing about it myself a few minutes ago, but I must admit it does not have quite the same effect on me. So, in future, please give me a word of warning if you feel that your ecstacy is going to overwhelm you."
The path led them to a narrow-planked bridge with two handrails for protection. It was just wide enough to allow one person to cross the creek. Jimmie sought permission to cross and when this was granted he was quickly pursued by Trip. Skip continued walking the river bank and then settled himself down on a small headland beside the ford which enabled cattle and carts to cross from the surrounding farms to Tabrums. Jimmie soon took his place beside his guide, letting his legs swing over the bank. Cattle that had been grazing on the fen were now being driven over the ford before the rising tide, to be milked at Tabrums Farm. Trip quickly volunteered his assistance to hasten the process, only to find that not all cows appreciate a fox terrier around their hocks, and beat a hasty retreat. He was commanded to lay at Skip's feet and not interfere where he was not wanted. All was quiet until Jimmie broke the silence. "Ain't much to look at 'ere."
"That may be your opinion, young man, but I entirely disagree." Skip pointed, "How far do you estimate the distance of that hedgerow on the other side of the creek to be?"
"Firty feet," came the quick reply.
"Well, I will double that. Now, tell me what you can see between us and

the hedgerow."
Jimmie thought for a few moments. "Water an' grass," he said.
"Are you certain about that?"
"Yeah. There ain't nuffin' else."
"Now listen, Jimmie. I don't blame you for that reply, you are no different from ninety per cent of the public who walk about our country and only see ten per cent of what there is to be seen. Now, take notice of what I am going to tell you. Remember and learn. Do you realise that between us and those bushes there must be around sixty species of plant life?"
"Wot's species?"
"Good question. Never be afraid to ask for explanations. By species we mean different types or variations. Just take a close look at that clump of green plants there and see for yourself. They all have their own botanical names. How many different birds do you know, tell me now?"
Jimmie scratched his head. "Robins, pidgeons, seagulls, starches, sparrers ... ow an' that fing we saw this mornin'."
"I don't suppose you see many more in your particular part of London, but in the country here, if one looks hard, you will find over a hundred different birds. Do you realise that in that grass live and crawl hundreds of different creatures. In that mud along the river bank are thousands of worms and crabs. Even in the air around us are millions of insects and germs. For many, you need a microscope to see them, and you tell me there is nothing to see or look at! It is not always important what you see, it is what you are looking for.
"In this part of the country, where fenland and sea water meet, the natural country environment abounds with life. That is why I consider the fens at Woodham Ferris my favourite hunting spot."
The sun shone, bringing the temperature into the eighties. Skip had dropped off to sleep and Trip appeared to be doing the same at his master's feet. Jimmie sat contemplating what Skip had been saying.
"Grandad was right: he is a clever chap, and he makes you want to know more about fings."
For a while, he watched men busy loading hay on the carts in a nearby field, then turned his gaze upstream. The river did a sharp turn. What caught his eye made him freeze in his position with bated breath. His eyes became fixed on the approaching creature, stealthily making its way downstream. Despite its size, its movement hardly disturbed the water.
It came to within twenty feet of where he sat, then stopped. Jimmie watched as the bird drew its long neck back over its body. With its long beak and tufted feathers, it looked a fearsome creature. Then, like an arrow leaving the bow, its head shot forward into the water, and returned holding an eel some eighteen inches long in its beak. Jimmie gripped the grass with his hands. He was mesmerised by the scene before him. He watched the bird swallow the eel in three gulps and could restrain himself no longer.
"You bally guts!" he shouted.
His voice caused the bird to flap its large wings and take off upstream, quickly pursued by Trip barking furiously along the bank.
Skip sat up straight in time to see the bird.
"Now what is all the fuss about?"

"That fing just swallered an eel, two-foot-six long."
"Are you sure it was two-feet-six?"
"Well, it ware a biggun."
"Fish and eels are its staple diet, so I'm not surprised. Do you know what sort of bird it is, Jimmie?"
"Not really, Skip. The only fings I know that 'ave long legs and necks are wot Grandad calls orstriches, so I suppose that was a baby one."
Skip laughed. Jimmie felt a little hurt.
"That, my boy, is a Frank Heron. They are found in most salt water creeks. I wouldn't be surprised if it hasn't a large nest somewhere in one of those trees over there. I brought you along this side of the fens hoping to see a special bird. Its favourite haunt is among those trees I just pointed to. Let's make our way along and find out whether we are in luck's way."
Large elms spread their branches over the narrowing creek, which at low tide was just a few feet wide, but when high, spanned some twenty feet or more.
"If we sit behind this hawthorn bush, and have patience, we may be rewarded."
It was not long before Jimmie and Trip showed signs of restlessness, especially not knowing what to expect. Suddenly, Skip's hand twisted Jimmie's head upstream, "Keep still, and watch. It's coming."
A shrill mechanical sound rent the air. A flash of blue and orange hit the water in front of them, submerged and then broke water a few feet further on, rose and settled on an overhanging branch.
"Now watch carefully," whispered Skip.
Jimmie trembled with excitement. The bird held a small fish in its beak. Then, with the skill of a conjuror, it flipped its head, threw the fish into the air, opened its beak full width, caught and swallowed its prey. The bird flapped its wings and continued along the creek.
"Cor lummy! I ain't seen nuffin' like that in my life afore. Wot d'you call that?"
"First you must try and describe it to me, then I will tell you."
"Well, it ain't very big, abawt six to eight inches, I reckon. Blue wings, and I fink it were orange on its front, and it 'ad an 'ell of a whistle."
"That's a fair description, although the naturalist would prefer a more refined version. It is known as a kingfisher: a most interesting bird."
"I'd like to catch one of them and take it 'ome to me Mum. She likes pretty birds and would give it plenty of fish."
"Why put it in a cage, Jimmie. It's happy living here, in its own environment. Don't you realise that?"
"I fink you're right, Skip. It would be cruel, p'raps she 'ad better come 'ere one day an' see it for 'erslf."
"Our next port of call," said Skip getting to his feet, "is the Whalebone Inn. I need a drink."
They collected their belongings and headed for a road that skirted the limit of the fenland.
"This road will take you back to London if you choose to leave me now."
"No, Skip. I want to stay with you on the 'Maywell' for ever."
The feeling in the boy's voice touched the man's latent emotions. He made no reply, just led the way over the stony road. A few cottages on the left

showed signs of local people, and to the right, almost lost among high trees, Jimmie could see what appeared to be a farmhouse and buildings. However, what attracted his attention most was a continuous rat-a-tat-tat in a nearby tree.

"Wot's that noise?" he asked.

From his shoulder-bag Skip drew his small telescope. "I thought this might be of some use."

He quickly focussed it and picked out the culprit, then directed Jimmie's eye onto a beautiful green and black bird, hanging by its feet onto the trunk of the tree. Through the telescope, it appeared but a few inches away.

"Ain't it a beauty, Skip. Wot's it keep banging its 'ead against the tree for? It's a wonder it don't knock itself out."

"It's not really banging its head. That rat-a-tat is its beak digging into the bark searching for wood lice and other insects. It is called a green woodpecker, and we have been very fortunate in our sighting of it today. In fact, in seeing so many different varieties."

Within a few minutes they had crossed a red brick hump-backed bridge.

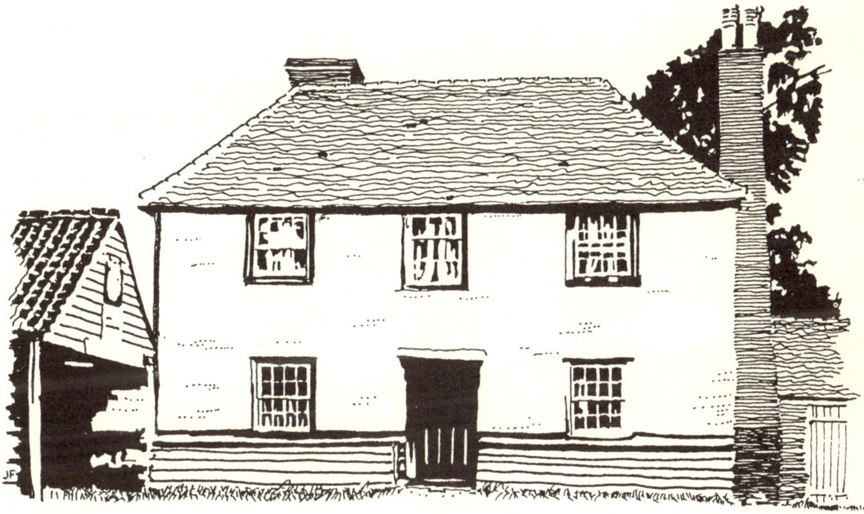

THE OLD "WHALEBONE" WICKFORD ROAD

"Here we are at the 'Whalebone'. We can quench our thirst here."

Jimmie surveyed the scene. Farm buildings were the predominant feature: Fenn Farm, on the 'Whalebone' side of the road, and Shaws Farm on the other. "Like the pub, they have all been around for two hundred years or more," explained Skip.

"They all look as though they need repairing," thought Jimmie. "Suffink like our 'ouse."

Dislodged tiles and loose boards exposed the heavy oak timbers on the pub. On the forecourt stood a couple of farm wagons, their horses enjoying a well-earned meal from their nosebags, while the drivers supped their beer inside. Around and in the pond to the side of the pub, ducks, geese and chickens seemed to abound. All were then disturbed by two boys leading a pair of horses into the water to have their fetlocks scrubbed clean of farm refuse.

"Is this Wudum Ferrus?" asked Jimmie.

"In a way, yes, but the real village is a mile further on. We shall get there one day, but for the moment let's go inside."

As they entered, they received a welcome from Mrs Hill, the landlady, "Hello Todd. No Paddy today? But who is this smart young fellow behind you?"

"I'm afraid you will not be seeing Paddy for a long while. He is returning to the Emerald Isle, and Jimmie here is my new mate."

They sat themselves down on a form beside a long table which appeared as old as the building. The heavy timber had been scrubbed until the knots protruded, while the edges had been worn round and hacked by many a farmworker's knife. At the far end of the table, his head laid on his folded arms, sat a typical local, fast asleep. He was dressed in corduroy trousers with leather buskins, a well-worn smock covering a coarse shirt, a red spotted kerchief round his neck and his shiny hardtop was lying on the table before him.

The arrival of Skip and Jimmie caused him to cock one eye in their direction. Then a scuffle broke out below the table. Trip and the local's dog decided to battle it out as to who should sleep where, and it was obvious that Trip was getting the worse of the bargain. Urgent commands brought the offenders laying coyly at ther masters' feet. Skip apologised profusely for the fracas.

"He know'd I were asleep, he own't let anyone come nigh, let alone a dawg. He oen't cause any more trouble, master."

Then, once more, the stranger placed his head on his arms. Skip ordered his drink and home-brewed beer for Jimmie plus some ham and pickle sandwiches.

"I'm certain our friend with the dog could drink another pint, Mrs Hill."

"I'm certain he'll not refuse," was her pleasant reply.

Skip placed the tankard down in front of the man's folded arms.

"Thank yer, sir, I reckon I knows you from somewhere, leastwise the Paddy Mrs Hill spoke about. He flitched me at dominoes a couple of year ago at the 'Anchor', Hullbridge. I'm awaiting to have my revenge."

"Yes, I also recall that evening. I'm afraid that Paddy had few scruples when it came to playing cards or dice. So, you must be the drover."

"Ay, that's me. I were jest ketching up on a few minutes shut eye."

"How far have you plodded today?" enquired Skip.

The drover took from his trouser pocket a large watch suspended on a heavy chain, and pointed, "It were jest turned half-past-four when I left Rayleigh this morning. I took six coos to Brentwood, then I collected a score o' sheep from a nearby farm; I be taken them to Southminster, they're in the 'bone paddock. I shell be sleeping in the barn opposite tonight and orf again around four tomorrow, so, looking at my watch, around twenty-five mile."

"What is the record distance you have walked in your profession?"

"Jest over forty, from Cambridge," then he winked, "but ten of they were

on horseback."
"You and your dog do a tough job, of that I'm certain," said Skip.
Jimmie had meanwhile palled up with an older lad who had produced two ferrets from his jacket pocket and tried to sell them to him. He was mystified by the creatures, with their long wriggling yellow bodies, pink eyes and long bushy tails. That they were for catching rabbits intrigued him. He had great respect for their needle-like teeth, but a great dislike for their putrid smell, and told the would be salesman that there was not much use for them on a boat.
Sandwiches and drink all consumed, Skip wished the drover, Mrs Hill and customers, "Goodnight" and, followed by Jimmie, left the 'Whalebone' for the 'Maywell'. Jimmie became interested in a large piece of bone hung under the sign of the pub and had to run to catch Skip and Trip up. "Why do they call that pub the 'Whalebone'?"
"Well," said Skip, "from the information I have gathered from the older residents of the area, it would appear that somewhere around a hundred years ago, a baby whale was marooned on the fens, and the bone you were looking at, and the number displayed inside the pub, are some of its remains. It is not for me to confirm the story, but it certainly is a feasible reason for giving the pub that name."
Once back on board the 'Maywell', Jimmie was given one more job to do before supper. While Skip visited Mr Millard, he filled the water storage tank on board. This involved releasing the brake which allowed the sails of the wind pump in the farmyard to clank round and draw the precious water up from a source some two hundred feet below ground. Then, through a small trapdoor on the deck, he was able to pour the contents of the buckets into the ship's tank.
When Skip rejoined the 'Maywell' the sun had set, displaying a gorgeous picture of red and gold.
"That's a fair indication of good weather for our trip tomorrow," said Skip, as they drank their evening cocoa.
"Are we returning to Lundun tomorrer?" asked Jimmie excitedly.
"No, tomorrow you will be in charge. I'll be your first mate!"
Jimmie looked puzzled.
"Can you drive Kitty in the trap? We are going to do a tour of the area."
"Cor, good. I can manage 'er."

Chapter Seven

Woodham Ferris Church and Area

At seven next morning, Jimmie was in the stableyard. A horseman had shown him where Kitty's harness was to be found, and said, "I'll be with you in ten minutes."

But for Jimmie ten minutes was a long time. He threw the harness over the pony's back, drew the trap up near the stable door and backed the pony between the shafts. Soon he buckled up and patted Kitty as he finished the job.

Sitting eating his breakfast, Harry Millard watched with interest. "Good gracious, Mary," he shouted, "that boy could show half my workmen a trick or two in fastening up."

He left the table and made his way out into the yard, to where Jimmie was standing.

"Good work. I saw you do that. You have obviously done it before."

"Yes, sir. Two 'undred every mornin' at me father's stables. You've only got furteen pair, that don't take long," Jimmie laughed. "I didn't do 'em on me own, guv'nor. I 'ad someone to 'elp me."

"Yes, I quite believe that, Jimmie. Another hundred and fifty at least! Right, take her nosebag into the granary and fill it. She'll need some food during the day."

"When do I feed 'er, sir?"

"Don't worry, Jimmie, she'll nip your arse if you forget, and don't forget to tell your skipper."

"Right, sir. I'll remember that."

Proudly Jimmie drove Kitty out of the yard and up to the 'Maywell'.

"Your carriage awaits you, sir," he shouted to Skip, who was talking to a workman making the final touches to the loading.

"Thank you, my boy," replied Skip, as he climbed up onto the trap.

Off they set, turning right over the hill. They followed the hedgerow, meeting a hard track in half a mile.

"If we turn right we shall arrive at Hullbridge Ferry, but we need to turn left."

Other than a pair of wooden cottages, from which about twelve children rushed to greet them, there were no signs of dwellings or people until they joined the Burnham to Wickford road. A wooden signpost in the middle of the road indicated the way. Once more they turned left. A row of cottages made a change from the giant elm trees which had enclosed their view for the previous three-quarters of a mile.

"That's the Manor of Champions Hall, which is the most prominent house of the area," pointed out Skip.

"By the look of the gardens they must be stinking rich," remarked Jimmie.

"Not necessarily so. They are often only tenants of the Manor, and farming is not the most lucrative of industries at the moment, but they will be important people." Pointing to the west of the Manor, he continued, "That

area on the far side of the paddock is where they practise archery."
"Blimey, they don't still fight wiv bows an' arrers round 'ere do they?"
"No," said Skip, "but that's no reason why the art should cease. To continue my description of the Manor - the depression on the side of the road and leading up to the rear of the Manor, is considered by locals to be the remains and extension of the moat, allowing shallow boats to come from Fenn Creek to bring merchandise to the Hall. Whether it be a fact I cannot be certain, but it could be feasible."
By now they had approached another signpost in the centre of the road.
"Which way?" asked Jimmie.
"Can't you read the words in front of you?"
"No, I only wish I could."
"We turn right, or starboard when on the sea."
Jimmie quickly brought Kitty around and to the edge of a shallow pond. "I reckon she needs a drink wiv it gettin' so 'ot."
"Had we carried on, we should have arrived at the 'Whalebone', but now we are heading for the real village of Woodham Ferris," explained Skip.
On the approach to a steep hill, Jimmie suggested they should walk.
"Good thinking. The exercise will do us no harm," agreed Skip. They made the hill, then walked down the other side. A few cottages and a wind pump, which Skip said was all part of the old village workhouse, drew their attention.
"Me Dad reckons he'd shoot 'imself rarver than go into one of them places."
"They certainly have a bad reputation and we can only hope the system will change for the better."

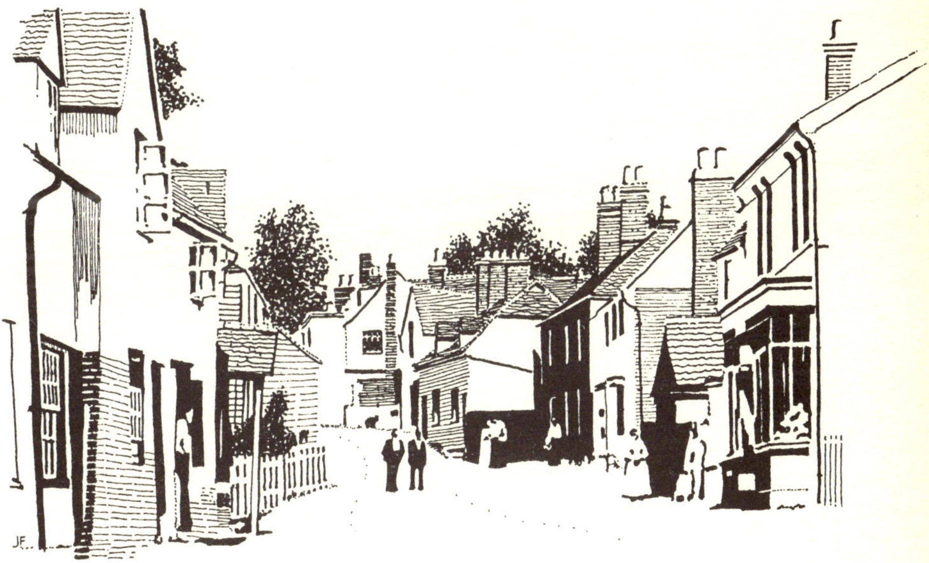

WOODHAM FERRERS VILLAGE

Their arrival in the village brought out a few spectators. They came to a halt at the village blacksmith's: one of the reasons for the day's trip. Kitty was to have a new set of shoes. Jimmie slipped the reins around a post and

Skip walked into the smithy. Within moments, Jimmie was surrounded by children.

"Where you from? Who are you? I know the pony and trap but I don't know you," said an older boy.

"I'm from Wappin'."

The answer made the children laugh.

"There ain't no such place," they screamed.

"Well, Lundun then."

"Where's that?"

Jimmie suddenly felt he was a veteran traveller. Once again he raised himself to his full height.

"Ain't you kids been anywhere uvver than Wudum?"

They in turn looked at the smart young man as being someone important.

Skip returned, "We have an hour to spare, so let's have a wander round."

Women standing in the doorways of their houses watched as Skip and Jimmie walked back down the street, followed by a dozen children.

"Ain't they seen no one from Lundun before?" asked Jimmie, keeping close to Skip.

"I will send that lot packing in a few moments," said Skip. "Anyone who is not local is a total stranger to them, and they become suspicious. Villages, like this, are one big family and they now have strangers in their midst."

They turned from the road along a gravel path. "I'm taking you for a visit to the church," continued Skip. Then, stopping suddenly, he turned to face the followers. "Now, be off with you!"

His voice was loud and sharp. The children looked at each other, turned, and ran.

"This is a typical village church, and has an interesting history. Let's walk to the rear of the building. There are a couple of stones which tell us a little of its past."

"It looks a nice old church, Skip. It seems to be about the right size for the village."

"Yes, it's befitting to the area. I am sure my sister would enjoy painting a picture of the scene."

They walked to the rear of the church and stood overlooking the valley.

"Crikey! You can see a fair way from up 'ere. There's a few fousand trees an' all."

"Yes, Jimmie. It's a pleasant view. Our predecessors chose some nice spots to build their churches. But it was not my intention in bringing you here to admire the view. I wanted you to look at those stones, Jimmie."

The boy gazed at the slabs fixed to the west wall. They meant little to him, being unable to read.

"Do you know anything about Church history?" asked Skip.

"Nuffink. I've never bin to church. My Mum goes now an' agen. She reckons it makes 'er feel better."

"Then you would not know who the Archbishop of Canterbury would be."

"No, Skip. I never 'eard of 'im."

"Well, Jimmie, he is the Primate of the Church of England. He is one of the highest ranking people in the land, and the Archbishop of York is the next in line to him. Now, that particular Archbishop," explained Skip, pointing to the stone, "had a special connection with this church, and the area, in the sixteenth century."

"Why, did 'e build it?"

"No, Jimmie. A certain Robert de Ferrers built it in the twelfth century. That's seven hundred years ago, or four hundred years before the man I was going to tell you about. The de Ferrers family were the owners of the Manor of Woodham, and it all ties in with the story you were telling me the other day on the 'Maywell', about the men with horns on their heads."

"Lumme! Do you mean those fellers came 'ere and built it?"

"No, Jimmie. Don't presuppose. Just listen to what I have to tell you, then try not to get it muddled up with your own fantasies."

Jimmie remained silent. He was not quite sure whether he had been told off in a nice way.

"In 1066, William of Normandy (that's part of France) invaded England and defeated the English king, Harold II, and England came under his rule. Among his army were men who were barons and knights. Many not only assisted in the fighting, but helped provide the capital, or money, for the invasion. So, in return, William the Conqueror gave areas of land to his special men, and he gave the Manor of Woodham to Henry de Ferrers. It was some hundred years later that his descendant, Robert, built this church."

"Ain't that marvellous, Skip, to fink a feller should come all the way from France an' build a church in this dead an' alive 'ole."

"That, Jimmie, is an unfair statement to make about this village, one that is commonly used by townsfolk describing village life, and all because it does not line up with their ideal."

"I'm sorry, Skip, I won't say it again."

"Right, now let us get back to the subject, namely the Archbishop of York. You may recall that on our way here this morning, you drew my attention to the large house on the high ground," he said, pointing with his stick, "over there. That was built by the gentleman, Edwin Sandys, Archbishop of York, in 1550. Inside the church is a memorial giving a number of details of his family. It is also reported that the said gentleman spent a time in exile in the Tower of London."

"Well I don't fink they put parsons in the Bloody Tower. I do know where that is. I fort it were for bad people."

"Not necessarily, Jimmie. History will prove the misdemeanours of men."

They walked inside the church and Skip read the wording on the memorial.

"What I want you to understand, Jimmie, is that because your first impressions of Woodham Ferris were disappointing, it is far from being a dead and alive hole. When you begin to study its history, you find these important people of the past have been associated with the area, and places we think are quiet and of no consequence are often places of great interest. It would appear from this memorial that Cecilie Sandys, or Mrs Sandys, was respected by rich and poor alike and, like Aunt Nell, was a fine Christian woman."

"Well, I don't know about 'er on that fing, but I know Aunt nell is a cracker."

"I'm not certain my sister would approve of your description of herself, but I realise it's well intended. But we came in here to talk about the past, not the present, so let us now make our way back to the smithy."

After calling in a small general store to replenish their larder, they returned to the smithy, hitched Kitty to the trap, and were soon on their way.
"Well, what did you think of Woodham Ferris after all?" asked Skip.
"I s'pose it's a nice place, but I'd rarver live on the fens wiv Mr Millard. I couldn't stand all their eyes watchin' me".
"I'm inclined to agree with you, Jimmie, but I don't think there is much chance for us to make a living on the fens, so we must stick to the 'Maywell' and the sea."
Little cottages, large houses, even a fairly new Congregational church, lined their route, then, half-a-mile on, they arrived at the Butcher's Arms.
"Let us stop here, Jimmie. The day is hot and some form of refreshment is necessary."
They dismounted and, as Jimmie led Kitty to a horse trough to drink, Skip became engaged in conversation with a local man holding a gun and carrying a huge canvas bag over his shoulder. Politely Jimmie waited. Kitty, having quenched her thirst, became restless on her feet and moved forward. A sudden shout broke the peace.
"That animal has just bitten my arse! You should keep the thing under control, driver."
"Funny fings, 'orses," said Jimmie, turning his head away to prevent Skip from seeing him laughing. P'raps we ought ter give 'er summat to eat."
"Then do something man. We can't have her eating us!"
Jimmie removed the nosebag from its hook as Skip and the stranger walked into the pub. He gave Kitty a pat. "I'm glad you chose Skip instead of me," he told her.
The rest of the day took them to Bicknacre Priory, East Hanningfield, Rettendon, and finally to Battlesbridge and the water mill. Here they collected seed for Mr Millard. Jimmie was quite surprised to find the river, with barges tied up alongside. Their return to the Fenn bridge and Eyotts Farm ended the grand tour.
Jimmie unhitched Kitty, hung her harness on its hook, and gave her a brush down. Then he put his arms around her neck, "Fank you for givin' me such a lovely day." He now had another friend.
Being their last night at Eyotts, dinner was at the farm. It was a happy occasion.
Jimmie had now overcome his embarrassment of feeding with his hosts and was enjoying the meal.
"I take it you had an enjoyable day, Todd."
"Yes, my driver performed in great style. When he can handle a barge with the same skill, I shall be delighted. There was just one bad spot. Kitty, I regret to say, is prone to cannibalism."
"Pray, tell me more," enquired Harry.
"She succeeded in getting her teeth into my rump."
Laughter went up all round the table. Jimmie refrained, but gave a confirming smile. The farmer gave a discreet look at Jimmie who, out of Skip's sight, mouthed only the words, "I forgot to tell him." Harry recognised the messsage with a broad smile. "Well, Todd, you surprise me. I trust your injury will soon heal, but I'm sure you will agree with me, horses are like barges: not always predictable."

"Yes, I'll agree with that," answered Skip.
Jimmie mused quietly to himself, "The farmer's a real sport. He could have dropped me in the muck over that."

Chapter Eight

Grandad

Three days later, having spent one night at Aunt Nell's, Jimmie stood in the foc's'le as the 'Maywell' nudged its way between ships and tramps into Sutton Dock. Within the hour, dressed in his best rig, a canvas bag on his shoulder, he left the barge for Number Twelve, Riverview Cottages.

His approach to the house was recognised by Bingo, who raced around him in ever decreasing circles, bringing Jimmie at last to a halt. He dropped the bag, picked up the dog and hugged him. From the house came his brothers and sisters and, last of all, Mum and Dad. Never in his thirteen years had he felt so embarrassed. For an hour they talked, laughed and ate. Suddenly, Jimmie rose, put on his neb cap, and walked to the door.

"Where are you off to?" asked his Mum.

"To see Grandad before he goes to bed."

His Dad intervened, "No, Jimmie, by the time you get there he will already be asleep. You can have the day with him tomorrow. Tonight you spend with us."

Reluctantly the boy obeyed. The younger children were sent to bed and Jimmie sat with his parents around the table. In a strange way he felt ten years older than his real age. He had already presented his mother with flowers from the Fen, and had given his Dad a pipe from Burnham. Now he handed an envelope from Skip to his mother.

When opened, she found it contained one golden sovereign, and a note, "For your co-operation. T.S." She pushed the coin towards Jimmie.

"That must be for you."

"No, Mum, I've bin paid me wages," and from his pocket he drew two half-crowns.

Without hesitation, she threw her arms around her son and kissed him.

"Jimmie, I don't reckon I've ever said it before, but you're a darling."

Jimmie blushed, "And you an' Dad are crafty. You never let on the day I joined the 'Maywell', but I really did miss you."

By eight o'clock next morning Jimmie had polished his boots, washed, and tidied his hair.

"By Gawd! Yer Grandad will be proud of yer, dressed like that," said his mother. "Remember to salute, 'cos he taught yer the way when yer were two years old."

It was twenty minutes walk to the cottage, and Jimmie decided to walk along the riverside. He could watch the boats and water that were now an important part of his life.

Mrs Dixon, the local midwife, who lived next door to Grandad, was watering the plants in her front garden. She kept an eye on Grandad, and noticed now as his grandson approached the front door.

"Hello Jimmie," she shouted, "Walk right in. Your Grandad is expecting you. He saw the 'Maywell' come up yesterday evening, and waited up for you.

He was certain you would come last night."
"That's a pity, as I wanted to come. Don't matter, I'll go an' cheer 'im up now."
Jimmie walked in. His Grandad sat in his usual chair, his head resting back on the horsehair head rest.
"Cor, 'e's gorn to sleep again. 'E spens most of 'is life sleepin'," thought Jimmie. On tiptoe, he crossed the room, stood smartly to attention in front of the old man and raised his hand in a perfect sailor's salute.
"Jimmie Brown reportin' for duty, sir."
He saw his grandfather lift his head, and waited for a grand welcome. Instead, Grandad's head dropped forward onto his chest and his mouth opened slightly.
Jimmie dropped down onto his knees and took his Grandad's hands into his own.
"Come on. Wake up Grandad. It's me, Jimmie. Come to see you."
The old man lifted his head. His mouth opened and shut a number of times. Jimmie felt the thin hands grip his, and the word, "J-J-Jimmie," come from his lips. His head dropped once more onto his chest and his hands fell from Jimmie's to his side. The boy rushed to the door.
"Come 'ere, Mrs Dixon. Come quickly. Grandad's ill," he shouted.
Swiftly, dropping her watering-can, she made her way to the door and into the cottage. She rushed to the chair, knelt down, felt the old man's pulse and looked into his eyes.
Jimmie stood agast. Slowly, Mrs Dixon rose, turned to Jimmie and gripped his hands tightly.
"Now, be brave Jimmie. I am very sorry, but your grandfather is dead."
For a few seconds, which could have been hours, he stood like a statue. His whole being had come to a standstill. Softly, the voice of Mrs Dixon came through to him, "Now Jimmie, you must run to the stables and tell your father to come at once. I will go round and fetch the doctor."
Down the cobbled road, over the small green, past the market stalls, his feet crashed down, his heart thumping like a piston in a dockside engine. People shouted as he bumped by them, but he was oblivious of his surroundings. Through the large gateway into Sutton Yard, past the checker's office, down to Block K, his father's stable. Down the centre track which separated the horses' stalls, he ran, to collapse on a bale of hay near his father, who was throwing a large forkful of muck onto a barrow.
"Wot the 'ell's that entry for?" asked his father, hardly turning his head towards the panting boy.
Suddenly, his father saw the boy's state.
"Calm down, Jimmie. Take a deep breath and tell me wot's 'appened."
With stops and starts the boy told his father.
"Right, Jimmie, you sit there and get your breath back. I will rush over to Grandad's. Then, you must go to Bob Taylor's, tell 'im where I 'ave gone, and that you will finish muckin' out till I return."
Slowly, Jimmie made his way to the company office and told the story. Bob put his hand on the boy's shoulder.
"I'm sorry, Jimmie. You make your way home. I'll soon get someone to do your Dad's job."
Telling Mum was no easy matter. He refused to cry: he was now a man.

Towards midday, Jimmie was making his way towards the 'Maywell'. He explained to his mother that Skip had planned to visit Grandad that afternoon. It would now be necessary to stop him.

All was quiet on board. No one had even started to unload. He went down the gangway and tapped on the door.

"Come in."

Jimmie's entry caught Skip's eye. Something had definitely misfired. The ruddy, energetic youth looked haggard and lifeless. He sat down on the bench without saying a word.

After a pause, Skip spoke, "Do I suspect that you have decided, or perhaps been detailed, to relinquish your post on the 'Maywell'?"

The answer was not what Skip had expected. The boy could contain his emotions no longer. He thrashed his arms in the air and then banged the table.

"I 'ate 'im! I 'ate 'im!" he shouted, then dropped his head and arms onto the table, and sobbed his heart out.

The situation was somewhat embarrassing to the hardy seafarer - a boy lying heartbroken on the mess table. He put his hand on Jimmie's shoulder, "Let it all go, then you'll feel better."

"Men shouldn't cry," came the weak reply.

"Don't you be so sure about that. It's nature's way to give relief."

Skip poured out two cups of tea and put a drop of brandy into each. He needed a noggin himself.

"Drink this up, Jimmie. You appear to be in a state of shock, and I need to know what it's all about."

Tears flowed freely down Jimmie's face into the tea as he drank, but the brandy had the desired effect. He put the cup down, wiped his face and sniffed. Still staring at the table, he said, "Me Grandad's dead."

The words hit Skip below the belt.

"Your Grandad's dead! But what's that got to do with 'I hate him', Jimmie?"

He sat at the table opposite the boy and took hold of his hands.

"Now tell me all that has happened since you left me yesterday."

"'E never sor me, Skip." Another burst of tears told Skip of the anguish the boy was enduring. He must take the lead.

"Did you go and visit your Grandad this morning, or last night?"

"This morning, Skip."

"Was he dead when you arrived?"

"No, he died in front of me."

"Well, I'm sorry. That was dreadful for you, but life is dreadful at times. But why do you hate him?"

"I don't 'ate 'im, Skip. It's me Dad I 'ate."

"Why, Jimmie?"

There was a long pause. Skip could see the mental rage expressed on the boy's face.

"Tell me, Jimmie. I want to know."

"'E stopped me from goin' to see Grandad last night, and 'e would 'ave bin orl right then, and when I went to the stable to tell 'im wot 'ad 'appened, 'e told me to carry on muckin' out while 'e went to Grandad's. I 'ate 'im! I 'ate 'is bloody stables! I ain't never goin' to forgive 'im!" The boy burst into tears again.

A couple of minutes passed before Skip spoke.
"We have something in common, Jimmie, but I cannot tell you what it is, only tell you what you should do."
"Wot's that, Skip?"
"First, we must pay homage to your grandfather, by that I mean respect, because he was a gracious man. Secondly, while it may not seem apparent to you now, I am sure your father acted in good faith. He is a very conscientious man, his devotion to duty may seem a little obsessive to you, but it comes out in you from time to time, because you too are determined in your ways. That is why I have taken to you. So please, Jimmie, please forgive your father, otherwise it will ruin your life. Thirdly, I knew your grandfather more than you realise, and your loss is my loss too. While I cannot replace him, I will try and make up for your loss in whatever way possible."
"Fank you, Skip. I knew you would help me before I got 'ere. I feel better now. Please may I go an' 'elp me Mum, 'cos Grandad was 'er Dad, an' she's gonna miss 'im."
"Yes, off you go. Tomorrow's Sunday, so come and see me on Monday, and keep your chin up."
On the following Thursday, Jimmie sat next to Skip in the local church. His mother had hired a black mourning suit for the occasion, but Jimmie had insisted that his Grandad would rather have seen him in his seaman's rig than a drab outfit. He followed the cortege, oblivious of the surrounding crowds.
He sat staring at the shining coffin, draped with a Union Jack. Four sailors stood nearby, looking very smart and serious. His eyes wandered around the high-beamed church, when gradually he lost all sense of what was going on. He could hear Grandad talking, "Up and down the gangway we rushed, Jimmie, jumping over the dead and wounded. The gunners were using the powder quicker than we could get it to them, and they kept on shouting at us to get more. Our bodies were covered in sweat, blood and smoke, but we carried on. When someone said "cease fire", we laid down on the deck exhausted. It took a fortnight to get the taste of cordite from our guts, but we won the battle. I learnt a lesson from that day, Jimmie. If you want to win, you must be prepared to fight as well."
A nudge from Skip brought Jimmie back to reality. They got up and left the church. In the churchyard, he watched them lower the coffin, heard them blow the bugles and fire the guns. He could see his mother weeping and felt Skip grip his hand. He looked up. He was sure that Skip was wiping a tear from his face with the back of his gloved hand.
"There's suffink funny abawt Skip," he thought. "I shall 'ave to try an' 'elp 'im."
On the Saturday morning the 'Maywell' set sail again. Paddy had left, and a relief man was to accompany them to Gravesend, but on this trip Jimmie would be leaving home for four months. The whole family stood by the quayside to wave him goodbye. His father had whacked him on his back as he jumped aboard, "You're a good boy Jimmie, keep it up." Those words worked magic for him; it was only the night before that he had condescended to forgive his father, and had told him so as he went to bed.
As he stood waving his farewells, he made up his mind. He would work to

raise the status of his family. His brief stay at Aunt Nell's, and at Eyott's Farm, had already given him ideas of a new and better way of life.

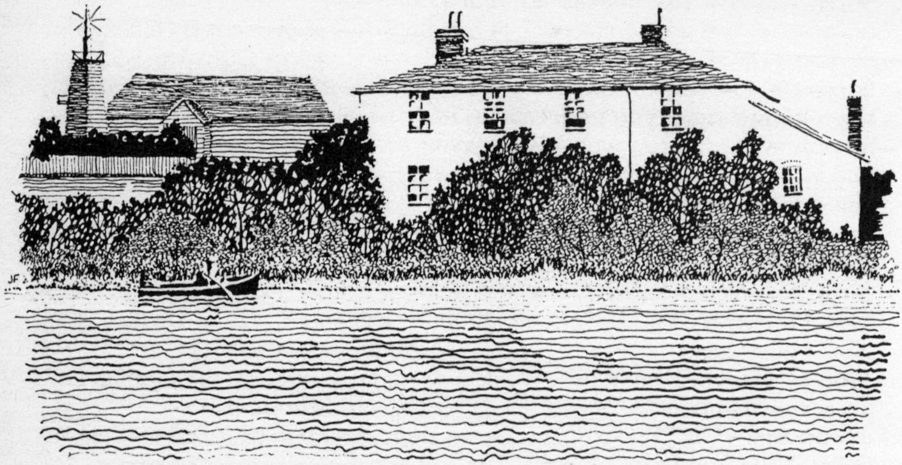

EYOTTS FARM AND FENN CREEK

Chapter Nine

Back to School

Benfleet Creek was their port of call. While the muck was being unloaded, Skip showed Jimmie around Canvey Island. The little round Dutch houses fascinated him but, the weather being wet, the surrounding marshland chilled his spine.

"I'd rarver live in the docks than 'ere," he told Skip.

A day touring Benfleet and Hadleigh Castle proved more exciting, and then, two days later, they sailed into Leigh, picked up a temporary mate, and made Burnham-on-Crouch late that evening.

Next day the 'Maywell' was sailed onto the blocks in front of King's boatyard. Jimmie and William, under Skip's instructions, spent the day transferring the kit and loose stores to a nearby shed. Many of the personal items were wheeled to Aunt Nell's cottage. The reason for this activity was that the 'Maywell' was in dock for a major refit.

It was after supper, when William had gone to bed, that Skip and Aunt Nell explained to Jimmie what his next four months' work would involve.

"In the short while you have been associated with the 'Maywell', you have expressed a desire to learn to read and write. Is that correct?"

"Yes, Skip. I'd luv to be able to do that."

"Now listen carefully. My sister and I have agreed, providing that you are willing to co-operate (and I am warning you that it will be hard work), that while the 'Maywell is being refitted, you will be taught the three R's, that is, reading, writing and arithmetic. Your programme has already been set out. You will rise at seven o'clock, wash and have your breakfast. From half-past-eight to half-past-twelve, you will be taught and given work to do, then, from half-past-two until four o'clock will be your afternoon session. Aunt Nell will be your teacher, and I will check your progress. Saturday and Sunday will be free days. I am sure you and William will find plenty to do. Any questions?"

A large smile came over Jimmie's face, "Fank you, bowf. I'll promise you I'll do me very best."

Sitting on a chair at a table was Jimmie's hardest task. He looked forward to half-past-twelve, when he could run to the river for an hour, but he was determined to succeed. His previous sschooling was a help, but he regretted that he had wasted so much time while there. The weekends were wonderful. He roamed the creeks and marshes with William. They collected shells, eggs and flowers to be studied on their return to the cottage. The whole spectrum of country life became a challenge to the youngster from a dockyard slum. Often, Skip would borrow a small sailing smack and take them down the River Roach, up to Rochford, and along the various creeks surrounding the Islands of Foulness and Wallasea.

Wet evenings were often spent with Skip teaching Jimmie the elementary rules of navigation, names of many parts of the rigging of a barge, and nautical terms. In fact his whole life seemed to be taken up with learning, working, and eating good food. Aunt Nell became the apple of the young lad's eye.

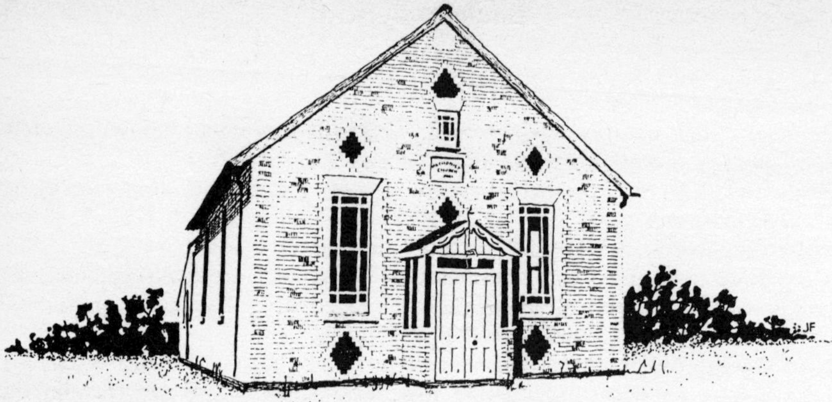

METHODIST CHAPEL, BURNHAM-ON-CROUCH

On Sundays he would attend the nearby Methodist Chapel with Aunt Nell and William. He enjoyed the singing. Aunt Nell had a lovely voice and would sometimes sing a solo. Jimmie would close his eyes and think it heavenly. Sometimes, the speaker ranted on a bit and he would find himself thinking about his lesson for the next day. Aunt Nell said that her brother had his own reason for not attending worship, but that he did not wish Jimmie to be deprived of the opportunity.

Late one evening, both Jimmie and William had retired to their rooms, Nell sat busy sewing, Skip smoked his pipe and was reading.

"Do you realise you have changed during the last couple of months, Todd."

Skip looked over his book at Nell.

"What makes you say that?"

"Because it's nice to see you smile again, and William wants to know why you are different."

"In that case I must watch my step or I shall lose my image!"

"You should not be ashamed of that Todd. Have you told the boy anything?"

The answer was abrupt, "No, and I don't see any reason why I should. I hope you have not said anything out of turn."

"No, Todd. I made a promise, and a promise I will keep, but you cannot stop boys from asking questions. I have said it before."

"And you will say it again, and again," nipped in Todd.

"Yes, I will. You are your own worse enemy. You are going through life punishing yourself just because you are too stubborn to make peace with your Maker."

"I'm fully aware that you are correct, but Todd Summers is Todd Summers, and that's how he will remain. The fact that Jimmie is working alongside of me is but a consolation. You have William, so let us see what we can make of them."

It was another hour before Skip retired to his room. He was conscious that he had hurt his sister's feelings. As he made his way from the sitting room, he stopped.

"Do you realise it's nearly fifteen years since we lost mother and father and, in some respects, we've been losing out ever since."

"Not exactly, Todd. Admittedly, life has not gone as we would have planned ourselves, but it has its compensations. We do not want for money. I have William, you now have Jimmie and surely we live in hope for the future."

"Nell, you are my only anchor to sanity. I admire you." He kissed her cheek and was gone.

As the weeks went by, Jimmie began to realise that there was no short cut in the art of reading and writing. Aunt Nell not only insisted that he did it correctly, but that he spoke correctly as well.

"Cor lummy. I dunno wot me Mum an' Dad'll fink of me talkin' like the people in the big 'ouse wen I get 'ome."

"I shouldn't worry about that, Jimmie, your rate of progress should not give them cause for concern. It's your future we are concerned about. If you are to be a captain on a passenger liner, then you will need to be able to converse with all types of people in society, and to be able to give instructions and orders to your crew in a manner that is recognised and acceptable to all."

"Yes, I know what you mean, Aunt Nell! 'Cos that's what the uvver men say about Skip."

Whenever possible, Jimmie would make his way to the boatyard to watch progress on the 'Maywell'. Often he was able to assist. Workmen played practical jokes on him, such as holding pieces of wood while they went to get a plane, then conveniently forgetting to return. They were quickly to realise, however, that Jimmie was no dullard. His experience of working with hundreds of men at the stables stood him in good stead, and he returned tit for tat.

Among the improvements on the 'Maywell' was a separate cabin for Jimmie, even though it was small, and a modern method of steerage: a wheel instead of a tiller. In fact, so much work was carried out that Jimmie questioned Skip as to whether it would have been better to buy a new boat.

"That was seriously discussed, Jimmie, but when you have sailed a boat for over twelve years, you have no heart to throw it into the breakers. The 'Maywell', when renovated, will serve us for another twenty years."

One day, as Skip left for the boatyard, at his usual time, his sister called him to one side. "I think it will be necessary for you to have a word with Jimmie. He tends to be slacking in his work, but please don't be too harsh."

"Say nothing to the boy, and leave it in my hands. I will deal with him later," replied Skip.

The climax came that evening, after Jimmie had spent a restless day with his books. Aunt Nell was, to say the least, on edge. At the evening meal, an uncanny silence pervaded. William asked to be excused as soon as permissable, followed quickly by Jimmie. Before Aunt Nell could grant permission, Skip spoke.

"William may leave the room now, but you, Jimmie, are to remain."

His voice brought a deathly hush. William scampered through the doorway. Jimmie was well aware of forebodings. This was the end. Skip lifted his gaze from his empty pudding dish, and looked sternly at Jimmie.

"Tonight you will go upstairs, clean and tidy your room, then pack your bag. Tomorrow you will rise at six o'clock, have an early breakfast, then I will accompany you to the 'Albert', and you will return to London."

Jimmie was flabbergasted. His lips quivered. Nell saw him grit his teeth. Sheer determination prevented him from bursting into tears. Nell turned on her brother.

"How ever could you be so callous, Todd? is there no pity in that soul of yours?" she cried.

In the few seconds that followed, Jimmie decided that on no account would he return to the stables. Todd slowly raised his good hand and placed it on his sister's shoulder. His face was severe, his voice forceful.

"Would you please let me finish what I was going to say. I will once more repeat. Jimmie will be returning to London tomorrow morning. May I continue?"

Nell nodded her head.

"He will return for ten days shore leave, or holiday if you prefer that description. He will return to Burnham, on the 'Albert', in just over the week."

With that he rose from his seat and left the room. Jimmie stared at Aunt Nell; she was crying, and it hurt him.

"Go home, Jimmie. Enjoy yourself and, if you return, you will find everything as you would wish. I apologise for my brother's sense of humour."

Jimmie rose from his chair, paused, then walked round the table.

"I will come back, Auntie, I promise." He looked into her tearfilled eyes. "Please may I kiss you?"

She hugged the boy as though he were her very own.

For Jimmie, the trip home and back to Burnham worked wonders. For Nell and Todd it was but another daunting experience they kept to themselves.

It was late October before the 'Maywell' was pronounced seaworthy again. Jimmie enjoyed the sea trials, even though he fell off the deck in the process. The shipwrights put her through her paces, racing her on full sail, turning her about at angles from which he considered it impossible to recover. Although Skip had explained the reason for all the erratic action, Jimmie had a sneaking feeling that the tip into the briney was the last of the long line of practical jokes that he and the workmen had played on each other during the renovations.

Chapter Ten

Continental Coast

It was within a week of the sea trials finishing that Paddy turned up in the town. Skip brought him into the evening meal, and he greeted Nell with typical Irish blarney. He took Trip into his arms and kissed him, then eyed Jimmie up and down. Being short of stature, Paddy virtually looked up to the boy.

"Be jabbers, Jimmie, if you grow much taller we shall be using you for the main mast!"

The evening was one of hilarity, as Paddy related the highlights of his four months vacation.

The renovated 'Maywell' was duly handed over with appropriate ceremony. Paddy exceeded his capacity, and was laid to sleep it off in the nearby sail shed, but he was fit and ready for duty the next morning. For the next few days, time was spent refurbishing the living quarters. Provision had been made for storage of books and writing materials in Jimmie's cabin. His education was to continue despite the arduous work ahead. All was set for a new episode in the history of the 'Maywell'.

It was Sunday evening, and on the table Skip had laid a quantity of navigation charts. "Tomorrow we sail to the Pool, Jimmie."

The boy's response was on impulse. "Cor blimey! You ain't gonna fill our luvly ship with 'orse dung are yer?"

"Jimmie, why ever have I spent four months training you, then you come out with a sentence like that?" chided Aunt Nell.

Skip laughed. "It will take more than four months to transform a true Cockney into an articulate Oxford Don! Now, Jimmie, re-phrase that sentence and restore my sister's confidence in you."

Jimmie apologised and thought hard. He was pleased that William had not been present.

"It would seem a shame to spoil that lovely paintwork on our first trip, Skip."

"That's better, but don't make too much hard work of your training. It will come naturally to you in due course. Now, the reason for all the charts is because we have taken on a new assignment. We shall be heading for the Continental ports in a few days - from Brest in the west of France to the Rhine ports in Germany. It should prove a new, and I trust profitable, experience, but do not worry, we shall return to England from time to time. The only member of the crew who will be shorebound is Trip. It will be fond farewells tomorrow."

At breakfast next morning, Jimmie found a small flat parcel on his plate.

"You may open it," said Aunt Nell. "It is for you."

To his great surprise, Jimmie found that it was a water colour depicting the 'Maywell' in its new rig, with Skip and himself sitting on the hatch covers.

"I thought it would decorate one of the walls of your cabin."

"Thank you, Auntie, I will keep it 'till my dying day, to remind me of you."

Their first freight consisted of pumping machinery for Antwerp. While it was being stowed, Jimmie was allowed thirty-six hours to make his way to Wapping. Though he enjoyed the family spirit, some conditions were repugnant to him after four months at Burnham. He left home the next morning with greater determination than ever to raise their standard of living.

And so, for nearly eight years, the 'Maywell' graced the coast and river ports of France, Belgium, the Netherlands and Denmark, and even up the Rhine and into Germany.

From his early teens and into his twenties, the awkward boy from Wapping matured into a quiet but extremely sociable young man. He learned that the sun did not always shine on the sailing barge. Rain, wind and storm meant battling for very survival. Often, after a storm, as they sought to regain strength, he would laugh at Paddy's apt remark, "Be jabbers, Jimmie, we only just won that round. The next toime oi'me sure he'll get me!"

Freezing snow, breaking ice from the rigging and the terrors of collision in fog, all helped to give the pale city boy a ruddy complexion, like his shipmates.

Meeting men and women of different nationalities widened his knowledge of what life was all about. Often, he recalled his grandfather's words, "If you think London is a dreadful place, you will find far worse as you travel around." How right he was. Despite the pressure of work on the barge, his education continued. Whilst Jimmie was not the material for Oxford or Cambridge, once he grasped a subject it was registered in his brain for all time.

The year was 1888, and Paddy decided to return to the Emerald Isle. Skip considered that a change of coastline would not come amiss after all this

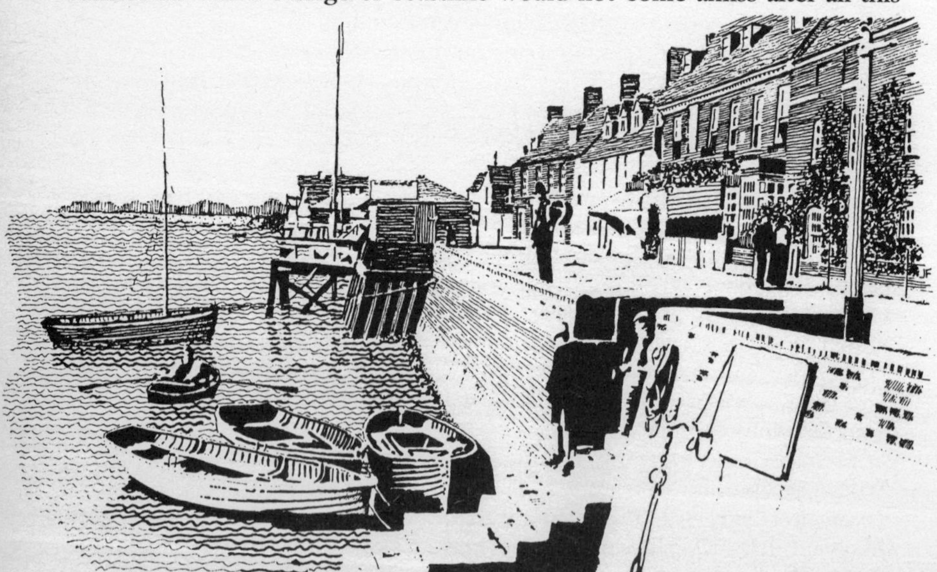

BURNHAM-ON-CROUCH

time, and returned across the Channel. Jimmie required more time for serious study so, on their return to Burnham, they left the 'Maywell' on the blocks for maintenance, and enjoyed a month's respite. William had left home to join the Royal Navy and Jimmie found the cottage quieter.

Paddy sold his share in the 'Maywell' to Skip, and made his way back to southern Ireland to set up in farming, promising that he would one day return to England to see how they were faring.

Chapter Eleven

The Second Visit to Woodham Ferris

The development of railways in the Eastern Counties led to the demand for thousand upon thousand of bricks. Brickfields in Kent required as many barges as possible to sail their materials up the Essex rivers to reach the ever lengthening rail tracks.

Once back on board the barge, Skip and Jimmie made their way over the Crouch estuary and down the Swale to the brickfields. Trip was now showing signs of old age, but was still extremely excited to be back on board. Barges lined up in convoy to take their turn at loading.

Having received their freight, Jimmie collected the documents from the dispatch office.

"Head of Fenn Creek, Upper Crouch, two hundred yards past Eyott's Farm. Do you think you will find that place?" asked the dispatch clerk. "I have a chart if you need it."

"No, thank you, my friend. It will be my joy and pleasure to renew my acquaintance with the area."

Two days later, they brought up at Hullbridge. After a meal, which had been prepared by Nell and re-heated on the faithful stove, they paid a visit to the Anchor Inn. This helped shorten the long November night. With three other barges moored alongside, there was no shortage of company, and no shortage of stories told. The outcome of their visit was that they re-joined the 'Maywell' at around midnight.

Jimmie instructed Skip that there would be no need for him to rise early, as they would not be able to get under way until half-past-one. Skip wished Jimmie goodnight. "Eight years have made a drastic change in the lad I brought here from Wapping," he thought, as his head dropped onto the pillow.

The morning hung heavy with mist. Thick white hoar-frost clung to the rigging, and Jimmie walked with great care over the frost-laden deck. He had a task to perform regardless of the adverse weather.

When they droped anchor the previous day, the winding mechanism of the windlass had failed. Jimmie now had four hours to carry out the repair. The spring flood had been running for an hour, and it created the only feeling of movement in the sea of mist.

Work on the windlass was proving difficult. Jimmie stood buffing his hands to regain his circulation. Looking upstream, he could just discern the ferryman rowing an early customer to the Woodham bank. At the head of the gangway, Trip appeared, put his head high into the air, and sniffed. From the straightness of his tail, Jimmie could tell that the dog found the atmosphere far from acceptable. Trip watched Jimmie continue his work until a seagull caught his eye. It circled around, then perched in the rigging, squarking for titbits. It was when one decided to rest on the rails that Trip came into action. Never in his ten years on the 'Maywell' had he permitted seagulls, or any bird, to settle on the deck. That was his domain.

From behind the cover of the hatchboard he made the pounce. But he had misjudged the icy conditions. Despite extending his claws, he skidded off the matching onto the deck, turning a complete somersault over the gunwhales. In doing so, he trapped a hind leg between the deadeye and rigging, and there he hung, head down and backwards over the lee boards. The ear-piercing howl brought Jimmie onto the scene, and Skip racing up from his bed.

Jimmie's hands were within three inches of rescuing the dog, and he cringed as Trip slipped into the water, his leg bare to the bone and pouring with blood. With supreme effort, Trip tried to swim to the barge, but the fast-flowing current swept the animal in its wake. Within seconds, Jimmie had discarded his seaman's boots, thrown his hat and sea jacket onto the deck, and dived into the swirling tide to recover the 'Maywell's' pet. The ferryman had also heard the commotion, and quickly bade his passenger farewell, and pulled hard on the oars to bring himself onto the scene.

The three converged on the centre of the river. Jimmie had grabbed the stricken dog, then clung with one hand to the stern of the boat.

"Tow me ashore," he shivered. "It will be a waste of time trying to get aboard."

Skip too had wasted no time. He jumped down into the dinghy and came alongside as they beached. Jimmie handed him the dog and raced up and down the causeway to induce some heat into his frozen limbs.

It was but a few minutes before Jimmie was sitting wrapped in a blanked before a roaring log fire in the bar of the Anchor Inn.

Skip, with Trip laid on his knees and covered with an old coat, was being taken by Tom Hitchen in the pony and trap to find the horse doctor. Despite all the effort and comfort bestowed, Trip was dead on their arrival at Rayleigh.

By twelve o'clock, Trip had been buried at the rear of the Anchor Inn garden. Jimmie changed into another rig and a hearty meal was provided for them by the landlady.

Having eaten their fill, Skip and Jimmie paid their respects to all concerned, and rowed out to the 'Maywell' to take the flood tide up to Eyott's Farm. Bricks were dead weight and it required all their skill to negotiate the tortuous turns to bring them to the riverhead. After tying up and furling the sails, they were able to relax.

"A strong cup of tea is what we need now." said Jimmie.

They sat in the cabin, their hands closed around the hot mugs. Skip broke the silence, "Hullbridge has a jinx on you, Jimmie."

"I'm sure you're right, Skip. Last time I was knocked out, this time I'm nearly drowned."

Skip reached out his hand and put it on Jimmie's. "Not only I, but Nell will be proud of what you did this morning."

Darkness was quickly taking over from the pale afternoon sunlight, and both men watched as thousands and thousands of starlings circled the spinney bordering Tabrum's Farm.

"There you are, Jimmie. When we are sleeping tonight we shall feel on our own, yet all those thousands will be there, heads tucked under their wings."

A little later, the noise of a trotting horse on the gravel track drew their attention from the starlings to the opposite direction. The rider brought his

steed to a halt.
"Someone has seen us bring up, and has come to make arrangements for off-loading," said Jimmie.
"Do I see Todd Summers standing there in the twilight?" came the rider's voice.
"Yes, Harry. Shall we come ashore, or will you come aboard?"
"No, Todd, I'm in a hurry, so you come up to the farm just after six. I'll tell Mary to put a couple of extra tatters in the pot."
He gave the horse a friendly slap, and was gone.
Their arrival at the farm, in the dark, woke the dogs from their early slumbers.
"Let's stop here," said Skip. "Dogs have played an important part of my life today. I don't want to be savaged by one to complete my day!"
Somewhere in the darkness, at least two dogs could be detected. Jimmie stood shielding Skip.
"Give me your staff. I will deal with them," he said, protectively. A shout from the farm buildings stopped the barking, and had the dogs running in that direction. As Jimmie handed back the staff, he felt the older man's hand trembling as he took it.
"Good gracious! I never realised you had a fear of dogs, Skip."
"I have a fear of the sea when it's angry, but I don't go around telling everyone."
Jimmie decided there and then that he would not pursue the point. The loss of Trip must have caused the unusual mood of melancholy. The advancing figure of Harry enlivened their situation.
"I'm sorry about the dogs. I was in the process of locking them up for the night and they were gone before I realised it. Come in. A stiff drink will revive us all. It's going to be another frosty night."
The evening was well enjoyed. Good food, wine and a good deal of talking about the bashed-up boy who had arrived there eight years previously, and who now had grown out of recognition. The railway then became the topic of the evening's conversation.
It was obvious that Harry was somewhat distressed by the project.
"Never in my lifetime did I expect those monsters crossing our fens. I can only foresee them disturbing the cattle, spoiling the milk yield, scaring the birds and reducing the number of eggs. I suppose for the younger generation it will provide an exciting way of life, being able to get from here to London and elsewhere, but for myself, I am content with my horse."
For Jimmie, much of the evening was spent with the now late-teenage family. Rosie, the maid, was now thirty, married and living on the farm with her husband and two children. She had joined the party for the evening.
It was late when Skip and Jimmie carefully edged their way over the gangplank to board the 'Maywell'.
"Jimmie, I'm not certain whether it was the pudding I ate, or coming out of the hot room into the frosty night, but that track seemed more undulating than when we went."
Jimmie laughed, "I don't suppose the wine would have anything to do with it!"
"I hardly think so, though, on the other hand, I did imbibe a little more than usual. I am afraid that the experience of the last few hours has had

rather a devastating effect on me, and I sought a little Dutch courage."
Jimmie dropped down the gangway and stood ready to catch the skipper, if the need arose.
"Goodnight, Jimmie. It's been a sad day, but thank you for all your help."
"Goodnight, Skip. I think I understand your feelings."
Skip turned away. "My boy, you will be an old man before you understand Todd Summers' feelings."
Jimmie rolled himself in the blankets. "There is something odd about Skip tonight," he said to himself, but he dropped off to sleep before his mind could dwell on the subject.
At first daylight, men began unloading the bricks. The shout of the ganger down the gangway had aroused them.
"Don't bother to come up, Skip. We'll have this lot off before you've cooked your breakfast."
"It sounds like Paddy's brother," commented Jimmie.
A convoy of tumbril carts, driven by boys, lined up to be loaded. Three teams of six men threw the bricks, five or six at a time, from hold to deck, deck to bank and bank to cart. They reckoned to be unloaded by twelve o'clock the next day.
Towards mid-day, Skip and Jimmie made their way between the convoy of carts to the Whalebone. They rested their arms on the protective rail of the bridge over the creek.
"Who would have thought that this bridge should suffer such use? I hope the contractors renew the structure when they finish," said Skip.
"Something of a contrast to my last visit," replied Jimmie, scanning the area.
Cattle in a nearby field stood close together for warmth; great columns of steam bellowing from their nostrils. On the fen, peewits stood huddled together, oblivious to the two men watching them, or the trundling carts.
"Do you realise, Jimmie, as we look at those creatures resisting the elements, at the trees bereft of leaves, at the absence of flowers and insects, that Mother Nature would appear to have come to a grinding halt. But not so, she is just resting. In a few months time, the birds will sing again, trees will be dressed in their new coats and flowers will grace the fens once more. The whole transformation will take place without the help of a single man. That is a miracle that should not be ignored."
Then, pointing with his staff, he continued, "Over there, we see man struggling against the elements to construct a means whereby people can rush from place to place at breakneck speeds, pulled by those monsters of steam. I can readily accept the arguments of our friends at Eyotts. The railway will certainly intrude on their way of life, although I have my doubts about their egg yield."
"I like your thoughts about Mother Nature, Skip, but I confess that I am hopeful of this new age of steam and even electricity. Why, one day I may have control of those combined powers in the form of a ship."
"Yes, Jimmie. You know, man is an aggressive creature. He craves power to create and to destroy, power to control and power to dominate his fellow man. I often lay on my bunk, speculating on the ultimate outcome of man's progress. I am certain that, if it was possible to get to the moon, he would have a try."

“Let us leave that to the future, Skip. I’m getting frozen to the marrow.”
With that remark, both men made their way along the track across the Fenn.
The scene was one of apparent confusion. Row upon row of men digging earth, throwing earth, wheeling earth. Tumbrils, barrows, even small steel trucks on a narrow gauge line, conveyed the rich Essex clay from area to area. Where Jimmie and Skip had once sat and watched the kingfisher, bricklayers were busy building a bridge over the stream. To the right, on the higher land, rows of timber huts formed the camp for hundreds of workmen.
Skip and Jimmie crossed what was to be the base of the rail track to deliver the consignment notes to the transport clerk.
“You have a fast-working gang,” remarked Skip, as the clerk returned the documents.
“You’re right there, skipper. Have you left anyone on board?”
“Not at the moment, but we can return.”
“That will be alright today, but they’ll be finished by mid-day tomorrow, so make sure you are both on board then, because they will otherwise strip the sails and take the bloody rudder as well!”
“Thank you for those few words,” said Skip, as he dropped a half-sovereign on the counter.
“You are in a generous mood this morning,” remarked Jimmie, as they proceeded towards the Whalebone Inn.
“Not so. I am conscious of my lack of attention for the well-being of the ‘Maywell’, leaving some eighteen Irishmen scrambling all over her. That will not occur tomorrow.”
“I feel guilty about it myself, therefore, I will pay for our lunch and drinks,” was Jimmie’s quick reply.
The approach to the inn gave little indication as to the period of prosperity that had suddenly descended upon the premises. Externally, it looked the same. The tiles on the roof still needed attention, as did the boards cladding the walls. Inside, all available space was used to house the hungry and thirsty men from the railway project.
Fortunately, mid-day in the inn still had a country air about it. It was in the evenings, especially on pay-days, that the locals stayed indoors, locking their wives and daughters in, while the brawling mass of workers either fought or slept their drink off in the area around the pub.
A couple of obvious locals occupied one corner of the bar and welcomed Skip and Jimmie.
“You be seamen. We oun’t mind yew sitting nigh us.”
Jimmie bought the drinks, including one for their hosts, and ordered a snack.
“Do I take it that you do not approve of the apparent invaders of your soil?” asked Jimmie.
“Approve bain’t hardly the word, sur. They bain’t men, they be wurs than beasts. You dursn’t leave a thing unlocked. They’ll swipe yer chickens and tatters from yer garden. I’m a’skard for me missus and girls. Our boss own’t even leave a coo’ out at night, and that’s saying summat.”
“I appreciate your predicament. Your only consolation is that they will be gone within the next few months, though I am sure you will enjoy the facilities the railway will provide.”

"I don't rightly 'now abawt that, sur. I've allus managed to feed and clothe my family without the use of one of they grit ingins, but I reckon we gonna have trouble wi' our youngsters, 'cos as soon as they're old enough, they're be on that thar train, leaving the farm and gallyvanting all over the place."
"I should not worry unduly," replied Skip. "In a few years time railways will be part and parcel of your way of living."
"O, that's as may be, but I'm moving out of 'ere to somewhere a bit quieter."
"So be I," chipped in his mate.
Having enjoyed their snack, Skip and Jimmie returned to the 'Maywell' via the track that led to Hullbridge ferry, past Champions Hall. The scene of activity that met their eyes was astounding.

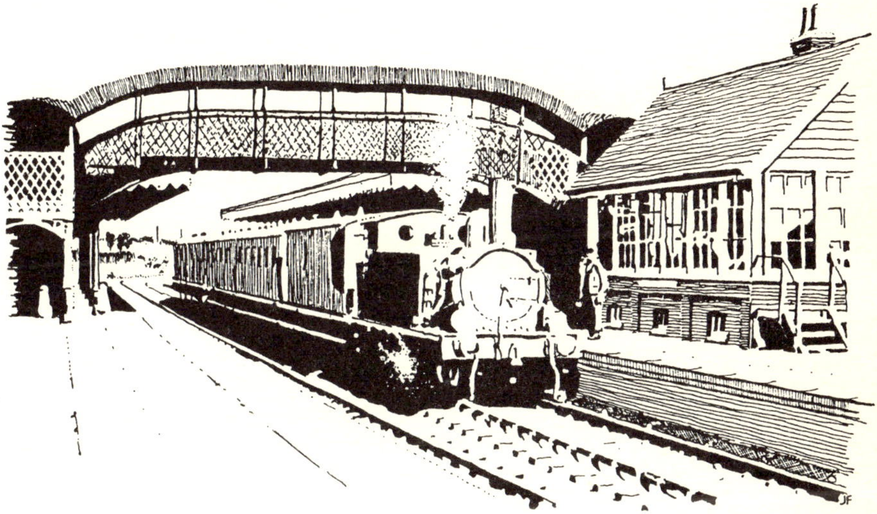

WOODHAM FERRIS STATION

"This must be Woodham Ferris station," said Skip.
"Not only the station, but a junction for Maldon, according to that notice waiting to be erected," added Jimmie. "I think a few minutes inspection of the vicinity would be interesting."
"I agree," said Skip.
The two men walked onto the beautifully laid paving that formed the platform. They asked the painters, busy working on the ironwork of the bridge crossing the track, their permission to pass over. Standing on the bridge, they viewed the makings of a goods yard. Men moving materials, men building a pair of cottages, men erecting signal posts and crossing gates, men working on a turntable for the engines – all scurrying about their work.
"If you could see this from a thousand feet up in the air, it would look like a swarm of ants working on their nest," remarked Skip. "Do you realise also, that while we are admiring the ingenuity of man, we are also viewing the means that will destroy the sailing barge."
"Not in our lifetime, Skip."

"It may be a slow process, but it will surely happen, my boy. The other fact that becomes apparent to me is that the planners of this project have not built this edifice in the middle of the Champions Hall Estate for the benefit of the Lord of the Manor, nor the sixty or seventy people residing in the area. If I were a gambling man, which I am not, I would bet my last sovereign that businessmen and politicians have already designated this area for radical change. But enough . . . let us not pre-suppose. The 'Maywell' could easily be in danger of being ransacked by Irish hoards if we are not aboard before dark!"

It took twenty minutes for them to cross the fields. The labourers were still busy at their task.

"If we haven't got you cleaned by noon tomorrow, we shall be monny out o' pocket. Sure, it is a hard loife we mortals endure," was their ganger's parting remark.

Another pleasant evening was spent with the Millards and the next day, unloading completed as planned, it was three in the afternoon as the 'Maywell' was brought about in the confluence of the fen creeks. With an extra hand loaned from Harry, she edged her way down the creek, with the aid of the ebb tide.

From 1888 to 1897 the 'Maywell' plied the rivers of the East Coast, wound its way up rivers and creeks, and hauled cargoes ranging from corn and salt to timbers, bricks and sheep. Occasionally, if freights were difficult, they would make up with London 'rough', or manure.

During this period, Jimmie, with a little financial assistance from Skip, purchased a new house in the village of Enfield for his parents. His father was employed as a groom and coachman for a local industrialist.

This enabled Jimmie, during breaks, to take the train from Burnham to Liverpool Street, for a few days with his parents. It was during one of these breaks that he took his mother and father to Woodham Ferris to show them his fens in full flower. He hired a pony and trap from Hambert's Farm, and gave them a conducted tour which included Hullbridge ferry and Eyott's Farm although, sadly for Jimmie, strangers now occupied the premises.

Over the fen bridge they went, on to the mass of flowering thrift. As they spent an hour wandering around, Jimmie pointed out the highlights of his earlier visits. His mother expressed her admiration of the scene.

"Jimmie, I never realised the mornin' you scared the wits out ov me, shoutin' 'Where's Wudum Ferrus?' that I would ever come 'ere as well. And to fink that my rough tearaway boy should lose 'is 'art to a field of flowers!"

"Not exactly, mother, but you must admit it is somewhat different from Wapping riverside."

"Yes, Jimmie. You did the family a world ov good w'en you went an' found out w'ere they took the dung, an' we're very grateful to yer."

That evening, they took the train to Burnham and spent a night and a day with Aunt Nell and Skip before returning to Enfield.

Throughout this period, Jimmie had continued his studies: engineering; electronics; science – much of which was beyond the help of Aunt Nell or Skip, but their interest and encouragement in what he was doing spurred him on.

Chapter Twelve

The last visit to Woodham Ferris

26th November, 1897

As the 'Maywell' left the Pool on the ebb tide, a heavy sullen sky seemed to enclose itself around them. Their cargo was a load of 'rough stuff' for the Woodham Ferris Brick Company, Clements Creek, Essex.

Both men had watched the barometer dropping to stormy weather.

Equally, both men had checked and re-checked the rigging and made fast all movable kit. Likewise, both men had agreed before weighing anchor that the prospect for their last journey together on the 'Maywell' could be a hard slog.

Jimmie gave her full sail, took over the helm and sent Skip to the galley to brew up.

Skip sat down, watching the heavy iron kettle come to the boil. This was going to be a rather nostalgic trip. Seventeen years was a long time, and except for a few differences of opinion, they had worked and lived together as father and son. There was no doubt about it, he was going to miss Jimmie. An overwhelming sense of loneliness came upon him, then a feeling of guilt. "Seventeen years, and I have never told him anything about myself, and he has rarely asked," he thought.

The lid on the kettle jumped up and down. Skip mashed the tea, filled the two tea cans, and made his way up on deck. "I must tell him before he goes to college," he said to himself, "and be hopeful that he will be a success where I have failed.

Meanwhile, Jimmie's keen hands on the wheel were edging the 'Maywell's' way past any craft likely to reduce their speed. He, too, was casting his mind back over the years.

"Seventeen years ago, I sat on those hatches nursing a sore neck, and my only known comfort was Trip the dog. And now, the man I thought to be a wicked ogre has turned out to be a perfect gentleman, although somewhat mysterious. I could never have wished for a better father."

They drank their tea in silence. From the tucker box, Jimmie selected a large onion to help down the cheese and bread. For a short while it appeared that each man was trying to read the other's thoughts. Jimmie took a large bite of the onion, but within seconds had disposed of the mouthful over the leeward side.

"Good gracious, Skip! Wherever did you dig those onions up from? They must have been on board since my first trip on the 'Maywell'.

Skip laughed, "No, Jimmie. I bought them yesterday from Grandio the Spanish onion man. He told me that his father, Pedro, grows them especially for men like us, to keep the cold weather out of our lungs when at sea. He assured me that we would be back for more, Senoro."

"If I had swallowed that mouthful, I would have had blisters from my mouth down to my guts, so tell him from me when you see him again, that just because Francis Drake wiped his forefathers off the high seas, he has no need to take his revenge out on the seamen of today by burning our guts out with these abominable fireballs!"

The gale increased and the rain came down. They donned their oilskins and re-checked the rigging. Given a chance, they would make for shelter off the Medway. Darkness had already fallen as they brought up. They cast anchor and stowed up for the night. After a meal, sleep was the only thing they needed.

Saturday morning broke clear. The wind was still south-westerly and fresh, but both men had sufficient experience to know that the lull would be short-lived. Providing the wind held its direction, they could make it.

They unreefed, weighed anchor and were away, followed closely by three other barges. Three hours should get them into the Whitaker Channel. However, within the hour they were fighting a westerly gale and soon the tide would be against them. Little by little, the four barges headed towards the Buxey, each crew watching the other's progress.

"A half-hour's lull is all we need, or we shall be blown over to Holland," shouted Skip above the gale.

"I'm sure Aunt Nell will be praying for us," returned Jimmie.

"Well, I'm certain He will answer her prayer on your behalf, but I very much doubt if He would bother about me," yelled back Skip.

"In that case you had better pray as well, Skip, then we can both get home."

There was not time for reply; a mighty gust of wind and a boisterous sea threw the 'Maywell' off course and heading towards the East Barrows sandbank. Jimmie was racing to the helm, to give assistance and bring her round, as another wave crashed over the barge, throwing him onto the deck and spreadeagled into the scuppers. Skip stood steadfast, his good hand gripping the wheel. With grim determination he held the 'Maywell', head against the wind, in an attempt to regain course.

Jimmie scrambled to his feet and took his place beside Skip. His strong young hands replaced his senior's on the wheel.

"Shall I turn her about?" he yelled.

"No, give her a minute, I've still got faith in Nell."

Then, as a cloud passing away from the sun, the wind ceased. The 'Maywell's' mast rose proudly skywards, she shook her sails as a dog leaving the water and rode the swollen sea. Both men looked around them. All four vessels, despite facing different directions had come through the ordeal apparently unscathed.

"Thank God for Aunt Nell," shouted Jimmie, as he shivered from his soaking, "I'll do a quick change when we round the Buxey."

They brought up in the Whitaker Channel and waited for the flood tide to strengthen. The last six miles of the Crouch estuary demanded the utmost skill of the seamen, but their determination was rewarded as they dropped anchor in the fairway of Burnham Quay.

The gales continued on Saturday night. By Sunday afternoon, they had settled in the north-west.

Jimmie rowed out to the 'Maywell' to ensure that all above and below deck was in order. Bargemen and locals gathered at the quay, as the afternoon tide rose above its normal height, and speculated on the outcome of the next early morning tide. With a full moon within twenty-four hours, the

prospect was causing alarm.
Throughout the afternoon, and all Sunday night, the gales increased in ferocity. Trees, haystacks and buildings all became victims of its fury. People living close to the river, and on low-lying land, waited anxiously into the night for the early morning tide to reach its peak, and ebb. Many became thankful that they were spared the misery of a flooded house.
For the next six hours, it became a battle of the elements: a conflict of wind against tide.
The increased volume of water, already forced up the Essex rivers by the North Sea surge, was doing its utmost to recede, but the wind had veered into the north and increased to hurricane force, thus preventing the normal ebb to take place. When Skip and Jimmie arrived on the quayside on the Monday morning, they had expected the tide to have completed its ebb. To their amazement, and to that of the many gathered there, it had only ebbed for about three hours. Within the hour, it began to flow again; almost two hours before its predicted time. It was obvious for all to see, that the next few hours would be critical.
Bargemen for Battlesbridge Mills, Hullbridge and Clement's Creek decided that it would be foolish to take the tide upstream. "We may be needed here before the day's out," said Skip, "and beside that, I don't fancy a trip over the marshes through a breach in the wall."
By early afternoon, the sea was flowing over the walls, breaking down the improvised barricades and flooding the houses and shipyards. There was still nearly two hours wait before the ebb. Helpless against the raging water, people in the High Street watched as the sea took possession of their homes. For some it was feet deep, for others inches. Children in the school climbed onto their desks as eighteen inches of water flooded through their classrooms. Every available man and rowing boat was commandeered to bring the marooned to higher ground.
It was about three o'clock in the afternoon when, before its time, the water began to ebb, and dropped some four to eight inches. Then, to people's surprise, it began to flow again. Pious people were predicting that it was a prelude to the end of the world. Others considered that, either the Almighty, or the Laws of Nature, had broken down, and the world would be flooded again. But for most, it was a case of "we have seen it before and we shall see it again: let's get on with the cleaning up".
At half-past-one on the Tuesday afternoon, the storm and gales having abated, the 'Maywell' weighed anchor and took the tide to Clement's Creek. The sight of the thousands of acres of marshland, inundated by the storm waters, had a sickening effect on the two seamen. They knew that farmers would have lost animals and crops, and that it would be months before the land would be capable of producing again.
They edged their way up to Saltcotes. Skip had been there before, with Paddy; it was Jimmie's first visit. Men waiting on the west bank, adjacent to the brick field, took the lines, put them through the pulley blocks and hauled the 'Maywell' into her berth. A gangplank was quickly thrown across and Tom Catt, the yard foreman, stepped on board.
"It's a good job you weren't here yesterday afternoon, Skip, because I reckon you and your barge would have gone rushing through that breach over

there. Had it busted this side, Skip, it would have been curtains for my house, six feet down below the water level."

With darkness falling, Skip and Jimmie retired to the galley to heat up the meal prepared by Nell. That evening, in the quiet of their cabin, Jimmie suggested the reason for the freak ebb of the previous day. "When you take into consideration the thousands of acres of land which were suddenly inundated with water, one ought not to be surprised that the level of the river should drop."

"I am sure you are right, Jimmie. Water has a unique way of finding its own level. The circumstances certainly provide a mathematical problem which should keep you busy for the rest of the evening."

"Thank you, Skip, for your comments. I presume you prefer to study the anatomy of the red spider than join me in my speculation on recent events."

"Not exactly, Jimmie. I prefer to go to sleep."

The morning brought the unloaders on board with forks and large wicker skips. Quickly, the skips were loaded, then placed on the carrier's shoulder. He then ran the plank from barge to sea wall, and tipped his load into the sifting area. This job was done by boys, who shovelled the rubbish against a wire-meshed frame. All combustible material was used to fire the kilns. Small ashes were used in the actual brick compound, and all articles of value were supposed to be handed over to the employers: Brake, Ward and Carter Limited.

During the summer season, some twenty to thirty men and boys were employed. Winter months were spent preparing for the next season's production. Tom Catt gave Skip and Jimmie a guided tour around the yard. Men dug the clay, then it was pushed in wheeled skips, which ran on narrow guage lines to the washmill. Here was the only piece of machinery operated by Tom, a steam engine which agitated large wooden paddles in an equally large wooden tub, turning the clay into a slurry. It was then let out of the washmill through wooden troughs into a compound called a washback. There it remained for three to four months, to mature.

Tom explained how, in the Spring, the brickmakers would team up into gangs of six, each with his own special job. Number one was the temperor. He took the mature clay and added the chalk and the black slime from the river bed, with water. He would mix them together to produce the right colour and consistency. He then wheeled the mixture to a workbench called a hand berth. Number two was the flattie. He would cut enough clay to make one brick, roll it in sand and hand it to the next man, the moulder. He was the head of the gang, and would press the clay into the mould and level it off.

"Although that sounds easy," said Tom, "it is a very skilled job."

He then passed it on to the fourth man, the off bearer, who tipped the newly formed brick from the mould, re-sanded the mould and returned it to the moulder. These two men would change their jobs every hour, so fast and strenuous was their task.

Number five was the barrow loader, who took the green bricks and loaded them carefully on a long flat barrow, thirty bricks to a load.

Number six was the off-pusher, who pushed the barrow with its two hundred pounds weight of bricks to the crowders, the men who built the clamps.

This team was expected to make around a thousand bricks an hour, and they aimed at making a million during the six-month production period.

"If they make their target," said Tom, "the guv'nors give them a new pair of boots, or the money equivalent."

"I reckon they need a new pair of hands, working at that rate," commented Jimmie.

Skip thanked Tom for the tour of the brickfield. "I suppose your employers expect to make their fortune, building a New Town in the area."

"Only time will tell," was Tom Catt's reply.

Having inspected the works, Skip and Jimmie made preparation to visit the village. A deadeye had become badly distorted because of the gales and it was now a job for Lewin, the smithy. They followed the cart track to the station. Many of the carts were using two trace-horses to get through the mud. On each side of the track was evidence of bungalows being built with the local yellow brick. Many were for the employers and employees of the brickfield.

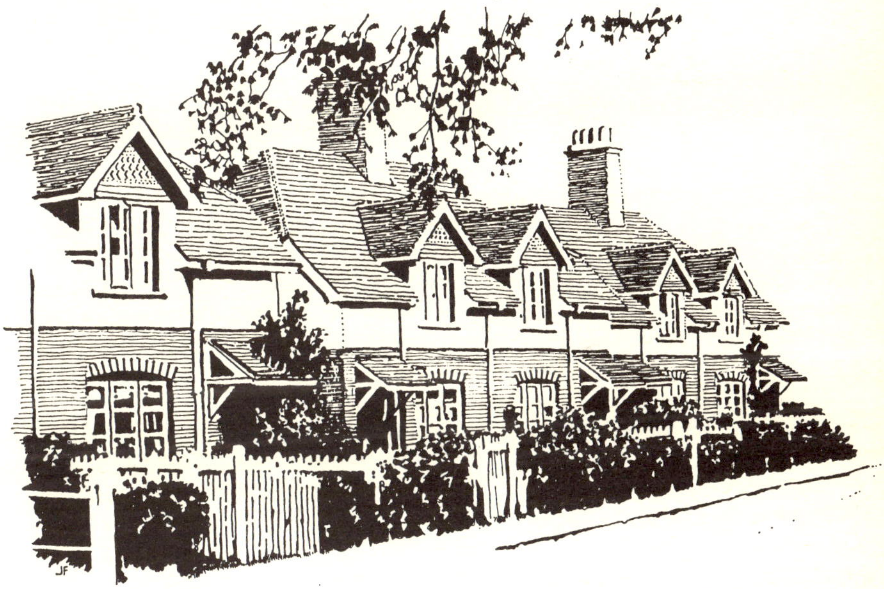

RAILWAY COTTAGES, HULLBRIDGE ROAD

"Build a railway and you can see what happens. Only ten years, and we can already see the change," remarked Skip.

The large, imposing Railway Hotel was the seamen's first port of call. They cleaned their boots of Woodham clay, with the help of grass and water, then entered.

It was just eleven o'clock. One solitary customer sat in the corner of the bar, a pint glass placed in from of him. This he had emptied on the sound of the door latch turning.

He doffed his cap, "Marnin' to yer, sirs. Yew be strangers."

The sound of his voice brought the landlord to the counter. Jimmie gave his order. It strangely coincided with the local banging his glass down in front of them.

"Thank'ee, sir. I were jest gooing to order mesel'."

With a full glass, he returned to his corner, a satisfied grin on his face.

Skip and Jimmie stood talking to the landlord about the weekend's storms. Then the bar door opened with a rattle and in peered another villager. Both of his hands were swathed in bandages. With difficulty, he shuffled across the floor, his legs as stiff as pokers. Then, with even greater difficulty, he dropped himself down on the form opposite the other local, but neither spoke a word.

"Give him a pint," said Skip, "he looks as though he needs something."

Jimmie placed the glass down in front of their new visitor.

"We'd better treat you both alike," he said.

"Oh, bless yew, sir. I nu' yew were gentlemen as soon as I came thru' the door."

"Let's hope you can drink it with those hands," replied Jimmie.

"Thar's noo need to be afeared o' thart, sir. Me throat be still in good condition."

Jimmie returned to the counter.

"What happened to that fellow, landlord?"

"Like you, sir, I am interested to know, but I imagine that we shall require patience before the story unfolds. Those two are the craftiest couple you could ever meet. Jess is the chap with his hands bandaged, and George is the fellow who greeted you. They have been working with a gang digging a trench from Danbury to Woodham to bring us a water supply, but Jess don't go much on the idea. He prefers his well water. "That blasted tap water fetches me owt in a rash," he tells everyone.

"Last week, we held a domino knock-out. By fair means or foul, those two finished up in the final. Last Friday night, they matched their wits against each other. Come the end of the night, neither would agree to the other's results, and so I was obliged to arbitrate. The prize bottle of whisky would be shared, I decided. Even then, they would not agree. Finally, they decided to come in on Saturday night and drink the bottle in front of each other. They took their place at the same table. "Can we 'ave summit with it, gaffer, 'cos that lot own't last us long?" asked Jess.

"Try some soda water," I replied, "that should eek it out."

"Not ifs we gonna pay," he quickly retorted.

"Then have water: that's free." And that's what they did. By the time half of the contents of the bottle were gone, they were getting happy. They can drink gallons of beer, but whisky has a different effect.

"George is not only crafty, but mean as well. "Jess," he said, "Yew had better not drink anymore."

"Why not?" asked Jess.

"Because yew jolly well know what thart tap warter will do to yew." He was obviously hoping to finish the bottle himself, but Jess was not falling for that.

"In thart case, we'll finish the bottle without warter." Which they did. When they left, just after ten o'clock, the fact that the wind blew a gale, and the

rain poured down, was the least of their worries. George called in yesterday, but this is the first we have seen of Jess."
Jess, holding the glass in his muffled hand, had succeeded in draining the last dregs. He then brought it down with a crash on the table, hoping to draw the kind hearted's attention to his need for a refill.
George at last broke the silence between them.
"Marning, Jess. 'Ow be yew, this marning, Jess?"
"Oh, Oi be orlright, Jarge."
"Thars didn't look thart frisky w'en yew do creep thru' thart door, Jess. War' 'ave yew bin since Saturday?"
"Oi've bin a suffering, Jarge, but thar's not troubled yar bloody 'ead to find out." There was silence for a couple of minutes.
"'Ow did yew git on arter I do leave, Jess?"
Once again there was silence. Then, "I wer orlright until I got to railway gates, then thart wind nearly blowed me head over tip, so I grabbed the railing and hoolds on. Arfter a w'ile, o'd Billy Norfolk, 'e come over to me from 'is 'ut and hoolds 'is lamp into me face, and says, "What's a matter with thee Jess?"
"Nutting," I say, "it's thart bally wind. It's upsetting me balance."
"Narsty, thar wind," he say, "I do get it at times." He put his hand in his parket, "Yew take a couple of my o' soda mints? They do me a power o' good."
"It bain't be thart sart o' wind, yew old faggot," I say. "It thart blasted nor'wester shrieking dawn the rood."
"Oo ar, it dew blow, don't it," he say. "Now let goo of the gate Jess, or thar ten-twenty will do more than upset yar balance."
"I let goo, so he could shut them, and I only went a couple o' steps and the wind do blow me flat on me face. I heard the owld goods goo rattling by. The ground regular shook. It frit the life out o' me. I try to get up, and dew yew know, I couldn't get on me feet. I went all sweaty and trembly. I shooted far Billy, but 'e don't 'ear me. I thart the train had gawn over me legs. It were really terrible, Jarge."
"Then how did yew get home, Jess?"
"I crawled 'ome on me 'ands and knees. That's orl I could do, Jarge."
"'Ow did yew get on then?"
"Oh! I managed orlright, Jess, but I had summat of a thick head on Sunday marning. 'Ow were your 'ead, Jess?"
"Oh, my 'ead were orlright. Thar whisky didn't bather me, it were thart blasted tap warter the gaffer do give us to put with it. Do yew 'no, it brought moi hands an' knees out in a most terrible rash. I couldn't even get ouwt o' bed next day."
Skip turned back to the counter.
"How far did he crawl, landlord?" he asked.
"Nearly half-a-mile. I reckon he will be claiming compensation from the Danbury Waterworks next!"
"There appear to have been a few changes taking place around here during the last few years," said Jimmie.
"Yes," replied the landlord, "and the next few years will show a drastic change. First, Champions sold out to Brakes Estate Agents from Farnborough

in Hampshire. They have divided it up into roads and hundreds of plots, and now Eyotts are doing the same."

"Well, I'm certain you can do with a few more people around here to keep this place going. Having said that, would you have a blacksmith in the area, to save us walking to Woodham village?" asked Skip.

"Not exactly a blacksmith, but we have a filemaker, he uses a forge."

"Good. Where do we find him?"

"Halfway between here and the river, in one of the original cottages. It's called 'Tazzi Mazzi', though goodness knows why. It's a Mr King you will be wanting."

"Thank you for your help, landlord. We must be on our way. I feel in a good mood, so give those two rascals another pint. Their story is one I shall remember with amusement."

Jimmie and Skip said their farewells and were gone. Their three-quarters of a mile walk down the tree-lined avenue of Hullbridge Road showed them signs of the weekend gales. Large elms lay prostrate on the ground. Workmen were busy clearing them from the gravel track.

Jimmie laughed, "I can just imagine Jess crawling along here on Saturday night, wondering what had happened to his empire!"

Here and there was evidence of building taking place, but no sign of any workers. Skip enquired the reason from one of the workmen cutting the trees.

"Oh, they be Londoners. They come orf the train and work weekends but they soon be orf w'en the weather turns sour."

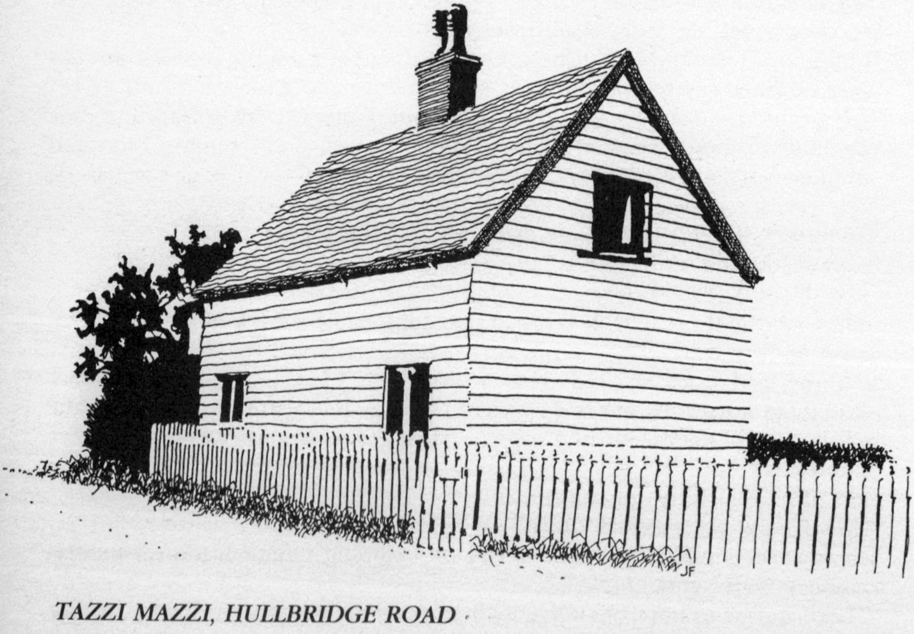

TAZZI MAZZI, HULLBRIDGE ROAD

'Tazzi Mazzi', a typical Essex cottage, was, according to Mr King, built on the edge of the Spring tide line. The track crossing the marshland, continuing to the river, had been raised in the distant past by digging large ditches and

throwing the earth to the centre.
"They tell me that this place was a regular smuggler's hideout a hundred years ago. From bits and pieces I find around here, I quite believe it."
Surrounding the cottage were a number of dilapidated sheds, and a low brick building housed the forge. Evidence of the materials for making the files lay in all directions.
Into the building, a lad of around sixteen years pushed a barrow loaded high with flat round discs.
"Well, I know what they look like, but do you mind telling me the truth and what they are for?" enquired Jimmie.
"They be cow claps, sir. I collect them in the summer, when the'ar dry, and store them in the sheds to use on the forge."
As he gave his answer, he stacked a load onto the smouldering forge, then stepped over to the large handle that operated the bellows, and began pumping. In a few minutes, the cow claps had turned into a white-hot seething mass.
"If you don't mind, gentlemen, I'll prepare this batch of files for the girls, then I'll attend to you."
"Go ahead, Mr King, we shall enjoy watching you work."
Deftly, he cut and hammered the metal into shape, while Fred the boy pumped the bellows.
"Pump, boy! Pump!" the employer shouted above the roar of the fire. Jimmie took pity on the lad, and put his hand to the bellows.
"Too many girls, that's his trouble," muttered Mr King. Fred gave Jimmie a thankful smile.
"Girls be damned! Arter a day on this bally 'andle I've 'ardly got strength to walk 'ome and eat me dinner."
The session of pumping completed, Fred carried a tray of red hot files into an adjoining room. Here were two young women, about Jimmie's age, sat, one each end, astride a long low trestle upon which was fixed a heavy metal bar some four feet long. They wore thick leather aprons and their hair was tightly covered with head scarves. They gazed in surprise as Jimmie followed Fred in.
"Good morning, ladies. I have come to watch the noble art of file-cutting being executed. I trust you will grant me that pleasure."
Fred, with tongs, laid a hot metal strip at each end of the long anvil. A wire loop was placed over the strips and the girls then pressed the loop down with their feet, to prevent movement. Then, with hammer and cold chisel, they cut the serrations. The speed at which the work was carried out so amazed Jimmie, that he called Skip. "There, sir, is truly a rural industry. It must be one of the first in this part of Woodham."
The repair of the dead-eye was expertly accomplished. Skip paid, and thanked Mr King. Jimmie slipped Fred a half-crown. "Take the girls out for a drink, they look as though they need one."
"Thanks, sir," was Fred's reply, "I be finding a way without their old man knowing."
Leaving 'Tazzi Mazzi', they turned left onto the raised track which led to the river and to Hullbridge. "I hope you know where you are leading me," said Jimmie, "because it appears to be away from the 'Maywell'."

"I am taking Mr King's instructions. I am certain he would not lead us astray."
In three hundred yards, they changed direction to port, over a foot bridge.
The bridge was made up of planks laid to a width of two-feet-six-inches, with a handrail on one side. It was some eighty to a hundred feet long, raised sufficiently high to enable pedestrians to cross the area of mud and water created by the back-up of the tides and surface water. Because of the recent floods, the water lapped the boards. As they continued and walked up the hill, a rough painted notice pointed to 'Gittens. Local Brickmakers.'
"That's not the same firm that we have delivered to," said Jimmie.
"No, according to Tom Catt, some of the local bricklayers make their own bricks."
They passed Broughton Farm and followed the muddy grass track to the sea wall.
Already, workmen had arrived with tumbrils, carts, planks, barrows and tools to repair the breach on the lower marsh. Some three hundred acres of land was still flooded. On the bank opposite the 'Maywell' another gang of men had arrived to do the same. At least six hundred acres of Stow Marsh resembled a vast lake.
"I do not begrudge those men their task," said Skip, "working up to their thighs in mud and water and with the risk of the springs overtaking them."
On Friday morning, at first light, the 'Maywell' drifted out of her berth on the ebb tide. With little wind, the progress was slow and painful. They needed to reach the main river before lack of water prevented them.
That obstacle overcome, Jimmie was able to relax. These were his last few hours aboard his faithful 'Maywell'. Now they were making their way past Fambridge and Jimmie took the tea mugs up on deck.
"What ever's this?" asked Skip.
"Best Jamaican rum, to celebrate nearly eighteen years service on the 'Maywell'. I felt my last trip was worthy of more than stewed tea."
"I will drink to that, Jimmie. They have been years of great comfort to me. Despite having Paddy back with me next week, the 'Maywell' will never be complete without you on board."
The weekend was a great time at the Browns in Burnham, with much coming and going. William had taken shore leave for the occasion; he was now training as a gunnery officer in the Royal Navy. Paddy had returned from his native isle, his farming enterprise a complete disaster, but his buoyant spirit and flair not quenched. On Skip's instructions, there were to be no speeches or emotional scenes, but when Jimmie and William left on the Monday morning to catch the train to London, it was Skip who, having shaken hands, did the quickest retreat to his room. Jimmie kissed Aunt Nell goodbye.
"I still believe that in your brother's hard heart there is a little bit like a soft boiled egg."
"You are quite right, Jimmie, but only a few have ever reached it. Goodbye and God bless you."

PART TWO Chapter Thirteen

Cannondore

January 1916

"Now, gentlemen, if you have no objection, I will catch up on some sleep."
"That is quite alright, captain. Please make yourself comfortable."
Sleep was not the true reason for the request. The other five occupants of the railway compartment were young naval officers on their way to join their first ship. That they were eager was evident from the many questions he had answered over the twenty to thirty miles they had travelled from Euston station. It would be another four or five hours before the train reached Liverpool, for war-time travelling was slow and unreliable.
Jimmie wanted time to think. So much had happened during the last four years. He stretched his legs over to the opposite seat, tucked his head into the corner rest and closed his eyes. "War, this bloody war, has turned the world into utter chaos," he told himself. "Throughout my life I have chosen what I would do and where I would go. Now, I am ordered to go here, go there, do this, do that: the operative words being, you will!"
The young lads had questioned him on the realities of war at sea, and respected him as a senior captain, be it in the Merchant Navy. Little did they realise that he was joining his first ship as its captain, and that his insignia had only been sewn on the day before, though it had received special attention to imitate the passage of time.
The motion of the train blotted out the chatter of his companions. He sank into a reverie all his own.
It was now nearly twenty years since leaving the 'Maywell' for Seaman's College. That was alright, but boring at times. Five years in Australian waters - not bad, but marred by that she-cat, Ruby. Five years on the west Pacific sea-board - great days. Four years on the Indian Ocean and South African coast - they had had their moments. Then war, and two years second-in-command on a troopship. "The most soul-destroying time of my life," he thought, "transporting thousands and thousands of men from Australia, New Zealand, India and Africa to be shot, bayonetted and blown to pieces on the fields of France. As soon as one shipload was disembarked, I returned for another, to receive the same treatment. Yes, it was little different from the old cattle drover driving his animals to the knacker's yard to be slaughtered." From the Mediterranean, he had left his troopship and travelled overland through France to England, enjoying seven days with his parents in Enfield, his first home leave for seven years. Now he had been promoted to Captain. He had a ship, a crew under his command, but what really concerned him was the assignment he would be given. He would readily accept anything except 'trooping'.
"Coffee or tea, sir?" Back to reality.
The train was standing in Crewe station and, to his surprise, he found he had been sleeping for at least two hours.
"You certainly know the way to relax, sir," remarked the red-headed lad

next to him.
"I trust that the instructors of the Royal Navy have taught you the art, because it is most essential when you are placed in a position of command," was Jimmie's encouraging reply.

"Captain Brown, we now leave the 'Cannondore' under your command, and trust you will find her a capable ship. We also wish you safe passage in her."
The late arrival of his train into Liverpool, and the mad rush by taxi to the dockside, had already tested his powers of composure. He had been greeted on board by his seniors, lunched and wined with them. They drank to his appointment and success in his future missions. In turn, he had shaken their hands and watched them leave the ship.
He made his way once more to the bridge, for a moment of quiet reflection. For late January the weather was quite reasonable. A weak, silvery sun tried to bring a ray of joy into the grey sombre dockland. Jimmie stood motionless, gazing over the superstructure of the ship now under his command, and into the restless sea ahead of him.
It was not quite the luxury liner which it was his ultimate ambition to command, "But let's get this war over first," he said to himself, "and the prospects will be more favourable."
The newly-named 'Cannondore' was some eighteen years old. She had been laid up for over three years, and was now completely refurbished and recommissioned, to help make up for the appalling loss of shipping through submarine warfare. It was not the largest ship Jimmie had served on, but eight thousand tons was no small craft. Tomorrow, the crew would be arriving. They would look to him for their safety, their instructions; in fact, almost everything. Inwardly, he began to realise the absolute responsibility he would now have as captain.
Two whistles on the speaking-tube beside him actually made him jump.
"That's a bloody good start," he said aloud.
"Second mate ... captain speaking," he corrected himself.
A beery voice, with an Irish accent, replied, "Oh, the saints be praised, we have the admiral himself on board, and I thought I'd be handling this tub on me own."
"Who the hell are you?" shouted Jimmie.
"They tell me you'll be wanting a Chief Engineer," came the slurred reply.
Suddenly, the voice seemed familiar.
"Report to the bridge immediately, you drunken coot, and I'll deal with you here."
It was five minutes before Chief Engineer McClean arrived on the bridge. They shook hands. Both men had served together for many years, and now circumstances had brought them together again.
"Congratulations on your appointment, Jimmie. I am certain you have deserved it for a long while but, by God, you are worthy of a better crate than this."
"How did you know it was me up here?"
"Well now, if you must know, when I saw that heap of kit on deck, I said to meself, I wager all the four-leafed clovers in Ireland that that's no other than Jimmie Brown on board."

"Thank goodness I have you at the working end, Mac. Have you any idea what we'll be doing?"
"Yes, Jimmie, about ten thousand feet in the air if we're hit amidships. They sure haven't put all that iron around her body to carry bananas!"
For the next hour, the two men toured the ship and discussed its potential.
"I'll give my verdict when we've had a trial run, but if it's as potent as the smell of the paint, it should perform quite well," said Mac.
It was three days before the thirty or more crew could be assembled on the mess deck. The men were a hotch-potch array of survivors of torpedoed ships, young lads, some only seventeen years old, and a few with more sea-years than their captain.
Jimmie viewed his crew. Many had their characters written clearly on their faces. One eighteen-stoner sat, his chin supported by two arms resembling telegraph poles, totally oblivious to his surroundings. When the duty officer called the men to attention, he did not even bat an eyelid.
"It will take all the T.N.T. in Germany to shift that bugger," thought Jimmie. "I shall have to keep a shrewd eye on him."
"Gentlemen, may I welcome you aboard the 'M.S. Cannondore'. To the more experienced among you, I am well aware that she does not qualify as a supership, but she does have a long history and we, fortunately or unfortunately, have been chosen to extend it.
"To the younger of you, I can well imagine you thinking that goes for her captain as well, and you are quite right. I was sailing the waves before this ship was built. My message to you today is the same one I received at the moment I put my feet on deck thirty-seven years ago.
"Firstly, do what you are told at once. Your life may depend on it. Secondly, always be on the lookout, and thirdly, remember what you see. If you do that, it will go a long way to making this a successful ship. Your work will be arduous and dangerous. Discipline will be strict, as far as discipline is necessary. Outside that, I want us all to live on this ship as a happy community. Every man will be respected for his position and rank. Senior seamen will be respected for their experience and, in return, I expect all ranks, officers and seamen, to encourage the juniors on board.
"On duty, you will refer to me as 'captain', in preference to 'sir'. Off duty, and that will be extremely rare, you may call me Jimmie. That's what my mother calls me, and I have always considered that an honour.
"Gentlemen, you may now dismiss."
Jimmie returned at once to his cabin. His reference to Skip's three instructions had raised a query in his mind. Where was Aunt Nell's painting of the 'Maywell'?
Within a few minutes, his cabin was strewn with papers and clothes, but all to no avail. Carefully he repacked. It was a complete mystery. He was absolutely certain that he had packed it at Enfield. The possibility of it being stolen could not be ruled out. Its loss would be a saddening blow for him.
That evening, in the mess, Mac challenged him, "Jimmie, I perceive you have a problem on your mind."
Jimmie suddenly alerted himself, "Heavens! Does it show?"
"Only to me, Jimmie. I have known you many years. I think you had better tell me what it is all about."

"Well, you may not believe this Mac, but I have lost my painting of the 'Maywell'. I have turned my cabin upside down looking for it."
For a full minute Mac was doubled up with laughter.
"Jimmie! You! The most methodical man in the Merchant Service, confesses to mis-laying a treasured possession!"
Jimmie stared hard. It was not a laughing matter to him. Mac saw his captain's reaction, "I'm sorry, Jimmie. I did not mean it to hurt. In fact, I am partly to blame. You will recall the other day asking me how I knew it was you on the bridge. I said it was because of all the kit on deck. That was not quite true. As I came up the gangway, I just happened to see a porter stuffing a load of papers in what was your case. He hurriedly told me that it had come undone. I informed him, in no uncertain terms, that if I heard of one thing missing, I'd boot him from one side of the Mersey to the other. As he left, I picked up a sheet of paper that was blowing across the deck. I took one look, and knew who was on board. I do apologise for not returning it at once. My ruse of being drunk at the time seems to have misfired against you."
"The knowledge that you have saved it from a watery grave astounds me. I have more reason to thank you than to accept your apologies."
Both men laughed, and drank to the other's health.
"I must learn to restrain my feelings at all times," said Jimmie, as they retired for the night.
The next day, the painting took pride of place on the wall of his cabin. As he fixed it in position, he wondered if Skip could possibly be still alive. He had heard about Aunt Nell's death, then nothing from that day onwards. He still had great admiration for his benefactor, and promised himself that, when the war was over, he would retrace his steps and search for him.
Three weeks later, after storing up, training gun crews, making trial runs and organising all the paraphernalia of war, the 'Cannondore' left Liverpool, destination as yet unknown.
It was four hours after leaving port that Jimmie knew for certain his new assignment. He had unsealed the orders in front of Andrews, his second-in-command.
"We shall not be trooping, which comes as a great relief. That remark applies only to me, Andrews. Sailing the ocean has always been a hazard and in wartime it becomes extremely dangerous. Under the conditions in which we are now being placed, it will become total suicide."
Andrews tried to read his captain's thoughts.
"Will you please enlighten me, captain?"
"I beg your pardon, Andrews. My thoughts were quite personal and selfish. Let us enjoy our sailing, while we may. Until further notice, or heaven calls, we shall be transporting some two thousand tons of gelignite and other high explosives from the shores of America to ports as yet unknown. We have now to train our crew on the importance and dangers of their task, bearing in mind that thousands of poor devils on those fields of France depend upon the efficiency of this ship."
The close proximity of being obliterated from the face of the earth at the slightest mishap had the effect of bonding the crew together. If one man goes, we all go, so let's be happy together, was their slogan.

The crew quickly found their captain to be a man true to his word, and by the time three Atlantic crossings had been completed, there were no applications for transfer. For the next twelve months, the 'Cannondore' sailed the ocean with her vital cargo. On the outward journeys, Jimmie enjoyed the comfort of the convoy escort, but on the return, he sailed well to the rear with, perhaps, a lone escort in the far distance.

When occasion permitted, Jimmie would often chaff his fellow captains on their reluctance to sail near him. Their replies were usually witty, "Would you cuddle up to a girl with two thousand tons of high explosives under her pinny?"

Jimmie would laugh, but to him, it seemed uncanny that the 'Cannondore' should have such a charmed life.

Chapter Fourteen

Breakdown and Tin Fish

November 1917

The 'Cannondore' was three days out of Boston. Jimmie had watched the sun rise. There was every sign of a fair day's weather, but for him, hopefully, a fair day's sleep. A message from the escort told him that the preceeding convoy had enjoyed an uninterrupted night, and had given him his recommended speed for the day.

However, as the day lightened, Andrews appeared on the bridge and Jimmie was able to confirm the suspicions that had been growing in his mind.

"Do my ears deceive me, or am I in need of sleep, Andrews, because we seem to have an extra 'clonkity-clonk' coming from the boiler room?"

Andrews rubbed his eyes. "I think you are right, captain."

He had hardly spoken when the boiler room tube sounded. Jimmie picked up the ear-piece. It was McClean.

"We're in trouble, captain. The wee folk are playing hell with the bearings on the main shaft."

"Then put that eighteen-stoner, Telegraph, in to sort them out before we grind to a standstill," was Jimmie's quick reply.

Fifteen minutes later, he stood down below with Mac. The situation was serious.

"How long do you need?"

"Could be ten hours. It's a major task, but I dare not drive her much longer."

"Right, Mac. Stop engines. Every available man will be at your disposal."

A message giving the situation was sent to convoy command. An escort was detailed to take a circuitous course around the stricken ship, which now presented itself a sitting target for the U-boats. Every spare man was posted at intervals, around the deck, to scan the water for mines or the tell-tale wake of a torpedo. All the lifeboats were lowered into the water. If a sighting was made, and impact imminent, the order to abandon ship would be given, but the only slender chance of survival was to jump into the sea, and the only ray of comfort for the anxious crew was the escort frigate. Throughout the day, Jimmie patrolled his ship. No sleep for him now, but there was little he could do in the boiler room. He had every confidence in Mac. Wherever possible, he put a senior seaman and junior on watch together; the younger had usually better eyesight and the elder the experience not to panic at every splash of a wave. Hot coffee and tea was in plentiful supply, but strong drink was forbidden.

During the afternoon, the wind blew strong and cold. Men on deck froze in their duffle coats and men in the boiler room sweated in their skins.

One hour, and the light would be failing. Jimmie was aware that it would be the most critical time. If they had been spotted during the day, it would be an ideal time for a submarine to attack and then escape from the escort.

Making his way into the engine room, he found the place unusually quiet. Men with black, sooty sweat running down their bodies, some laying, some standing, others crouching, were struggling and straining to free the jammed shaft.

"Please, pray for us, Jimmie. We need another sixteenth of an inch, then we can link it up."

Jimmie tapped his engineer on the shoulder.

"Put Telegraph next to the flange and try again."

Without question, Mac rearranged his men. "Right boys, when I give the word we'll show the captain it can be done."

Jimmie's eyes caught those of Telegraph's. He gave a wink which was returned by the burly man.

"One, two, three, LIFT."

"Grant them strength, Lord." That's what Aunt Nell would say, and expect an answer, "Please grant it to us, O Lord," said Jimmie. His prayer was quite audible, but the men were so occupied that they were not aware of his pleading on their behalf.

Every muscle strained. Faces were contorted with pain. Men stood motionless, waiting to insert the connecting bolts. The thought of failure was never far away. Jimmie's attention was on Telegraph. He watched, as he took in a deep breath, flexed his muscles, then braced himself. Every part of his body went into tension. He gritted his teeth and closed his eyes. Sweat poured from his body and face.

"Hold!" shouted Mac.

Telegraph's body quivered and changed colour from red to white. The men slid the bolts into position.

"You've done it boys! Relax!" shouted Mac.

Men cheered, groaned and threw themselves onto the deck. But Jimmie's eyes were still fixed on Telegraph, for he had collapsed into the shaft housing. While men quickly rallied round and carried him to the sick bay, others worked frantically connecting the shaft.

"Give me twenty minutes and we'll be under way," called Mac, as Jimmie made his way to the upper deck.

The news travelled around the ship in seconds. The feeling of being helpless on the high seas had been terrifying, but was now lifted.

Jimmie stopped to speak to a young lad scanning the seas on the starboard bows. He had a fearful expression.

"Am I right in thinking that this is your first trip?"

"Yes, captain," came the rather meek reply.

"Let me assure you that you always remember your first trip. I can still recall vividly my own, down the Thames, nearly forty years ago. It was the most exciting day of my life."

The fact that the captain talked to him at such a critical time gave David renewed confidence. His face glowed with relief.

"That's better. Now be honest with me, would you recognise a tin fish?"

"Yes, captain."

"In that case, keep your eyes trained on those waters. We are not out of trouble yet."

Jimmie watched as heavy smoke began to billow from the funnel. He turned to his second-in-command. "The moment for departure is at hand. Alert all stations to stand by."

It was but a few minutes before Mac's voice came up from the boiler room.
"Just say the word, Jimmie, and I'll get you back to Blighty."
"Thanks, Mac. I'll see you later. Take her away."
Slowly, as the engines began to turn, the mighty hulk of iron came to life and gradually began to move through the water. Flurries of snow swept across her decks, and a shout of 'Hurrah' echoed throughout the ship. Jimmie wiped the condensation from the observation window. Below, he saw the lad he had spoken to run to congratulate his fellow watch. Picking up a megaphone, Jimmie opened the window and yelled, "Get back to your posts." Both men scuttled back. Instantly, he saw the lad's arm pointing out to sea and heard the frantic cry of "Torpedo starboard!"
Jimmie slammed the Action Station alarm, while following the direction of the boy's arm. He saw two torpedo wakes, some four hundred feet apart, heading towards the 'Cannondore'.
"Hard to starboard," he shouted to the helmsman, and "full steam ahead" to the engine room.
The great bulk of iron forming the 'Cannondore' shuddered from the demands made upon it. Within seconds Jimmie countered the order.
"Slow astern, engine room."
The mighty propellor thrashed the water like a furious beast. The ship swung, head towards the torpedoes, and held its course. Men on deck watched with bated breath as each deadly projectile passed, first on the starboard, and then on the port side. Jimmie drew his forearm across his brow.
"The last two minutes have added ten years to my life, Andrews. Put her back on course, we have many miles to make up."
The dramatic moments had also been closely watched by the escort. The two torpedo wakes had been sighted. Quick asdic calculations estimated the approximate position of the submarine and the possibility that they would be the next target. Like a snake, weaving its way through grass, the frigate attacked its prey. Depth charges sent columns of water high into the darkening sky. Through his glasses, Jimmie saw the debris of their attacker.
"Another U-boat and crew who will never return to the Fatherland. Why must men be so callous towards each other, Andrews?"
"I don't think there's any answer to that question, captain. We all just live hoping to see another day."
Meanwhile, deep down in the bowels of the 'Cannondore', McClean was inspecting the outcome of the drastic action placed upon his replaced bearing. Fitters re-checked the work. As all proved satisfactory, a message to the bridge said, "Proceed, everything normal."
The crisis over, Jimmie left his officers to re-schedule the duties, and returned to his cabin to prepare a report. He had hardly sat down when a knock on the door broke into his thoughts.
"Come in." It was a weary call.
Mac entered.
"Thank goodness it is you. Anyone else would have been court martialled, but why look so miserable? I would have thought you could raise a smile on such an occasion. Let's have a tot. I think we deserve it."
Jimmie walked to the locker.

"I've lost Telegraph," said Mac.
"That's nothing to look miserable about. Put two men in his place. He will be back in a couple of days, shovelling his precious coal."
"Not so, Jimmie. He's dead!"
Both men stood quite still for a moment. Then, as Jimmie sat down, he broke the silence.
"I'm responsible for that man's death, Mac. It's a dreadful thought."
"For goodness sake, don't hold that against yourself, Jimmie. That man gave his all for the sake of us, and ruptured his heart into the bargain. That's war!"
Mac was in the process of continuing the tale of what had happened, but Jimmie raised his hand.
"Give me a moment, Mac."
They silently sipped their rum. What his engineer had said had disturbed in his memory familiar words of his boyhood days. Yes, it was Aunt Nell telling him about the one she loved. He could do with a little of her faith right now. He placed his hand on the table again.
"The doctor asked me to give you the information before the crew."
"Thank you, Mac. I will tell the men after dinner."
As Mac was about to leave, he turned. "I understand that the new lad sighted the tin fish after you had bawled him out. I trust you will deal with him accordingly. We don't want that sort on a ship like this!"
"Yes, Mac. You can depend on me to settle that score. As you go down, will you instruct the duty officer that I don't want any callers for thirty minutes, then he can send young Carter and Gibson to see me."
Jimmie lit his pipe, replenished his glass and laid back on his couch to relax. It had been quite a day, and the news about Telegraph had a devastating effect on him. Shortly, he was to consider what action he should take with Carter and Gibson. While he insisted on discipline, he was soft-hearted when it came to punishment.
Thirty minutes, exactly, passed before there came a sharp rap on the door.
"Come in, Carter," he shouted.
The door was opened by Manners, the Duty Officer.
"Shall I march them in, sir?"
"No, Manners. On my ship men walk in. And refer to me as your captain."
Like Carter, this was Manners' first trip on the 'Cannondore'. For reasons best known to himself, he had failed to get a commission in the Royal Navy, and had a nauseating habit of letting his fellow men know that what he was doing was only second best, and just temporary.
Gibson, an experienced seaman, followed by Carter, walked smartly in and stood with Manners in front of the desk.
"Shall I read the charge, captain?"
Jimmie fixed his eyes on the young officer, who suddenly felt as though his life's blood was running out of his boots.
"No, thank you, Manners. You may leave now. Your duty above deck is far more important."
Jimmie sized up the two men. It seemed remarkable that he should have Gibson, one of the longest serving men in the Merchant Navy, and Carter, the youngest serving man on the 'Cannondore', standing before him, for failing to carry out their duty.

He couldn't help admiring Gibson for his coolness. "Experience teaches men how to cope with situations like this," he thought. The lad looked petrified, and Jimmie could see his knuckles standing out white, as he tightly clenched his hands.

"Right, pick up a chair each, and sit down. I'm too tired at the moment to strain my neck looking up at you."

They had hardly sat down before Gibson jumped up again.

"Permission to speak, captain."

"No, Gibson."

"But I accept full blame. It was my fault, captain."

"I will decide whose fault it was, Gibson, and do not butt in again," shouted Jimmie.

The older man sat slowly on his chair, knowing that nothing he was going to say would change the captain's thinking. Jimmie turned to the boy, who had witnessed his senior shipmate put in his place, and had turned as white as the writing paper on the desk.

"Where is your home, Carter?"

The question came as a complete surprise to the boy, but it had the effect Jimmie wanted, although the answer gave him somewhat of a jolt.

"W-Wap-Wapping, sir," stuttered the lad.

"That's interesting, but I will speak to you about that later."

"Y-you-you saved our lives, sir," blurted out the boy amidst a waving of arms and the falling of tears.

Gibson grabbed the boy's arms and held them tight. "Calm down, David, and listen to your captain."

He sat shaking and whimpering, with the older man's arm on his shoulder.

"Give me a couple of whisky-sodden brawlers, and I could cope easily," thought Jimmie.

"Gibson, I know this is completely unconventional." Then, pointing to the glass left by McClean, "Give the boy a drink."

He passed his own glass, and the rum bottle, "And take one yourself. Then we can get some order into the meeting."

Both man and boy drank in silence. Jimmie watched the colour return to the lad's cheeks.

"Right. Now, let's get down to business. I have not brought you down here to read out the riot act, or decide as to who did what, and least of all did I expect to make a drinking party out of the occasion.

"I know, you know what happened, and I am certain that it will never happen again. No further words from me are necessary on that point, I am sure."

Both culprits nodded their agreement.

"But there are other matters which need emphasizing, and I will deal with you, Gibson, first. I appreciate your gesture to accept the blame, but fifty years good conduct is a lot of service to throw away. But then, perhaps, you are thinking that life on the 'Cannondore' is so uncertain that there is nothing to be lost, or that, perhaps, I would trade your fifty years good conduct as sufficient punishment. But I am old enough and, I hope, wise enough to know that was not your motive. You did it out of love and compassion for Carter, and I admire you for that."

Jimmie turned in his chair. "Now Carter, listen to me."
David had now composed himself, but realised that the captain knew the facts, and that he would now receive the full punishment for his misdeed. He lifted his head and faced his superior.
"What is your real age, Carter?"
"Seventeen, captain."
"I repeat, your real age."
"Sixteen, captain."
"When will you be sixteen, Carter?"
"Next week, captain."
"Thank you. I would have preferred to have known the first time around. Your secret is safe with me. I accept your courage in serving your country under-age, not realising the true consequence of war. I have little time for people who say they have no fear of death; it is a natural reaction. But I have less time for people who become hysterical, and that is a lesson you must learn before you become successful. Gibson has demonstrated how it can be done. Do you think you can develop the art of self-composure? If not, you cannot remain on this ship. Do you understand what I have said?"
"Yes, captain."
"Then I will give you one more trip to prove yourself. Now, you will both be punished equally. First, you will under no circumstances repeat what has transpired between us. Secondly, on leaving this cabin you will go to the galley and assist in the preparation of dinner, and remain on duty as long as the cook requires you."
Man and boy stood smartly to attention, turned and walked to the door. As he was closing it, Gibson looked back.
"The whole crew are sincerely grateful to you, captain."
Jimmie nodded his head in approval.
"Be off with you. I'm waiting for my dinner."
Later that night, after all had partaken of a filling meal, every available man gathered on the mess deck. Jimmie took his place at the table.
"Gentlemen, like many of you, I am dog tired. I will not delay you long. Already I have heard that the captain has saved our lives. I now wish to put that statement to a sudden death. Today has been exceptional for us, and it is easy to get the situation out of proportion. I do not have to remind you that we are always a slow-moving target for Jerry submarines. Today, we have been a sitting target: two thousand tons of explosives just waiting to be detonated."
"While we can be thankful that today has passed, and that we are still sailing the high seas, I cannot vouchsafe for tomorrow or the next day. Therefore, I see no reason why a few words of praise for our escape today should come amiss now."
"Because the Chief Engineer and his staff carried out a repair in only ten hours, when it would usually have taken twenty hours, they saved our lives."
"Because the galley crew provided an endless supply of boiling hot drinks for those freezing on deck or sweating below, they saved our lives."
"Those who paced the deck and scanned the seas for mines and torpedoes, they saved our lives.
"Young Carter, who recognised a tin fish when he saw one. He saved our

lives."

"The helmsman who slammed the rudder over at once. He saved our lives."

"For those in the engine room who reacted immediately to an incredible demand, they saved our lives."

"To our escort who circled us all day, and then went into action at the vital moment, they saved our lives."

Nods of approval, and murmurs of, "Hear, hear," endorsed Jimmie's remarks.

"There is still one man who I have not mentioned. He saved our lives."

"Three cheers for the captain," came from the rear of the mess deck.

Jimmie waved his arms in rebuke.

"It is not your captain, but Telegraph, whom we often treat as a simpleton. Today, he expended the entire strength of his mighty body to release the jammed shaft."

Once again, men interrupted their captain, "Three cheers for Tele, the lazy bugger."

Jimmie once again waved them down.

"Gentlemen. I have not finished. Will you please listen to what I have to tell you. Telegraph, in doing so, ruptured his heart and died. What you have already said about him may be perfectly true, but remember Telegraph in the words used today by our Chief Engineer. Today he gave his all to save us all. I ask you, gentlemen, to stand in silence in respect for him, and his supreme effort."

The whole company stood as one man, stunned by the news. Many felt guilty of the stick they had given to the hero of the day. The voice of Jimmie broke the silence, "God bless Telegraph, and all who give their all. To those of you on duty, and those who will be able to sleep, I wish you a good night. Gentlemen, dismiss."

Jimmie made his way back to his cabin, accompanied by Mac.

"If you will allow me to say so, I consider that you made a great impression on the lads tonight, captain."

"Thank you, Mac. I only wish to emphasize the importance of the fact that we all depend upon one another, but if you start calling me captain, I will consider that you and I are drifting apart."

"Jimmie, that must never be, although at times like this I cannot help respecting you for what you really are - our captain."

They reached the cabin door.

"One more question before I say goodnight. What made you change Telegraph's position?"

Jimmie opened the door. "Come in, Mac, then I can tell you in comfort."

He poured them both a drink, and sat down.

"It was purely a hunch. It occurred to me that Telegraph, standing in the middle, was matching his strength against the others, and the shaft was being raised horizontally and fouling its connection. Putting Tele to the jammed end, and encouraging him to increase his effort, would tip the angle of pressure and, hopefully, have the desired effect. I shall never forget the look on his face. It's tragic that he should bust his guts in the effort."

"I shall give him a good report, in fact, everyone will get a good report."

Both men finished their drinks and wished each other goodnight. Jimmie laid his head on his pillow. It was nearly thirty-six hours since he had closed

his eyes in sleep. His last vision was the painting of the 'Maywell', hanging above his bunk.
"You wanted me to be a captain, Skip. I trust if you are in the great beyond, looking down on me, that you will approve of the way I have carried out my duty today."
Their eventual arrival at Liverpool was a welcome relief, especially for Mac, who realised that there was much to be done to make the 'Cannondore' fit for further service.
The crew was given a well-deserved fourteen days shore leave, while a quick overhaul was undertaken.

Chapter Fifteen

A Sad Occasion

December 1917

For Jimmie, these days were spent at his parent's home in Enfield. Complete relaxation was his only wish.

Mum and Dad were now in their seventies and, because of their son's generosity, enjoyed a comfortable existence. Both were proud of him, and made his success known. Unfortunately, the war had been extremely unkind to the Brown family, as a whole.

Emily, Jimmie's eldest sister, had lost her husband during the early part of the war. There had been no children of the marriage. Rosy had never married, and was killed in a munitions factory explosion, at Woolwich. Fred, Jimmie's younger brother, was a prisoner of war, and Joe, the youngest, was also serving somewhere in France.

On the first Saturday after he arrived home, a party in Jimmie's honour was given. Other than Emily, it was mainly family friends, although they were mostly strangers to Jimmie. He amused the children with stories of Australia and remote parts of the world, like Woodham Ferris, where strange birds and animals lived. At the end of the party, Dad made a speech, which surprised Jimmie. They drank a toast to absent friends and a speedy end to the war. They rounded off the evening by singing 'God save the King'. No sooner was the party over than another tragedy struck the Browns in the form of the Black Flu. It attacked with a vengeance and, on the following Wednesday, Jimmie's father died. The very next day, his mother followed him to her grave. Whilst the shock was great to Jimmie and Emily, they had the one consolation that their parents were not aware of each other's death. They were both buried on the following Monday.

Jimmie returned to Liverpool on the Wednesday, after making full provision for his sister, now his only direct link with the family of his childhood.

The journey back to rejoin the 'Cannondore' was, for Jimmie, sheer agony. His usual ploy, of pretending to sleep, gave him an opportunity to go over things in his mind. He had almost reached the peak of his career when war had deprived him of his ultimate ambition. And now, since the beginning of the century, he had lost all those people dear to him who had sought to encourage his promotion in life.

No one could replace Grandad, the hero of his boyhood days. The tragedy and circumstances of his death remained in his memory as vividly as if it were yesterday.

Aunt Nell - well, if saints lived, then she must have been one. Skip - he owed him everything. Death could be the only thing that would finally part them, and if that had happened without Jimmie's knowledge, then all he could do was pay homage to Skip's memory. And now his Mum and Dad had died in his presence. He could accept that, and was thankful for the well-timed shore leave.

Rose killed, Fred a prisoner, Joey in Flanders. What hope had he of ever seeing them again, or they him, sailing the Atlantic with three seconds between life on earth and Eternity? Grandad may well have said, "Learn to overcome disappointment." At this point in time, there seemed no purpose or justice in living. In fact death, it would appear, freed one from the demands of this murderous world.

For two hours or more, Jimmie did battle with an acute attack of depression, an experience new to him. He at last decided that the future held nothing in store for him, but that in continuing the battle for peace, he might be providing a future for those children he had talked to at the party. Perhaps they would create a better world.

Once back on the 'Cannondore', duty overcame depression. They joined the convoy, and headed once again across the Atlantic. Despite the fact of being away from their loved ones at Christmas, the crew enjoyed the twenty-fifth, with roast turkey and all the trimmings, plus a liberal quota of drink. They toasted their families, each other, and in fact anyone they could think of. Jimmie was invited to make a speech, and he prophesied that the war would be over within the year, and that they would spend the next festive season with their loved ones. They all drank to that prediction, then sang 'For he's a jolly good fellow'.

Jimmie closed the festivities by saying that he found it difficult, under present conditions, to be jolly. He made no claims of ever being good, but that he did have the qualification of being a fellow.

The party over, life on the 'Cannondore' returned to its usual humdrum of daily duties.

For the next three months, they lived their charmed lives, sailing the Atlantic. According to the law of averages, they should have been sunk two years previously and, in fact, German reports had written them off on more than one occasion.

Chapter Sixteen

Mines and Meetings

In late March, the ship's destination was changed, and they docked in a south American port. Their cargo, on return, was much the same as usual, but it was late April before they actually got under way. It would be another three or four days before they tacked onto the end of the convoy.

The weather was blistering hot, and four days out they were fog-bound. Speed was reduced to a minimum as they estimated that their escort was in the vicinity. On the fifth morning, wireless contact was made with convoy control. They were instructed to reduce speed yet again, to enable the main convoy to get ahead, and to keep a look out for survivors of a ship recently sunk by a U-boat. The situation for Jimmie was far from pleasant. He disliked the fog, he disliked sailing so slowly, and he disliked the thought of being rammed or ramming someone else. The danger of submarine warfare had decreased, but this could be only temporary. Fog would most probably keep them down again today, as they too would be subject to being rammed. Every available pair of eyes was put on watch to try and penetrate the fog. Jimmie paced the deck, hoping for a sign of breeze, but it was late afternoon before his wishes were granted. Within the hour, they had visibility of two or three miles and gradually increasing, but still no signs of the convoy. Were they ahead or behind? It would be a great relief to him to know their whereabouts before nightfall.

The shout of, "Lifeboat adrift, five hundred yards, port bows", had Jimmie rushing to the bridge. He trained the telescope onto the stricken craft, where he could discern men waving to attract attention. "Poor blighters, it could easily be me," he thought as he issued orders. It required little diversion to come alongside them. He gave Gibson, because of his experience, instructions to prepare a rescue boat ready for a quick transfer of survivors onto the 'Cannondore'. Leaning over the rail of the bridge companionway, Jimmie was able to watch Gibson, with Chapman and young Carter, take his position in the boat and drop from the davits towards the sea.

The 'Cannondore' came almost to a standstill. Jimmie was on the point of shouting "Cast away" to Gibson when a cry, "Torpedo starboard!" rent the air. Jimmie turned and raced to the bridge.

Something in the back of his mind told him that he was travelling in space. It did not matter whether he opened or closed his eyes, he was enveloped in a golden orange mass. The sensation was quite pleasant. What was it that Aunt Nell used to say? "In the twinkling of an eye we shall be caught up to meet Him in the air." This must be it.

The sudden shock of darkness blacked out the already limited use of his brain, then, as it momentarily returned, he realised that he was thrashing the water with his arms. Gone was the golden glare and the feeling of weightlessness. Everything was black, and he felt as if he weighed a ton.

Again he blacked out, then a sudden pain as his arms crashed down on a solid object and jarred his senses into action again. He grappled frantically to secure a hold on whatever it was. Suddenly, he became aware that he was jammed between a cross spar and mast, and entangled in wire and cords. The moments of bliss were gone. It was now a frightening disaster and fight for life. With excruciating pain, he dragged his body over the cross spar. He tried to shout, but no sound would come forth. He tried to look around - all seemed darkness. He was blind: he must be. He vaguely realised that he had no feeling in his legs. "Blown Off". He hugged the cross spar, his only hope. The uncanny stillness terrified him. In moments of consciousness he tried to assess his situation. He must hang onto the mast.
Painfully, he twisted the trailing lines around his body and around the mast, then, putting his arms over and under the mast, he grabbed his jerkin with both hands and clung like a limpet.

Gibson passed his hand across his face to wipe away the nightmare he had just experienced. The pain was terrific. Was it blood or sea water? He found it difficult to decide. It was pitch black and deadly quiet. He was laying and not sitting in the boat, but where were Chapman and David? He called, but only the lap of the water against the boat replied.
He sat himself up slowly and tried to recall what he had last been doing. Someone yelling "Torpedo".
"Then we must be adrift," he thought. "Oh God! What do I do now?"
He called out a number of times, but again only the sea answered. Painfully, he crawled along the well of the boat to find his mates. His hand found a body, only to tell him with horror that it was headless. Could it be David? He rose on his knees and was violently sick. Then, recovering from this discovery, he crawled on to search for his other shipmate. This time his hand found a smooth face which confirmed to him that this was David, for Chapman's face was bearded. He put his head close to the boy's.
"Can you hear me David?"
He shook him gently, but there was still no response. He felt for the lad's pulse, but his own hands were too cold to detect any movement. With a feeling of despair, he accepted that he was the sole survivor on the boat. Squatting himself on a seat, he contemplated committing the bodies to the sea. It would be less heartbreaking in the dark. His first attempt proved to him that he was too weak to carry out the task. He would rest now and hope that he would have regained enough strength by daybreak, or else would join his mates in the mystery of death.
From a locker, he took a blanket and put it round his shoulders. Sitting, he tried to decide how long it had been since the torpedo had exploded. Had it sunk the 'Cannondore'? All was confusion in his mind. From sheer exhaustion he dropped off to sleep, but he awoke suddenly. Someone was calling for help, but he had little means of help. He shouted back, but there was no reply.
"Nerves, Steve," he said to himself, "I must control myself."
Once more he tried to compose himself, and gradually pain and sleep took over.
He roused again. Something had touched him. He rose to his feet and swung

his arms in panic, but only the darkness mocked him. He sat down once more, his whole body trembling, but gradually he regained his composure.

A tug on his trouser leg alerted him again.

"Is that you, Steve?"

The voice was David's. Instantly Steve dropped to the deck, beside the lad.

"Where are we, Steve? What's happened?"

"Don't worry, David. You are safe."

Steve helped the boy onto the seat beside him.

"Now listen to me. Do as I tell you and we shall be rescued. The explosion must have blown us away from the ship. It should soon be light, so we must huddle together to keep warm."

"I will keep calm, Steve. I feel safe with you," said the boy.

At first light, Steve found the boy asleep. He pulled the blanket over the lad's face, for the sight of Chapman's body was horrific. With a supreme effort, he managed to lift and roll the torn remains and commit them to the sea, and with a sea-bucket he flushed the deck of blood stains.

A slight movement in the air told the veteran seaman that the fog, which had again fallen overnight, would soon clear.

Quickly, he checked the lockers. Water was the essential commodity. His search satisfied him that they could sustain a fairly long period adrift. This being his third time shipwrecked, he would be able to put his experience to good use.

David's first question on rousing was, "Where is Chapman, Steve?"

The older man was slow to answer.

"If you recall, when we came down the side of the 'Cannondore', we were sitting, and he was standing. I'm afraid the blast must have thrown him clear of the boat. We, fortunately, were thrown to the deck."

Steve checked their injuries. Despite looking serious, they were all superficial.

A drink of water and a biscuit were the morning's rations.

"From now on, David, we must plan our programme of survival. While we hope that we may be picked up today, we have to accept the fact that it could be two weeks or more before we are sighted. If the 'Cannondore' blew up, we should find plenty of debris, so we must pick up anything that may come in useful."

Within the hour, the fate of their ship had been confirmed. Shattered crates, tins, cannisters and even pieces of shredded clothing floated by, but not a single survivor or body.

The one comfort was that the fog had receded and the sun shone hazily down upon them, giving warmth and drying out their clothes. David said that it made him feel better.

Steve replied, "Enjoy it today. After a few days you will curse it!"

They recovered a large, battered tin of jam from the sea, and enjoyed a liberal helping, spread on their next hard biscuit. Visibility they now estimated as six hundred yards.

Steve stood, scanning the water. There was always the hope that someone was there, just beyond that white cloud, waiting to help them or to be saved.

"Do you think you can row, David?"

"Yes, Steve, but will it help?"

"I'm not sure, but I am very interested in what is drifting on the port side horizon. Unfortunately, it is not getting any nearer."

Both man and boy, despite their injuries, took to the oars. It was painful and slow, but gradually they drew alongside their objective.

"Good heavens alive!" shouted David in an instant of recognition. "It's the captain! What do we do? He is obviously dead."

"Dead or alive, he's coming on board," replied Steve. "Whatever we do, we must not let him slip from the mast or out of our hands when we transfer him. While you fix a line fore and aft to the mast, I will try and sort out the confusion of rope and wire around his body."

Both men proceeded with their tasks. Carefully, Steve passed a line around the captain's body and tied it off to a seat in the boat, in case of any mishaps. Then, one by one, he severed the lines which apparently held his captain onto his means of support.

There was little that indicated any sign of life. Steve and David leant over the gunwhales and attempted to lift the body, but it was to no avail. Again Steve's hands passed under the mast and his suspicions were confirmed. Jimmie's fingers were clenched onto his jerkin, and set fast.

With a knife, he cut the jerkin away from the body and straightened the arms from under the mast.

With a supreme effort, they then succeeded in raising their captain from the mast and gradually lowering him onto the deck of the lifeboat. David cut loose the mast, as Steve examined the inert body. His faint hopes were dashed: again the ocean had claimed a victim.

"Thank God the sea has remained calm, or we should never have accomplished our task," puffed Steve. Both men sat down, humbly looking at the bedraggled body of the man they had come to admire.

"What do we do next?" enquired David, after what to him seemed an eternity. "All we have done is dragged a dead man on board."

The question remained unanswered, for Steve had suddenly left the seat and dropped down by the body.

"David, I am not certain that he is dead."

Quickly, he cut away the remaining clothes, baring Jimmie's chest. Then, placing his head near to the captain's chest, he listened carefully. For David these were moments of anguish.

"I'm positive he's alive. We must work fast. You massage his chest." Steve demonstrated the correct way.

"I must make a fire. Heat is essential."

He placed an empty cylinder into a large metal drum, which they had salvaged from the sea. The cylinder provided the firebox, and the drum an area to warm and dry clothing. From the emergency locker, Steve found the means to start a fire and, using any dry, combustible material he could lay his hands upon, achieved his aim. Removing his woollen pullover, he placed it in the makeshift oven.

"Right, David, let's change places. You have got to keep the fire going and watch that the clothes don't catch alight."

Carefully, Steve removed the sodden clothes from Jimmie, and replaced them with the hot pullover and blanket. Meanwhile, David had replaced Steve's pullover with his own. For two hours or more, the exchange of hot clothing and blankets continued, during which period Steve bandaged Jimmie's body and arms. Periodically, he listened, and was convinced that the heart-beat was improving.

It was during a lull that Steve noticed Jimmie's tongue slowly wipe his lips. He got out the flask he had found in his captain's pocket, and moistened the lips with rum. It was the first hopeful response they had seen for the two frantic hours' work. Throughout the day, man and boy continued their efforts to maintain life in the body.

Steve realised that Jimmie's legs were broken, and possibly his back, and that he was also suffering deep concussion. Warmth, massage and the wiping of the lips with rum were all that they could do.

The fear of the coming night was never far from their thoughts. How could they maintain the fire? Driftwood was now hard to come by. If recue was not forthcoming, the only satisfaction they would have was to have done all that was possible. So engrossed had they been in their duty that neither had realised that the fog had completely dispersed. The sun had dropped low in the sky and the wind had freshened. Steve scanned the horizon with dismay. His experience told him that stormy weather was on the way. He said nothing to David, but the feeling that they would not see another morning's light was definite.

"We will have two biscuits, plenty of jam, and a sip of the captain's rum. I am certain he would not begrudge us that," he said to David, and to himself, "then Fate can do the rest."

They enjoyed the jam. As Steve stoked the fire, David pulled at his sleeve and pointed to the starboard horizon. His mouth opened, but no words came forth. Within seconds, Steve had fired a distress rocket, and the boy had taken a burning board from the fire and was waving it furiously.

It was ten minutes before their signals were answered by the distant flash of a morse lamp, and a change of direction by the vessel. The action raised their hopes. Cloud and driving rain began to change the evening sky. It would take nearly an hour before their rescuers could be upon them.

"We must keep the fire burning, or we could be lost," stressed Steve. So, with an axe, they smashed the seats and lockers to extend the life of their beacon.

On board H.M.S. Newtown, men prepared the plan of rescue. With rising seas and darkness falling, it would be fatal to draw too near to the distressed boat. C.P.O. Broughton and six ratings left the destroyer to row the last two hundred yards. Their only guide through the rain and darkness was the failing light of the fire.

"I take it you're off the Mercury," shouted the chief petty officer, as the rescue boat drew alongside.

"No, sir," shouted back Steve, "M.S. Cannondore. The captain and two ratings on board."

"Hell's bells! How did you survive that lot? Anyway, jump across, we don't want to spend the night out here talking."

"You will have to take us in tow, sir. The captain has a broken back."

"Oh, bloody hell! It's hard enough going without towing your craft!"

"Take the lad to help you. I can manage to row to the ship without your help," yelled Steve.

Without further ado, a line was made fast, and slowly the three ship-wrecked survivors were towed toward the destroyer. Once alongside, C.P.O. Broughton stepped into their boat. Quickly, a bosun's chair was dropped from the 'Newtown's' deck.
"Jump in," snapped the C.P.O.
The boy hesitated.
"Off you go, David," said Steve.
Down came another chair.
"Get in," shouted the C.P.O. to Steve. His tone of voice made Steve feel like knocking his rescuer overboard. Swallowing back his feelings, he shouted back, "Not until the captain is safely aboard, and you'll need your surgeon down here to supervise that."
"I'm responsible for your rescue, sailor. I give the bloody orders."
"And I'm responsible for my captain's well-being," retorted Steve, "so get your medic down here."
Eventually, this being done, men gently lifted the captain of the 'Cannondore' onto the stretcher, surpervised by the medical officer, Doctor Hartly. Very slowly, he was raised to the deck of the 'Newtown'. Only Steve and C.P.O. Broughton remained. The rain and wind swept hard into their faces.
"I'll say this for you, sailor," shouted Broughton above the storm, "you have an obvious appreciation for your captain. I can hardly imagine anyone on this ship would show me the same respect."
"If you ever had the pleasure of meeting a man like him, I'm sure you'd do the same."
"Don't you be so cocksure. They are all the same if you like to be their lackeys. What's his name?"
"Captain Brown," said Steve, proudly.
"Brown! Good Gawd! All Browns are either captains or commanders. I must have been born with the wrong bloody name!"
Steve's temper was now at boiling point, "I don't know who the hell you are, but I do know you are a heartless bugger to insult a man you don't even know."
Down came the bosun's chair again. "Would you do me the honour of getting in that chair, and getting out of my bloody way," shouted Broughton.
Steve took hold of the seat, "It gives me the greatest pleasure to part company with you," said Steve sarcastically.
It was later that evening that Steve and David sat at a table in the commander's quarters. They were now dressed in the uniform of the Royal Navy, swathed in bandages, but clean, warm, well fed and reasonably happy. Also at the table sat Commander Brown, the medical officer, Dr Hartley, and a naval clerk.
"Now where the devil is Broughton?" the commander cried. He turned to the clerk. "Go and find that man. He should have been here fifteen minutes ago."
Looking at the surgeon, he continued, "That man's a pest, doc', you will have to do something about getting him off the bottle."
The commander turned to Steve and David, and welcomed them aboard.
"I will not delay you longer than necessary. I am well aware that you need sleep, but because your captain is unable to make a report, I must ask you

to give an account of the last thirty hours."
C.P.O. Broughton arrived with the clerk, and reported the cause of his delay, which the commander ignored.
Both David and Steve told their stories. C.P.O. Broughton gave a report of the resue, which had a notable bias against Steve. Dr Hartley stated that Captain Brown was in a deep coma and had severe injuries to the spine. Both his legs were broken, and his chances of survival were minimal. He congratulated David and Steve on the emergency first aid that they had carried out. Doubtless, without their help, Captain Brown would have died.
Commander Brown briefly summed up the evidence, while the clerk quickly wrote down the report.
"It would appear, gentlemen, that the charmed life of the 'Cannondore' came to an abrupt end while carrying out a mission of mercy. Whether there are any other survivors has yet to be discovered."
He confirmed the doctor's remarks on the conduct of Steve and David, and agreed that their remaining alive to tell the tale was little short of a miracle. Meanwhile, they would remain guests of the Royal Navy until reaching port.
"Now, I assume you wish to get away for some well-earned rest."
Both men rose to go. "May I have permission to speak, sir? I omitted to hand over this envelope with Captain Brown's clothing, sir. I realised it could be important when I undressed him on the boat, and retained it in my own security pocket. I apologise for my forgetfulness, sir."
"I am certain that, under the circumstances, you may be forgiven, Gibson," said the commander.
Steve placed an oilskin wallet on the table. The commander picked it up and studied it.
"Somehow, I think this could be a private matter, therefore, I will open it before you all."
He undid the seals. The contents were perfectly dry, and he laid them on the table.
"There is no official matter there, so I will replace them forthwith."
One folded paper remained, and the commander opened it out.
"That, gentlemen, is a water colour. It depicts what looks like a Thames barge, with its skipper and rather young mate sitting on deck. There is also a monogram in the left hand corner, N.E.B. I presume it must have a connection with Captain Brown's younger days."
Carefully, he folded the painting and looked up.
"That is all, gentlemen."
Steve, who had sat next to C.P.O. Broughton throughout the meeting, had been conscious of the man's total disdain of the proceedings. He now watched with amazement as the man's face suddenly turned white. He watched, as he dropped his head into his cupped hands, elbows resting on the table.
"What the devil is the matter with you, Broughton? You have been on that bottle again!"
Broughton lifted his head and faced his commander.
"No, sir. Would you permit me to look at the painting, sir?"
"I see no reason why I should, but if it will satify your curiosity, then please hurry up. We are all waiting to get our heads down."

He pushed the painting across the table towards his C.P.O.
Broughton sat, his head supported by his hands, his eyes fixed on the paper. All was silent.
The commander spoke sharply, "Well, come on man! What have you to say now?"
Broughton's hands covered his eyes. All attention was focussed on him. Very slowly, with a breaking voice, he spoke.
"Sir, my mother painted that picture. The skipper of the barge is my uncle, and the boy ... is Captain..."
His voice broke. Tears ran down his face onto the table.
"The boy is Captain Brown, my boyhood hero and friend. Tonight, sir, I have brought him to this ship, despised and insulted him."
The information stunned his listeners. For a short while, the silence was broken only by the sobbing of Broughton.
At last the commander spoke, "Well, all is not lost Broughton. We trust your schoolboy hero, now Captain Brown, will recover from his ordeal, then you will be able to apologise. Meanwhile, I suggest that you return to your cabin, compose yourself without the aid of spirits, and then offer a prayer to the Almighty on his behalf, and feel justified that you, at least, were called to take part in his rescue."
Broughton rose and asked permission to leave. Steve and David were led by the clerk to their sleeping quarters, where they soon slept like logs.
For C.P.O. Broughton, however, the night was quite different. The experience of the last few hours had stopped him dead in his tracks. It was twenty years since he had last seen Jimmie, and seventeen years since he had last spoken to his mother. Sixteen years had passed since he had last heard of Uncle Todd. Tonight, sailing in the Atlantic, the impossible had happened. He had actually helped rescue Jimmie Brown, that tearaway from the London slums. And he was carrying on his person the painting of the old 'Maywell', with his own mother's signature upon it, and he now lay on the verge of death, within a few feet of him. His own behaviour towards Jimmie and Steve had been despicable. Just how could he obey his commander's order, "Pray for him?" He had profaned the name of Christ since his late teens. How do you go back to a person after that?
His life was a complete failure. He had resolved, at the age of eighteen, that if Jimmie, a slum boy, could train as a sea captain, then he was of the material that makes a Navy admiral, but it all went sadly wrong. His early weakness for drinking and gambling had lost him his opportunity of Officers' Naval College and a commission. His present rank was only given him because of his years of service and the demands of war. In five years, he had squandered the money left to him by his mother; his marriage had been a complete failure; and his only son had been drowned at sea.
He had long decided that, as you couldn't make good from bad, he would content himself by being plain disagreeable to all he met. The sudden appearance of the simple painting in his mother's hand, and seeing the total admiration of Steve for the boy he had once idolised, devastated him. He paced his cabin: he tried sleeping; it was useless.
"More things are wrought by prayer than this world dreams of, William." It was as though his mother was there speaking to him. At last, in desperation,

he threw himself to the floor. "Oh God, I'm not worthy to ask you anything, but for the sake of my mother, who loved you to her dying day, and loved Jimmie as her very own, please give Jimmie his powers of reasoning, and restore him to health."

The mental strain had reduced the six-foot-three-inch giant to a helpless lamb.

He made his way to the galley for a large mug of tea, and spent the remainder of the night on the mess deck.

For the next two days, Steve and David took turns to sit by their captain, waiting anxiously for signs of him regaining consciousness. C.P.O. Broughton had already apologised to Steve, and was asking as much information concerning Jimmie as was possible to give. When off-duty he too would take his place by the bedside, talking to Jimmie in the hope that he might hear him, even if he could not answer.

It was on the third evening that David had the excitement of seeing Jimmie open his eyes. David stared, but said nothing.

"Aunt Nell, you're wonderful." The words were clear.

"I'm David," said the lad, but Jimmie just closed his eyes and was again silent.

The news was rushed to Doctor Hartley, Steve and C.P.O. Broughton. They waited another hour by the bed before they heard Jimmie's voice again. Vaguely, he recognised Steve and David, but just stared blankly at Broughton and the doctor. Whilst Broughton was inwardly disappointed, the M.O. expressed his delight.

"Tomorrow we should see an improvement, so let's go to bed and be thankful for small mercies."

The next morning, though, brought great disappointment. Jimmie had returned into a deep coma. He was running a high temperature and his heart was failing. Melancholy seemed to pervade the whole ship. Doctor Hartley discussed the situation with the commander.

"The only chance of extending Captain Brown's life is to get him to port, and hospital."

Commander Brown sought, and was given, permission to leave the convoy and make for the nearest port. It was estimated that they would make landfall in three hours. David conveyed the news given to him by Broughton to Steve, sitting by Jimmie.

"Three hours and we shall be in England." The excitement radiated from his whole being.

"David," came the cool answer from Steve, "have you never realised that since we joined this ship we have been travelling back towards America? For goodness sake, don't mention what you thought to any of the crew, or we shall be the laughing stock of the Royal Navy."

David blushed, "Thanks Steve. I don't know why, I just took it for granted we were sailing home."

"Don't worry, my boy, you are learning a tremendous lot in a short while."

Steve and David stood on the top deck. The feeling of a destroyer cutting its way through a choppy sea at thirty knots was somewhat in contrast to the 'Cannondore' plodding away at eight to twelve.

"If I was not so concerned for our captain, I could enjoy this. In my fifty years at sea, I have never covered the water so fast. I must admit it's exciting, but I've no intention of joining the Royal Navy at my time of life, but it does give you an insight into the life if you wish to change, David."

Chapter Seventeen

Hospital and Disappointment

It was early evening when H.M.S. Newtown drew alongside dock. Jimmie was transferred to an ambulance and whisked away, along with Dr Hartley, to a nearby hospital. Steve and David were taken to another hospital for treatment of their wounds. Throughout the night, american doctors and specialists examined and tested the mutilated body of Captain Brown for reactions. An eminent bone specialist was secured from New York. Late the next evening, Jimmie regained consciousness. The specialist sought to explain to him what they intended to do to promote his recovery.

"I am quite prepared to die, sir, but if you can prolong the day, by all means go ahead." His voice was very weak.

Next morning, a team of doctors and nurses carried out the delicate operation of realigning Jimmie's vertebrae. Finally, he was encased in a plaster cast, so that his hands and face remained the only visible parts. Two days later, Jimmie was still unconscious following the operation. Broughton, who had been granted shore leave, sat by the bed. In fact, he had waited patiently for about six hours, hoping and praying inwardly for a miracle to happen. In forty-eight hours, they would be sailing again to England. The opportunity to speak to Jimmie was all he wanted in the world. From the tomb of plaster, he saw the eyes open. They stared at the ceiling. Broughton rose and stood over the living effigy. The eyes of Jimmie now stared directly into his own. Broughton waited. His patience was rewarded.

"What are you doing here, William?"

The words were quite plain and, without hesitation, Broughton immediately bent down and kissed his hero's cheek.

"Jimmie, you know me," he cried and, unashamed of his tears, he left the small ward to fetch the medics.

Specialists and nurses surrounded the plaster cast containing the Englishman, Captain Jimmie Brown.

"How do you feel, sir?" was the first question asked.

"I think I have chilblains," was the low reply. "My toes itch."

"That is splendid news. Your operation has been a success. Time will see you back on your feet again," were the words of the medical team leader.

The following day, William spent as much time as the doctors would permit with Jimmie. Being told the circumstances, they had granted a special favour. Little by little, the two men exchanged information. Jimmie tried to thank William for rescuing him and he, in return, explained that Steve and David were worthy of the thanks, not him. Briefly, they agreed that, when the war was over, they would make a concerted effort to find out the demise of Skip, but meanwhile, William must return to duty, and Jimmie must return back to health.

The time for saying farewell was extremely emotional inwardly, but outwardly it was a credit to their ranks. On his return to ship, William realised that he had been unable to tell Jimmie of his own disastrous life. Even his reference to their different ranks had been over-ruled by Jimmie. "Real friendship outweighs rank. The feel of your hand is all I want, William."

Ten days later, the charge nurse announced that two men wanted to speak to Jimmie.

"Send them away, nurse, I'm tired of newsmen and officials begging information from me."

"They are far too important for me to do that, Captain Brown."

"I don't care if it's your President himself, tell him to talk to someone else," was Jimmie's quick reply.

"If that is your wish, I will do so, captain."

It was but a matter of minutes before Jimmie heard the rustle of screens and the shuffle of feet. He gazed in the mirror, high on the wall before him and adjusted so as to give him a view of what was going on around him. Standing smartly to attention, their hands in a seaman's salute, stood Steve and David.

"Look into the mirror there, then I can see your faces," were Jimmie's first words of greeting.

The shock of seeing their captain in his plaster cocoon, and the sound of his voice coming from it, stunned the two men.

"You may hold my hands, boys. They're the only part of me that's touchable. Seeing you two is the greatest surprise I have had since I came to realise that I was actually alive, and apparently I owe that to your ingenuity. Now, find a chair and sit down. Look in the mirror. It saves you craning your neck over the bed, and I can see you in comfort."

They placed a chair on either side of the bed.

"Before you sit down, I will make one request. I am not usually subject to this sort of impulse, but the situation in which we three are now placed demands it. Hold my hands, and let us remember we are the only survivors of the 'Cannondore'. I may be utterly wrong in thinking this, but I believe the Almighty must have some specific reason for extending our lives. May we use them for good, in memory of our shipmates and their families."

Jimmie gave a slight squeeze to their hands. It was all the strength he could muster, but it registered.

"I will say 'Amen' to that, captain," was Steve's firm reply. Doing his best to swallow back his emotion, David managed a quiet "Amen".

They stayed in silence for a few moments, then sat down. The art of talking via the mirror was soon acquired.

"To think that I told the charge nurse to send you away makes me shiver, but now we are all here, so let's catch up from where we suddenly parted company. I have already had newspaper reporters wanting to photograph me and get my story and, of course, representatives from the company have come to visit and grill me. I have told them all that I have little to say until I have met you."

In sessions of thirty minutes talking, and one hour resting, they passed the day. The next day, Steve and David would be joining another ship bound for England. After their hospital treatment, they had enjoyed a week as guests of a farmer in the rolling countryside of South Carolina.

This was now their last session with their captain, and farewells were imminent. Jimmie had thanked them for the part they had played under his command, and for their devotion to his personal needs at such a critical time.

"Now, David. If I remember correctly, we have something in common. We are both Wapping born and bred, and I am sure you are as proud of your place of birth as I am. It has made many a high-ranking officer raise his eyebrows during my lifetime, but it does not deter me.

"In the locker beside you are my few possessions; not many, I admit, but because of your honesty I still have them. In there, you will find a sailor's knife, one which I treasure. I want you to accept it as one Wapping boy to another, on the same condition as it was given me in 1879. Never sell it, or give it away until you have no further use for it. It was given to me by my grandfather, another Wapping boy, and he served with Nelson at the Battle of Trafalgar, as powder boy. My career at sea is finished. Yours has just begun. Take it with my blessing and heart-felt thanks."

Very quietly, David thanked his captain and made the same promise that Jimmie had made thirty-nine years previously. He turned his head away from the mirror to hide his tears.

"Steve, I realise that I owe my life to you and, if I am any judge of character, you would hardly be offended if I did not thank you. To you it would be devotion to duty. You will be returning to England tomorrow. I have already agreed with the company that your knowledge is far more useful to the war effort in the teaching of young intending seamen than working on a tramp steamer.

"You may object, Steve, but I say three times adrift on the ocean is enough for a man of your age. Enough is enough, Steve. Don't tempt Providence any more. In the little bag on the shelf, you will find a rather dirty looking ring, shaped from a cow's horn. That was also given to me when I was thirteen, by Rosie, a girl a little my senior, who helped nurse me through a difficult patch.

"Actually, I had been fighting three boys and came worse off. It was in a little village called Hullbridge, in Essex. I was afterwards taken to a farm called Eyotts, in Woodham Ferris, nearby. I had a soft spot for her but, when I returned a few years later, she was married. I felt she saved my life and now you too have saved it. Please take it, there's little else that I can give you that is important to me."

"Jimmie, if you will pardon my familiarity, I will accept it with the same sincerity as it is given, and I will humbly accept your recommendation for shore service."

The next morning, Jimmie asked the charge nurse how the two men were able to enter the ward, despite his instructions to her. She smiled, "Captain Brown, the elder of the two politely told me that it gave him great pleasure to countermand his captain's instructions, and that only a fatal heart attack would prevent him walking the last few paces to report to you."

"Thank you, nurse, it's men like him that make wars worth fighting."

With the return of William, Steve and David to duty, Jimmie was on his own in a far country. It took a few weeks before a letter was received from Emily. Even that brought bad news, for their youngest brother had been killed in France. It made a bad day for Jimmie. The ravages of war began biting into his soul. Here he lay, in his almost motionless state, while the world fell apart around him.

“A useless freak of humanity, that’s all I am,” he thought.

”Good afternoon, captain.”

Jimmie now recognised the voice so well that he knew just what would be said next. ”Ah, yes, I detect a slight improvement. Give it another week. Be patient, captain, we will have you back in England before long!”

For Jimmie, eight weeks lying looking at the ceiling was not getting him back to England in record time.

“Ah, yes. Tomorrow we shall have you outof your plaster, captain, but don’t get too excited, we shall be giving you a new case, but you will have more freedom of movement.”

“Thank God for small mercies, my Aunt Nell would say, doctor, but in the mood I am today I want the largest slice of the cake.”

“Captain Brown, you are an extremely good patient, and I can assure you that your patience will be rewarded. I am certain we can excuse you a day off-colour, now and again. I understand you have had bad news this morning.”

“Yes, doctor, I’m afraid so. My youngest brother.”

“I too have received notice this morning, but for me it’s my eldest brother. So we can commiserate with each other.”

The new plaster cast gave Jimmie freedom for his legs, movement of his arms from the shoulders, and a slight freedom of the hed. To him, it was like a new lease of life after the tortuos coffin he had endured for two months.

Chapter Eighteen

An Unexpected Guest

It was late July before Jimmie had any visitors of consequence. By now, he was able to be elevated to a postion whereby he did not have to rely on the mirror. He could now read and write with a modicum of comfort. He had received one letter from William, two from Steve and three from David. Emily's letter came regularly each week.

The sudden tidying of the bed clothes by a young nurse raised Jimmie's suspicions.

"And who have we visiting today? Another film star? Or a general?"

"I don't really know, sir. Sister just said to make you look presentable."

"In that case, you had better whitewash my plaster. I spilt my coffee on it this morning," laughed Jimmie.

The sister walked in, followed by a tall Naval officer.

"Commander Brown to see you, captain." She turned and left.

Both men extended their arms and shook hands. Their greetings and compliments over, the commander took a chair and made himself comfortable beside Jimmie. "Captain Brown ..."

Jimmie intervened. "I apologise for interrupting, sir, but I would consider it an honour if you call me Jimmie."

"In that case, let us be even. I am Thomas. I will now start again. I am very sorry, Jimmie, but I am the bearer of bad news. C.P.O. Broughton (William to you) was killed on duty four weeks after we left you here."

The commander gave Jimmie time to take in the sad news. He watched as he cupped his hands over his face as though in prayer.

At last, Jimmie spoke. "The destiny of man is a secret known only to his Creator. Were it otherwise, I feel we would be the most miserable of the species."

"That is a very serious observation, Jimmie, and I value your opinion. I would like to add, on this occasion, that happy is the man who is prepared to meet his destiny."

"Do you believe William was prepared, Thomas? I felt he was a very troubled man, although I do accept that I was not in a fit state to judge."

"My visit today, Jimmie, is a two-fold one. I now know sufficient about you to have a great respect and admiration for you. I also consider it a privilege to sit and talk to you. I could have written and explained what happened to William, but the information that I wished to pass on required more than a letter. Your last question confirms that I was wise in my decision."

There was a pause. "Please carry on, Thomas. I feel you have something important to tell me."

"About two days before he was killed, William asked if he could speak to me in private. I knew little about the man, having only taken command of the 'Newtown' just prior to the sinking of the 'Cannondore'. He was no doubt a disgruntled and often inebriated man, but what was obvious during the period between you coming on board, and his death, was the radical change in his way of life. He told me how he was the son of a Methodist minister, and that his mother could only be described as a saint."

"I would confirm that description," said Jimmie.

"He confessed that he had completely disregarded all the ethics of his upbringing, with the result that he lost his chance of a commission, and was also reduced in the ranks. His failings being drink and gambling.

"On the night he came to your rescue, he resented me for giving him, as he called it, such a menial task. His attitude to your surviving crew, and likewise to yourself, was despicable. Steve Gibson's devotion to you, and his duty, angered him immensely, and he totally disdained the short inquiry I held that evening. So you see, Jimmie, he was a troubled man.

"Then, as he carried on talking to me about himself, he apologised for breaking down when he discovered the identity of the man he had rescued, and on seeing his mother's signature on the painting. He said that, after my advice that he should go and pray for your recovery, he had spent a night of conviction and confusion and finally, in desperation, he had cried to God on your behalf. While he told me considerably more than I have conveyed to you, his main requests were that, if the fortunes of war went against him, would I convey to you his great admiration of you as a boy, and also as a man.

"He deeply regretted having spurned the love and teaching of his parents, and his greatest wish was that you may be granted a full return to health and strength. He also hoped that you would be successful in the discovery of what happened to Uncle Todd. His last request was, I feel, for both of us. "Sir," he said, "many would say that the meeting of Jimmie in the Atlantic was Fate, or sheer coincidence. Were it not for the deep conviction of my mother's presence throughout that night, I would agree with them, but on deep reflection I now give the benefit of the doubt to Providence, and I have since sought to reform my ways." I must admit, Jimmie, it did seem uncanny to me that within forty-eight hours I would be required to carry out his requests. I confess that I quickly recorded his story in the event of a similar accident myself."

"I must thank you, Thomas, for giving me this information. William and I were great pals together, totally unalike, from such different backgrounds, yet we had a grand time during our teens. I realised he grieved his mother, but not to the extent that you have told me. It comes as a consolation to know that he came to revere his mother and her instructions in his last few weeks. Please, would you now tell me what happened to cause his death."

"Yes, Jimmie. I intended to leave that 'till last. We were making our way towards Portsmouth. It was early morning, and a wet mist hung heavy over us. With limited vision, we surprised two Jerry torpedo boats. One we almost rammed, but the other circled and let go a tin fish, which by-passed us at a safe distance. William's gun crew slammed the ship out of the water, but the ship we almost rammed let go with its own machine guns, as it raced away into the mist. William was the only casualty. He died within seconds."

The news being given, the two men enjoyed a good meal together, speculated on the possibilities of an end to the war, and then made their farewells.

"I look forward to the day when we can meet in England under more favourable conditions," were Commander Brown's last words.

Chapter Nineteen

Welcome Home

So the weeks and months passed by. Little by litte, Jimmie was able to extend his activities. Still in plaster, he was at last able to be helped into a wheelchair and be taken around the hospital grounds. The hope of ever being able to walk again hardly ever entered his mind. He frequently tried to plan his future. Writing was not his forte, and coming to grief on an ammunition ship hardly constituted the grounds for a spectacular story. Undoubtedly, he would finish up smoking his pipe, reading a book and trundling his wheelchair into the park to be pitied by the passers-by. When in that frame of mind, he wished he had gone the same way as McClean and the rest of his crew. That he should be an encumbrance to other people bothered him considerably. November 11th, 1918, found him with mixed feelings. While he wanted to laugh and rejoice, he also wanted to cry. Other than Emily, there was little, if any, reason for him to return to England. Fortunately, the hospital staff lifted him from his doldrums. As the only Englishman in the hospital, he was to take part in a concert. He could name his own act, and after great thought Jimmie announced that if they provided the music he would do the Sailor's Hornpipe.

This request brought confusion to the staff. On no account must he dare ruin six months nursing. Even the specialist was brought to convince him of that, but Jimmie remained adamant.

"Have no fear, doctor. In no way will I destroy the good work you have carried out. Come and enjoy the fun."

The victory celebrations continued all day. That night, sitting in his chair behind a table draped by a Union Jack, Jimmie performed his act. The band played the Sailor's Hornpipe, very slowly at first, and with his hands in a pair of boots, a sailor's cap on his head, he tapped the dance out on the table. Gradually he increased the tempo, and had his audience and fellow patients dancing and clapping around the floor. That evening, he was again their hero.

Easter 1919 came, and with it the news that Jimmie would be returning to England. He could now manage a few steps with the aid of crutches, though he still had to wear a staightjacket. His departure from America was not only a great occasion for the sea captain, but the hospital staff as well. For some twelve months he had graced their wards, his cheerful stories never ceased to amuse them, and rarely did he grumble or criticise.

The staff presented him with a beautiful silver watch, inscribed 'For you, 12 months pain – for us, 12 months admiration. God bless you, Jimmie'.

Even the boy who brought the newspapers round the ward each morning put his arms around Jimmie's neck and hugged him.

"Do you have to go back to England, sir? You can come and live with us."

"I would love to live with you, Robert, but I have a lonely sister in England, waiting for me."

"In that case, sir, I guess you had better return", he said, and ran from the ward crying.
As Jimmie was piped aboard the ship that was to take him home, the band played 'Will ye noo come back again?' Sitting proudly in his wheelchair, Jimmie waved his goodbyes.
His trip back to England was sheer luxury. Even the seas behaved kindly. Sitting in his chair on the deck, enjoying the sun, he revelled at the sight of the vast ocean. He spent many hours with Captain Weeks on the bridge, and it gave him a feeling of satisfaction to look down on the deck and watch men working. He was able to imagine that they were working under his command, though knowing full well his career had come to an end.
The arrival at Southampton was an extremely emotional one. Led by Captain Weeks, men carried Jimmie carefully in his wheelchair for the last few yards from the ship onto the soil of England. Emily was the first to greet him, followed by representatives of the shipping line, and local dignitaries.
An ambulance took Jimmie to the shipping line's reception hall, where a formal dinner and receiving party awaited him. As the doors swung open, Commander Brown stepped forward to welcome him, closely followed by Dr. Hartley. After informal greetings and drinks, Jimmie was wheeled to his place at the centre of the dining table. To one side of him sat Emily, and on the other, Commander Brown. The guests each took their respective seats but three seat opposite Jimmie remained vacant. The chairman of the line welcomed the guests of the day and then said that it was his great pleasure to announce the two men who had made the occasion possible.
"Would you please stand and welcome Leading Seaman Steve Gibson and Able Seaman David Carter".
Both senior and junior seamen marched proudly to their seats, to loud applause. With outstretched hands, they were greeted by Jimmie, and then took their places behind their chairs. Once again, the chairman called the guests to their feet.
"Before we partake of our welcome home banquet, I pray your silence as we remember the crew of the 'Cannondore', of whom thirty souls lost their lives, and C.P.O. Broughton, better known to some of you as William, who lost his life in action on H.M.S. Newtown. From the rear of the hall, two men, one a naval rating, the other an able seaman, carried a large anchor shaped wreath of flowers and placed it in the one vacant chair.
They then stepped back, stood smartly to attention and saluted. Clearly, the chairman's voice broke the silence.
"Ladies and gentlemen. We will remember them."
The words were repeated around the table. "We will remember them".
At the end of the delicious meal and several speeches, Jimmie was asked if he would care to add a few words to the occasion. He raised his hand.
"Mr. Chairman, ladies and gentlemen. Forgive me for not standing, but to do so would be my greatest pleasure. Not all surprises are pleasant, but those I have been given today have been truly delightful. That a man who loses his ship, and almost his whole crew, should receive a hero's welcome bewilders me. Throughour the war, I have read of the heroism of men and women, in and out of uniform, which makes me feel that my contribution to the war effort is insignificant.

"To say I am delighted to meet Commander Brown and Doctor Hartley again would be an understatement, after the effort they went to in order to secure a place in an American hospital for me; to meet again my dear sister Emily has a special significance of its own; but the meeting again of Steve and David is something beyond my powers of explanation. I have no intention of embarrasing them before you, but I just wish to say publicly, Steve and David, I thank you. You have served your King and Country faithfully, and were a credit to your captain and crew."

The remark brought red faces to the two men and a loud response from the guests.

"Once more, I thank the shipping line for the welcome they have given me and, in fact, all who have made this a great occasion. And that, Mr. Chairman, concludes my speech."

Later that night, Jimmie, tired but in good spirits, was taken to an officers' recuperation hospital near Watford, where he was to stay for another two years.

It was 1921 before he eventually returned home to Enfield to live with Emily. He was fifty-four, and his recovery, although slow, was almost complete. He accepted the fact that he would have to wear a spinal corset to prevent further injury to his spine, and that he must restrain himself in the art of walking and working.

PART THREE Chapter Twenty

Jimmie Retraces his Steps

By grim determination Jimmie mastered the art of walking again. Day by day, he walked the streets and parks, and gradually increased the distance. At times, Emily was concerned by his physical state on return.

"Why must you walk so far, man? There is no compulsion to do it."

"I agree with you, Emily, but Jimmie has promised himself that, by next summer, he will be able to walk five miles and still be fresh, and I don't like breaking promises, even to myself."

By May 1922, he had accomplished his target, not once, but quite a few times. Local men and boys would often accompany him, the men to share the friendship and the boys to listen to the stories he would tell, plus the coppers they would receive for finishing the course.

It was now early June: the weather was fair, and Jimmie's intuition told him it would remain so for the next few days.

"I shall be taking a few days in the Essex countryside," said Jimmie to Emily, as they ate their supper.

"When?"

"Tomorrow."

"Why?"

"Because the weather is favourable, and I wish to find out what happened to Skip."

"So that is why you have been pushing yourself these last twelve months."

"You could say that, Emily, but on the other hand, I have enjoyed doing it, and I certainly feel fit. Tomorrow, I shall take the train to Burnham and spend a day or so there, then call at Woodham Ferris and Hullbridge. I would like to have a last look around the area, and pay homage to Skip. It is nearly twenty-five years since I was last there. One wonders how much it will have changed."

At ten o'clock the next morning, Jimmie arrived at Liverpool Street from Enfield Town and, with a ticket for Burnham-on-Crouch in his pocket, stood on platform sixteen, awaiting his train.

A cheery porter spoke to him, "Did you say you were going to Woodham Ferris, sir?"

"Yes," replied Jimmie.

"Then you must be a very brave man, because they tell me they still fight and stalk their food with bows and arrows there!"

"Have no fear, my good man, the natives will accept me."

"Would you be a missionary, sir?"

"Not quite! I'm on my way to sell them my latest self-returning arrow!"

Both men laughed, and the porter realised he had met his match for wit. The train came in, and he closed the carriage door for Jimmie.

"Good hunting, sir."

"Thank you," shouted Jimmie, as the train moved away, "I hope to catch my prey."

The train left town and rushed through the countryside, stopping now and then for breath at the various stations. Jimmie amused himself by trying to estimate the number of milk churns spread around the platforms. There could be hundreds, more likely thousands, if fully totalled up. That was one thing that had not changed: he had carried out the same exercise when he used the line in the nineties.

"Wickford, this is where I change." He picked up his Gladstone bag, and stepped carefully onto the platform.

"I'm afraid yew have just missed the connection to Burnham, sir," said the porter, "Yew have to wait another hour for the next. Yew have time to look around the market, if yew wish."

"That's a clever trick," laughed Jimmie, "I suppose your wife has a stall there?"

"Yes, sir, the second on the right. She sells home-made jam."

"I'm sure it's very good jam," said Jimmie, "but under the circumstances, and it being a hot morning, I will sit here, eat my sandwiches, and watch the world go by."

From his seat overlooking the market below, he watched the milling crowd of villagers, heard the sound of lowing cows, bleating sheep, and the squark of the pigs, as the drovers prodded them with their sticks into the pens. Added to that, the constant cluck and cackle of chicken and geese created a truly rural symphony. Trying to make their voices heard above the commotion, were the market vendors and the auctioneers. Somewhere in the back of Jimmie's mind was a feeling of satisfaction. The scene he was looking at was a part of the British heritage, something which men will fight to preserve.

"Do you mind if I sit next to you, sir?" The speaker placed two large wicker baskets onto the seat beside Jimmie, then sat himself down and wiped his brow with a red spotted handkerchief.

"I'm just about knackered, if you will pardon the expression, by this heat," said the elderly man. "Some fourteen hundred eggs have I carried in those baskets this morning. That's nearly a hundred-weight-and-a-quarter. Not bad for a man of sixty."

"If you will pardon the expression, I think it's bloody marvellous. I would be pleased to carry a quarter of that weight," replied Jimmie.

Some thirty minutes later, the two men boarded the local train. Soon, every carriage was full of women, children and baskets. With a blast of the whistle, and a snorting of steam, the little engine left the station as though it had only two minutes to get to Burnham, some fifteen miles away.

"It's certainly full steam ahead on this line," said Jimmie.

"Do not be carried away, sir. It may be necessary to get out and push before we reach the top of the hill!"

As the stoker frantically refuelled the engine, black smoke enveloped the carriages. At any moment, it felt as though the engine would capitulate.

"What happens if we don't make it?" asked Jimmie of the egg man.

"We run back and have another go," was the cheerful reply.

However, the hill finally surmounted, the engine chuffed with glee and raced its way to its next objective, Battlesbridge. This was, for Jimmie, his first view of the River Crouch for twenty-five years. He could just detect

the masts of three barges laying in the mud alongside the mills. He was so engrossed in his thoughts that he was hardly aware that the train had stopped and re-started again from the little station. Within minutes, the engine was racing down the long gentle slope towards Woodham Ferris. Jimmie's eyes scanned the surrounding fields and the river banks.
"It's still there," he said, accidentally speaking aloud.
"What's still there?" enquired the egg man.
"Eyott's Farm."
"Well, I suppose it is. They tell me they have been farming that site for nearly a thousand years, so I would not expect any sudden change now."
Jimmie nodded his head in agreement. The sight of the blooming thrift on the fenland aroused his attention.
"Good, I have planned it just right," he said quietly to himself.
"Woodham Ferris, change for Stow Maries, Cold Norton, Barrons Lane and Maldon," shouted the porter. Jimmie helped the egg man out with his baskets and wished him farewell.
Saltcotes Farm, the brickfields and the Red Hills which Skip used to get so excited about, were the next things for him to look out for. To his surprise, the farm was still there, although in a somewhat dilapidated state. The Red Hills remained the same, as though time had no meaning for them. The brickfield cottages were also there, the workings and signs of past industry were obvious, but there was little evidence of actual activity now.

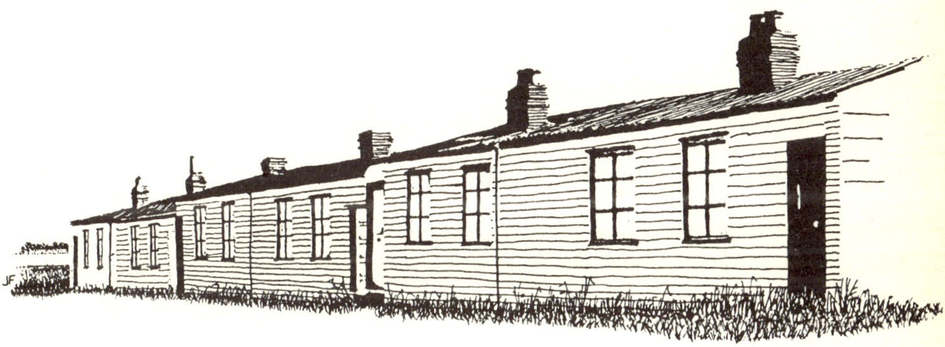

BRICKFIELD COTTAGES

"Another enterprise gone to waste," thought Jimmie to himself.
His arrival at Burnham, soon after one o'clock, was uneventful. He left the station, and was offered a lift by a man with a pony and trap, who then refused any gratuity when he dismounted at the 'Star' pub, on the quayside. Something to eat and drink was Jimmie's first requirement, and after being duly nourished, he booked a room for the night, had a wash, and set out for a tour of the town and shipyards. Before making any real enquiries, he wanted to just look and reminisce.
The cottage, where he had spent his first night in Burnham, looked much the same, perhaps not quite as trim as Aunt Nell had kept it, but for Jimmie, the sight of the little dormer window in the roof was nostalgic. His walk along the quayside raised the question, 'Where are all the barges?' There

were certainly less than he had been accustomed to, and there were definitely more pleasure boats.

His arrival in King's boatyard gave him his first contact. Working on a mast, was a shipwright he recognised.

"Good afternoon, Walter. I am pleased to see you have not forsaken your craft."

The man, well into his sixties, looked up. "How do you know my name, sir?" He stared hard at Jimmie. "Somehow, I think I should know you, but when you get to my age, you're apt to forget, sir."

"If you stop calling me 'sir', and just call me Jimmie, it may come back to you."

The old man scratched his head again.

"You're Todd Summers' boy." He took Jimmie's hand. "Forgive me, sir, for not recognising you."

"I'll not forgive you if you insist on calling me 'sir'."

"But you are a captain, sir, and I must address you accordingly."

"To blazes with the captain bit! Jimmie is what my mother called me, and Jimmie I wish to be called by people I know."

"I presume you wish to see Mr King, but he'll not be back till six or seven."

"Yes, I would, Walter. Meanwhile, what do you know about Todd Summers?"

Walter sat down on the mast and invited Jimmie to do the same. "It was all a bit of a mystery. I would prefer Mr King to tell you, he seems to be the only person who knows the real facts, and he always covers up when the subject is raised, although, I reckon it is twenty years since I last heard his name mentioned."

"Not to worry, Walter. How many men can you round up who knew Todd and me twenty-five years ago?"

"There not be many, perhaps a dozen or so."

"Right, then, can I rely on you to arrange that they meet me at the 'Star' by eight o'clock? Tell them the evening's at my expense, and be certain that Mr King is with you."

"That will be done, Jimmie."

"Thank you. I will now leave you to your work, and enjoy a further walk along the front."

By eight-thirty, some ten men had re-made their acquaintance with Jimmie. Despite his protests, 'captain' was their favourite way of addressing him. Mr King arrived last. He extended his hand.

"I'm very pleased to meet you, Captain Brown."

Jimmie shook his hand. "I give up. Why all this captain stuff?"

Tom dropped the rank, "Jimmie, you must realise that we can read. If you get yourself plastered over the front page of the daily papers, what else can you expect? We have a great admiration for you, the cockney boy who played hell with my tradesmen, commanding a thundering great vessel loaded with T.N.T. across the Atlantic. That does not go unnoticed."

By closing time, every man had had his fill, not only of beer, but of sandwiches and pies, of which the supply seemed never-ending.

They exchanged stories, and sang 'For He's a Jolly Good Fellow'. Then, they made their way home, or back to their boats, in great spirits. Only Tom King remained.

"I understand you want to talk business with me, Jimmie."

"Yes, Tom. Would you like to come up to my room and we can talk in comfort."

Upstairs, they sat down in the quiet room. "It would appear that Old Walter had warned my guests not to refer to the demise of Todd Summers," said Jimmie.

"Yes, I feel he did. I was hoping that no one would stir up mud tonight. They did that out of respect to you. As you are well aware, Todd was a most secretive person, although I always had great respect for him. I think he talked to me more than anyone else in this town."

"I do know he had the same respect for you," said Jimmie. "A mystery man he certainly was. I lived and worked with him for twenty-four hours a day, for seventeen years, and learnt very little of his past, other than that he must have come from good stock, and was well travelled. But what you do not know is that, after Aunt Nell, his sister, died, I lost all contact with him. That was in 1901. I did meet up with William, Nell's boy, who told me that his uncle had retired from bargeing, but he had no idea where he had gone. It is those last years that I wish to find out about."

"You surprise me, Jimmie, with that information. I always considered that you and William were his contacts. We all knew around here that William was somewhat of a tearaway, and I could understand Todd writing him off, but to cut himself off from you astounds me. After his sister died, which Todd took very badly, he became an almost aggresive man. I know he and Paddy would argue over the slightest thing. Then came the tragedy of the 'Maywell'. Did you know about that, Jimmie?"

"Whatever you tell me about events after Nell's death will be news, so please carry on."

"Well, she capsized in a freak storm, just off the Naze, during June 1901. Paddy was drowned and his body never found. Todd was picked up on some wreckage later. As you know, Paddy was at heart really devoted to Todd, although he mixed with the roughest of men. It was from them that the rumours abounded, but from my last dealing with Todd, I concluded it was just an accident, and nothing more could be read into it.

"When Todd returned to the cottage, he was a broken man. He shut himself in and would only speak to old Mrs Wilson. He then sent for me, and instructed me to convert an old fishing smack, so that it would be comfortable to live in. I was to tell the men that it was for a London businessman, for weekends up the Thames.

"We completed the job in record time. Then, for a few nights, I helped him load his goods and chattels on board. He told me that the cottage and remaining contents would be sold by an agent, who would also settle up with me for the trouble he had caused. I asked him where he intended to go. His reply was, "I know a very nice berth around Canvey Island, Tom, where I can spend my last few days in comfort and peace. That is all I require of this life." It was late in September, 1901, that we shook hands, and I watched him by the light of the moon, sail the old smack on the last of the tide, down to the estuary. I had a sneaking feeling that his destination was much further afield. He had talked quite a lot about Holland during our last contacts. Other than that, Jimmie, I know no more, except that he paid me about three times the money he owed me."

"Aha! Holland. I have no doubts, Tom, your suspicions were correct. "Walkshun." I know the exact spot. When we were sailing that coast, I was a lad of thirteen, fourteen, or so, and whenever we sailed up that channel, he would say, "That is where I will retire to Paddy." It was absolutely no-man's land, and Paddy would always say, "Build a half-dozen pubs, and I will stay with you Todd!" The crafty old man! Why should he tell you Canvey?

"I am very indebted to you, Tom, for this information. I intend to spend the day at Woodham Ferris tomorrow, before returning to Enfield. Then I shall make arrangements to visit Holland."

It was very late when Tom left Jimmie's room. They shook hands.

"Before I leave, Jimmie, please do not build up your hopes too high. I well remember, in fact it haunted me for weeks, that by the time Todd would have arrived at the open sea, a deep depression had settled over the area, and we had three days of wind and storm, but I never heard of any wreckage being found."

"Thank you, Tom. I have got the message. It must have caused you great concern, but I am certain he would have been happy to go that way."

It was ten o'clock the next day, when Jimmie stepped onto Woodham Ferris station, and it was a pleasant fresh morning that welcomed him, as he crossed the footbridge. He paused awhile, to watch the activity in the goods yard. It was thirty-three years since he had last stood on the same spot, admiring the transformation of the area, with Skip. The Railway Hotel would be open, so a quick refresher before he set out on his planned tour would be beneficial, he thought.

The only occupants of the bar were two men. One had a smiling red face, and a fine set of white teeth. The other was dour and looking despondent. Jimmie placed his glass on the table and sat himself down. On the floor stood two wicker baskets, with cloths covering their contents, although from the aroma, Jimmie had no difficulty in deciding that one of the men hawked fish.

"Yew be a stranger to these parts, sir," said the red-faced man.

"Not exactly," replied Jimmie.

"Well, yew wer'n't aroond here afore me, so I count yew as a stranger."

"I question that assumption," replied Jimmie.

The two locals looked at each other and nodded.

"Bet yew a pint we were aroond here afore yew, sir."

"That's on," was Jimmie's quick reply, "but you will tell me first when you arrived in Woodham."

"1893, with my father, when they started work on them there brickfields. Now beat that!"

"1879. Eyott's Farm," grinned Jimmie.

"Oh, hell! That's afore I were born. There, it were worth a try. Can I sell you some kippers, sir. Fourpence a pair, I caught them fresh in the Crouch this morning!"

"No thanks, I don't fancy walking around Woodham today with kippers in my bag, but let me have the pleasure of filling your glasses."

The landlord laughed as he refilled them, "You may be good at catching kippers, George, but not so good at catching out our guest."

Jimmie bid the fishmonger, and his partner, farewell and made his way over the level crossing and headed for Hullbridge.

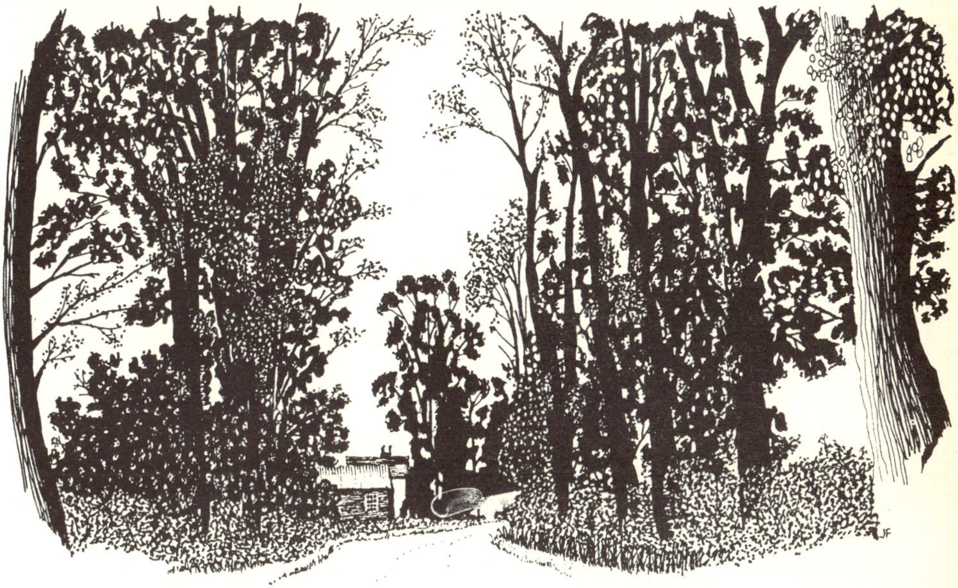

HULLBRIDGE ROAD NEAR THE CONGREGATIONAL CHURCH

Though still a country lane, bordered by large elm trees and deep ditches, houses of all shapes and sizes had been built. Large poultry farms had been established and spread out over the adjoining fields. On his left, he passed a Congregational chapel, built of corrugated iron and painted red. A little further on, a Church of England mission, complete with belfry, again built with corrugated iron cladding. "At least the settlement has good intentions," thought Jimmie to himself.

He paused awhile at the old cottage, 'Tazzi Mazzi'. The old forge looked closed up and disused. Further on, to the right, quite a modern shop graced the area. F.W.DEAVIN - GROCERS AND CONFECTIONERS was the signboard displayed above. He stepped inside and treated himself to a large bar of chocolate, served by a pleasant young lady.

The lane now crossed the low marshland. To his surprise, bungalows and houses were now bordering the lane, but what appeared more conspicuous to him was the fact that, although it was summer, there was a lack of leaves on the trees and hedges. Many looked dead.

His query was answered by a man filling ruts in the road with flint stones, and who soon introduced himself as Charlie Cundy, the local roadman.

"That, sir, is the result of the river busting its banks over there."

He pointed with his shovel to the Fenn creek almost half-a-mile away.

"Came across they fields like a roaring lion, sir. There were three feet of water through our houses before you could say "Jack Johnson". We all take a chance, living on the low land, and the sea has a nasty habit of

reminding yew, noo and again, how far it can goo when it wants to."
Jimmie sympathised with the roadman over the circumstance in which they had to live.
"I trust they have made a good repair of the breach, so that you can live again in comfort."
"We shall jus have to keep our fingers crossed and hope for the best," was his reply.
Within fifteen minutes, Jimmie was sitting on the sea wall, viewing Hullbridge. The tide was flowing fast. Three barges were moored: two at the Hullbridge jetties, and one unloading stones on the Woodham hard. Other than the row of boarded cottages missing on the Hullbridge side, all looked the same. Because he wanted to walk around the Fenn Creek to Eyotts Farm, Jimmie abandoned the idea of calling the ferryman. Hullbridge, after all, had a 'hoo-doo' on him. He re-kindled his pipe, and set off again along the sea wall. The grass was long, and progress was slow; the rising tide rushed up the creek, as though it were urging him on towards his goal. Within the hour, he had reached the repaired breach in the part of the wall responsible for the flooding of the lower part of the village.
He was hungry and thirsty. It was one-thirty by his watch, and in another hour, he estimated, it would be high tide. From his Gladstone bag, he removed the sandwiches prepared by the landlady of the 'Star Inn' that morning, made himself comfortable on the grass, and enjoyed his picnic lunch. A small bottle of beer completed the meal.
A slight poke in the ribs brought him suddenly to his senses. He looked up. A tall man, wearing a battered straw hat, knee breeches and gaiters, and with a stick in his hand, stood towering over him. A large collie dog sniffed at Jimmie's boots.
"I am very sorry to have to disturb you, sir, but you have been here rather a long time, and I began to fear the worst."
Jimmie drew his watch from his pocket. Four-fifteen.
"Good heavens! I've been asleep for nearly two hours."
"I happened to see you arrive when I was working in the top field, this morning. I assumed that you were an inspector, dealing with the cost of repairing the wall. Seeing you laying there, nearly three hours later, had me concerned. Perhaps I should introduce myself. My name is Steve Donaghue. I live at Eyotts Farm: the building you can see in the curve of the creek."
Jimmie scrambled to his feet. "Well, I am very pleased to meet you, and grateful for your concern as to my well-being. I am Jimmie Brown, from Enfield, and you may be interested to know that it was my intention to call at the farm when I had partaken of some light refreshmen, but sleep obviously overtook me."
"In that case, Mr. Brown, let me have the pleasure of escorting you to the farm. I am sure that my sister can provide a cup of tea, or something stronger, if you so desire."
Within ten minutes, Jimmie was sitting under the verandah of Eyotts overlooking the river, and enjoying the scene that he knew so well. Each was interested in the other's story of what had happened to the farm in the last thirty years.

"I now have seven acres of poultry; the rest of the estate has been sold off as plot land. People arrive here, building little asbestos huts for weekend homes. I'm afraid it will not be as you remember it, Mr. Brown.
They talked until nearly six o'clock, then Jimmie made his farewells, thanked them for their hospitality, and told them that he would stay the night at the 'Whalebone', if he could get a room.
"It will not be the 'Whalebone' you knew in your day, sir. That was burned down in the 1890s."
"I am sure that if it had not burned down, it would have fallen down by now," replied Jimmie.
"Just keep to the track, sir. You will not find that any different. You are not likely to see anybody, unless it's old Nobby Clark, the railway guard. He lives in an old boat, near the bridge."
"I can hardly imagine one could get a boat that far," said Jimmie.
"It's not on the water, Mr. Brown, it's on the land, surrounded by a tall hedge. He is generally known as the 'Hermit of the Fenns'. He is more likely to see you, than you him, and if you get into conversation, he can only talk about his life on the railway. If you want to see the 'White Lady of the Fenns', then you will have to visit after midnight. Locals reckon that she's his wife, come to haunt him."
The walk along the track, the sight of waving thrift, and the song of the skylark overhead, all had a peculiar effect on Jimmie. It was as though Skip was walking beside him. "Why should boyhood memories linger with such reality?" he asked himself.
He was not interested in the asbestos shacks built alongside the first part of the track, the sight of peewits and seabirds scavenging in the mud creeks and fens was sufficient for him.
He pushed open the gate, and walked onto the old wooden bridge. At a glance, he could see that it had been repaired, again and again, but to him it was the same Old Wooden Bridge. He rested his arms on the guard rails. Below, in the water and on the stones, large green crabs were fighting. It was all as he remembered as a boy of thirteen. The only thing missing was Skip. At least, if it was possible to find his old mate in Holland, he would be able to refresh the old man's mind of the scene they both enjoyed.

Chapter Twenty-one

The Hermit of Woodham Fenns

Jimmie looked at his watch. "I must press on."

He picked up the Gladstone bag, hooked it onto his walking stick, and threw it over his shoulder. He opened and passed through the second gate, then turned, and took one last glance along the creek to Eyotts Farm. He had a strange feeling inside himself that he did not want to leave the bridge. "How the devil did I pass that clump of bushes where the old 'Hermit of the Fens' lives? I don't recall seeing it," he mused.

He hesitated. "I don't know why I should bother. My mother always said, curiosity killed the cat. At least I could ask him the time of the last train to Liverpool Street."

He re-crossed the bridge. It was but two hundred feet or so to the hedgerow. Like a little boy, scrumping apples, Jimmie parted the bushes, and peered into the Hermit's domain. Sure enough, there was the boat, supported by a timber gantry. On a wooden bench alongside, lay the Hermit, apparently asleep. Jimmie placed his bag on the ground, and walked along to where there was a gap in the hedge, opposite the sleeping Hermit.

Now he could study the old man properly. He lay outstretched, his head resting on a stuffed sack. His railway guard's uniform looked worn and faded, his peaked hat shielded the evening sun from his eyes, and his long white beard lay spread across his chest. He looked so peaceful, it would almost be sacrilege to disturb him, thought Jimmie, but at least I can now say, with authority, that I have seen the 'Hermit of Woodham Fens'.

He turned away from the lonely figure to head towards the 'Whalebone Inn', but a slight sneeze from the recumbent form made Jimmie turn again. It did not seem to wake the old guard, but Jimmie saw the old man's hand drop casually to the ground from underneath his beard. What he saw caused him to freeze to the spot. There was only one hand in all the world like that, but what he was thinking was absolutely impossible. Surely Donaghue's home-made wine must be having a bizarre effect on him. But still he stood, his eyes transfixed on the guard's hand resting on the ground beside the bench.

"There must be scores of men with their hands shot off during the war," he thought to himself.

Jimmie coughed. Perhaps it would arouse the guard. But it had no effect. "If I shout, it could give him a heart attack." Was it possible that the old man was feigning sleep? There was one acid test that would satisfy his curiosity. He took a few steps and stood behind the hedge. Then, in an ordinary pitched voice, said, "Ahoy there, Skip!"

He waited with a tense feeling of excitement, not quite certain of what to expect. He watched the old man turn on the bench, and then sit up. He raised his feeble arms towards the sky, as though expecting something to descend from heaven.

Jimmie trembled. "Oh God, what am I looking at?" He felt a cold sweat running down his face. He could see but an apparition of his former employer: the result of his drinking too much of Donaghue's wine, and his own vivid imagination. He cursed himself for encroaching on the old man's privacy, so he turned, and once again made his way towards the wooden bridge, in total confusion.

"Jimmie ... Where are you, Jimmie?"

The feeble cry stopped Jimmie in his tracks. Even his heart stopped beating. Then it began to pound away again. Instinctively, he walked back to the gap in the hedge, and then, in a faltering voice, said, "I'm here, Skip, standing in front of you."

The old man stood up, glared at Jimmie, then with outstretched arms, he tottered forward.

"I knew you would come, I knew you would come, Jimmie," he cried, as both men's arms locked together.

Jimmie could feel Skip's body shaking like a leaf, as he sobbed like a little boy. The only words that he could decipher were, "Jimmie, my boy. Jimmie, my boy."

Suddenly, Skip's body went limp and slowly sank to the ground, out of Jimmie's grasp. At once, Jimmie dropped down beside him and put into practice his First Aid knowledge. Within a few minutes, Skip regained consciousness. Carefully, he was helped to his feet and guided to the bench, where Jimmie sat beside him and sought to help him overcome the shock.

Skip grasped Jimmie's hands. "How did you find me? Who told you that I was here?"

His voice was weak, but it betrayed his excitement.

"That is a long story, Skip. Can we just say, for the moment, that we are together again? If you feel strong enough, I have a small flask of your favourite rum. Perhaps we could celebrate the occasion."

"That is very thoughtful of you, Jimmie," said Skip. Then, pointing with his hand, "Go through that door into the galley, and you will find two mugs hanging in front of you."

Jimmie walked to the door and stepped inside. To his great surprise, everything was clean and tidy. Skip was still the perfectionist that he had known as a boy.

Slowly, they drank to each other's health and their meeting together again.

"There is one thing you have forgotten, my boy. I may be old and doddery, but my memory is still good. If I am not mistaken, it's your birthday, the thirteenth of June."

"That could be so, Skip. I have been so busy in my pursuits that the event has been completely overlooked. This means that it is forty-four years since we first met."

"It may be forty-four years since then, but waiting for you to return has seemed like an eternity to me."

Suddenly, Jimmie stood up.

"You are not going already," said Skip.

"No, I've just realised that I have left my bag along the hedge."

"Don't worry. You could leave it there for a fortnight, and no-one would touch it."

"There are some ham sandwiches in it. I am sure we could enjoy them."
"In that case, I will make a pot of tea," said Skip.
It was eight o'clock when Jimmie presented his quickly formed plan to his old shipmate. He took hold of the old man's hand.
"Skip, I am not running away. I shall be sleeping at the 'Whalebone' tonight. I will be back here with you between eight and nine in the morning, and spend the day with you. Don't prepare anything in the way of food, I will bring it with me. Today has been a strenuous day, even for a youngster like me. May I suggest that you have an early night. I can tell that you have not yet recovered from the shock, so take a stiff drink, and sleep well."
"On one condition, Jimmie: I shall escort you to the bridge."
"Granted, Skip."
They said goodbye, and Skip watched Jimmie walk the track and cross the railway line before he returned to his boat.
In the 'Whalebone', Jimmie was taken up to his room.
"I need nothing other than to sleep, ma'am. I have had a very busy day, but I shall look forward to breakfast in the morning."
Sleep did not come that easily. It was not only the excitement of being re-united with his old ship-mate and benefactor. There was also the stark realisation that, having come so close to his discovery, he had actually been in the process of walking away, to leave Skip to die of a broken heart. Then, he would have searched the waterways of Holland, or maybe the marshlands of Canvey Island, in vain.
He mulled the circumstances over, again and again, in his mind. His final conclusion was that, however illogical it seemed, the 'White Lady' (or was it Aunt Nell) had been the unseen influence that had prevented him from leaving the treasure undiscovered.
Finally, from sheer exhaustion, he fell asleep.

Chapter Twenty-two

Skip's Story

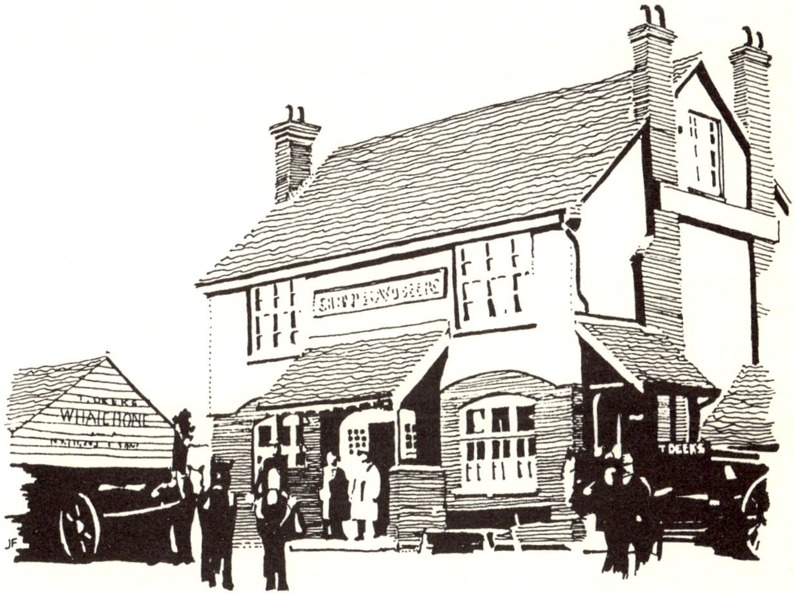

THE NEW "WHALEBONE" WICKFORD ROAD

The clatter of horses' hooves on the gravel outside the inn woke Jimmie. It was six-thirty, and he had slept solidly from about midnight.

At seven, the landlady rapped on the door.

"Come in."

"Your tea and hot water, sir."

She placed the tea on a small table, and left the jug of hot water on the washing stand.

"If you can wait 'till eight o'clock for your breakfast, all the hustle and bustle will be over, sir."

"Very good, ma'am. I will rise, wash and take a short walk before breakfasting."

Breakfast gave Jimmie time to talk to Mrs Deeks. He explained that he would be spending the day with an old friend on the fens.

"Not Nobby Clarke, sir?"

The name seemed strange to him, but he intended to go along with it.

"Yes, ma'am, we have known each other for many years. How do you find him?"

"Well, I know they have nicknamed him the 'Hermit of the Fenn', but to me he has always appeared a reserved and respectable man. He comes in once a fortnight, buys his matches, his tobacco, his bottle of rum, and wishes us a good day. He never drinks in the bar, but is always polite. That, I would say, is all anyone knows about him in Woodham, other than his wide

knowledge of the railways."
"Yes, Mrs Deeks. Now I wish to ask you a favour. Could you prepare me something in the way of a cold meal for around one o'clock. I shall be going over to see him in a few minutes. I could return and collect it at any time you say."
"I will be pleased to do that for you, Mr Brown, but you have no need to return. I will send the lad who does the garden and odd jobs with it."
Jimmie arrived at Skip's enclosure just after nine. To his surprise, he found Skip dressed in dark blue serge trousers, a seaman's pullover and his old bargeman's bowler.
"Ahoy there, Jimmie," he shouted, as he made his way through the gap in the hedge. "I can see that I have surprised you."
"Ahoy there, Skip. But not as much as you did in that gash uniform yesterday."
"I do change as befits the occasion, my boy. Now, let me first escort you around my estate, Jimmie."
The area was some sixty by three hundred feet, surrounded by a tall hawthorn hedge. Inside, was a variety of fruit trees, a kitchen garden, a few chickens and a nanny goat.
"As you can see, I am self-sufficient here. Rabbits abound for meat and the water box is just ouside my patch."
He then showed Jimmie his boat. The main body made a cosy living room, and for'ard was the sleeping quarters. A short corridor had been built from the stern to a small shed, which Skip called the galley. Despite external appearances, the inside was all clean and tidy.
Once more Skip led Jimmie outside. "I have prepared a place where we can talk in comfort. It will be a warm day, so I have put the awning up for shade, and I am sure you will enjoy the comfort of my self-designed sailcloth chairs."
They both sat down, filled their pipes, and were silent for a while. Each was wary not to start off on the wrong slant. After their initial greetings the day before, they had avoided direct questions.
"Right, Jimmie. It's got to be done, so would you care to fill me in on your last twenty years?"
For an hour or more, Jimmie explained his progress and experiences in the southern hemisphere, including his foolishness and disappointment in his short-lived marriage in Australia. He told of his days as second-in-command on troopships and last as captain of 'M.S. Cannondore'.
He gave a brief account of his meeting with William, and how his old pal had died. Then he spoke of his visit to Woodham for old time's sake. He purposely left out their lack of correspondence, and his previous day at Burnham, until he heard Skip's story.
Skip sat up in his chair and removed his pipe.
"First, may I congratulate you on your appointment. It would have given great satisfaction to those who have now passed on to know that their hopes and plans had been fulfilled in you, Captain Brown.
"I consider your report somewhat conservative. I am certain, knowing you as I did, it was far more exciting and dangerous than you have cared to tell, but I hope to extract a little more from you, in due course. But for the present, we will indulge in a mug of coffee and some buttered scones, which I purchased from Davidson's, our local store, earlier this morning."

They ate and drank, then re-fuelled their pipes. Jimmie laid back in the comfort of the deck-cum-easy chair.
"Now, Skip, I think you owe me a few years' explanation."
The old man thought for a little while. "Not a few, Jimmie, but many. I have always been guilty of denying you the knowledge of the part you have unknowingly played in my life. You accepted me in a way I could never have believed possible, and fulfilled your role completely. I am totally indebted to you, and am now obliged to tell you the truth about Todd Summers. I am sure that you will fit yourself into the story, as I go along."
Skip laid back in his chair and rested his feet on a small wooden stool, then closed his eyes.
"First, Jimmie, I have to confess that, throughout my life, I have been a failure because of selfwill and obstinacy. But I have dearly paid the price.
"I was born in a little village in Oxfordshire, in 1844. I grieved my parents by arriving prematurely, while they were visiting friends. The honourable thing was to be born on your own estate, so I began life on the wrong foot, in fact, I must have been an embarrassment to them till their dying day.
"My father was a government official, and was appointed to a position in India. At the tender age of six months, with Nell, my older sister, we sailed to Calcutta. That was in 1844. I enjoyed my boyhood days with Nell in the luxury of the legation. As I grew older, I began to realise the injustices of mankind to his fellow man. While we enjoyed every comfort, and received the highest of education, the natives who cleaned our shoes and did our every chore, received but a pittance in return.
"When I reached the age of eighteen, my father decided to send me back to England, to be prepared for Cambridge, but I rebelled against my parents' wishes, and the society in which I lived. I left the safety of the legation, without giving any indication of my whereabouts or intentions, and joined a tea cutter to Australia, as a galley boy. It was extremely hard work, but I enjoyed it.
"I stayed aboard that ship, under a false name, for over twelve months. Because of my education, the skipper had me on deck, as he considered I was wasting my life in the galley. When the excitement of my new way of life began to wear off, I began to regret my conduct and treatment of my parents. It was in December, 1863, that we sailed into Calcutta. I told the skipper that I would be leaving ship and would rejoin him, if he so wished, on a later trip. I returned to the British legation with fear and repentance, only to be told of the death of my parents, and that Nell had returned to England. It appeared that, because of the shock of my disappearance, my mother failed in health; that my father took her to the hill country for a holiday to recuperate; and while there, they were both killed in the crossfire of tribal riots.
"It was the first real bombshell of my life, and not to be the last. No one was able to convince me that I was not responsible for my parents' death. I have carried that conviction throughout my life. My only consolation was that Nell was safe in England. Other than short holidays, of four months or so, when I was seven and fourteen, I had never had any experience of living in my homeland. Now, I could not get back to England quick enough. Nell was two years my senior, and had taken a teaching position in a village near

Oxford. She was all I had, as far as family was concerned. We shared the loss of our parents, and the joy of being reunited, as only those who pass through similar circumstances can fully understand."

"My parents' estate had been more or less settled before I arrived back in England. Nell and I went to the solicitors in London for the final details. The outcome was that we were reasonably well provided for, but my share of the money was held in trust until I was twenty-one years old."

"I spent three months with Nell, trying to decide my future. She wanted me to apply for Oxford, to finish my education, but the lure of the sea had already gripped me. I applied, and was accepted by a Hull shipping company, for training as a junior navigation officer. I promised faithfully that I would write frequently, and return to Oxford on every shore leave. I joined ship, and sailed once more for Australia. Despite the constant feeling of remoteness, I enjoyed my life at sea."

"It was in February, 'sixty-five. We were racing north for Hull, off the Suffolk coast, when we ran into a north-westerly which stripped us of rigging and masts. We were swamped by high seas and sank within minutes. There were but six of us who escaped, rescued by the crew of a fishing smack, making its way through the storm to Yarmouth. A scotsman named McKinnon, one of the crew, took me to his home for the night. It was there I met Moira."

Jimmie suddenly became doubly alert. It was the first time he had heard Skip refer to a woman intimately, other than Aunt Nell.

"Whether it was the Scottish lilt in her voice, or the infectious smile she gave as we met, I could not really say, but it was love at first sight. Four days later, I returned to Hull and severed my contract with the shipping company."

"I returned to Yarmouth, and was accepted into the McKinnon's home. Both Moira and her mother worked in the fish market. For two months, I spent the life of an independent man, going out on the fishing smacks, often with Moira's father. Within three months, Moira said she would marry me and, to my surprise, her father consented. I was to learn later that he had an ulterior motive."

"I returned to Nell for a few days. She thought, at first, I was marrying below my station, but agreed later that if it would make me happy and stop me racing around the world, she would give her blessing."

"It was after the wedding that her father made the proposition. He knew a man, lower down the coast, at a place called Maldon, in Essex, on the River Blackwater. He had a cottage and a fishing smack for sale and was wanting to return to Scotland. Could I help him raise the money? We could then be in business together, he said. Mac was a good fisherman, sometimes foolish, but I agreed. I arranged for the purchase of the boat and cottage. Within two months all their belongings were loaded onto a barge and we sailed down to Maldon."

"For the next twelve months, Moira and I were on top of the world. I got on reasonably well with her father, and he taught me a lot about the sea and fishing, but it was not long before I became suspicious. He was jealous of me. Moira's mother absolutely adored me, and I sensed the danger. By early 'sixty-six, we were expecting our firstborn. Our joy knew no bounds. On the twelfth of June that year, Mac and I sailed down the Blackwater to spend a night's fishing off the Buxey Sands."

"It was about seven o'clock when the 'Beatrice', heading for the Crouch, hoved to, to tell us that Moira was in labour. I shouted to Mac to pull in the nets. His reply was sharp and cutting, "I make the decisions. I give the orders on what we will do, young man. I'm not losing a night's fishing because of you two. Women can have bairns without our help. If you want to go, jump on the 'Beatrice'. She's bound for Burnham. You can make your way across land. You'll be there before midnight."

"Without hesitation, I jumped. That short trip to Burnham was my first experience of sailing on a Thames barge. The skipper made certain it would be a lasting memory. Every yard of sail lay open to the wind. The 'Beatrice' rushed up the Crouch, like a coach and four."

"I told the skipper not to take unnecessary risks, but he whacked me on the back, saying, "Don't you worry my boy. After hearing the remarks of your ungrateful father-in-law, I am in the mood to do anything. If the wind had been favourable, I would have sailed straight back to Maldon."

"When we brought up at Burnham, I was to see, for the first time, the townscape that I was to see so many times: a picture of the place that was to have such a great part to play in my life. The skipper insisted I shared a drink at the 'Star' before I set off overland, and got one of the locals to give me precise details of the way I should take."

Chapter Twenty-three

Dark Days

"The evening was hot and sultry, and darkness was beginning to fall, as I made my way along the lane leading away from Burnham. My instructions were to take the first turning to the left, and head for Latchingdon, then right, to Mundon. I enjoyed the first half-hour. The expectation of being a father spurred me on, but the distant flashing of lightning began to cause me concern. Heavy clouds soon blotted out the light of the moon. The storm broke overhead, and I was lost in darkness and drenched with rain. I plodded on, the crunch of gravel underfoot being my only guide as to what was the road."

"The sound of a trotting horse raised my hopes. I stood aside as a pony and trap drew level. Someone shouted, and told me to jump in and get under the small tarpaulin. I asked my host how he could see where he was going, under the cover. "I can't, but the horse knows the way," he replied. He was good company and raised my dampened spirits. He had obviously been drinking heavily. His answer to my question, about why the road was so twisted, was that his forbears, when building the roads, always worked with their backs to the wind, and never cut down an oak tree in case of bad luck!"

"The storm had passed and the moon now shone brightly. "This is where we part company, sir. You have only two or three miles to go. I turn left, you take the right, through Mundon. I wish you all you wish yourself and thank you for your company."

"No, sir, it is I who should thank you," I replied, and set off again happily, having shared my host's whisky. I would soon cover three miles, and be with Moira. I did hesitate on the way, whether to turn slightly left, or follow what appeared to be the main track straight ahead. The sight of a farmhouse looming in front of me made me realise I had made the wrong decision.

"I turned to retrace my steps, but the sound of feet pacing the gravel, and the snorting of a beast made me turn again to face the commotion. Was it a bull, or a herd of cows? I had no time to decide. The beast sprang upon me. I plunged my fist full in the attacker's face. The weight of its body thrown against me made me stagger backwards. A hot, boiling pain seethed through my body as its teeth engulfed my hand. I screamed in agony, then kicked with all my might into its lower parts.

"The beast gasped, dropped to the ground, taking half my hand with it. From a window close by a gun fired. I heard the pellets riccochet on the farm buildings.

"Stay where you are, or the dogs will get you." I cringe, even today, at such an ironic statement. As I stood, blood pouring from my hand, I could hear the beast slobbering and groaning before me. In moments, two men arrived, carrying guns, and yet another dog.

"Put your hands up and walk to the door!"

"Father, the man's wounded. How can you be so cruel?"

"Shut up! You can't take chances," was the curt reply. I stumbled into the doorway. A woman holding a lamp stood nearby. She screamed as I collapsed to the floor. They dosed me up with brandy, and wrapped my hand in bandages. I explained, the best I could, what had happened and where I was going. They were, I think, genuinely sorry. Thieves had been rustling their sheep, and they were taking precautions. The two great mastiff dogs saw to that."

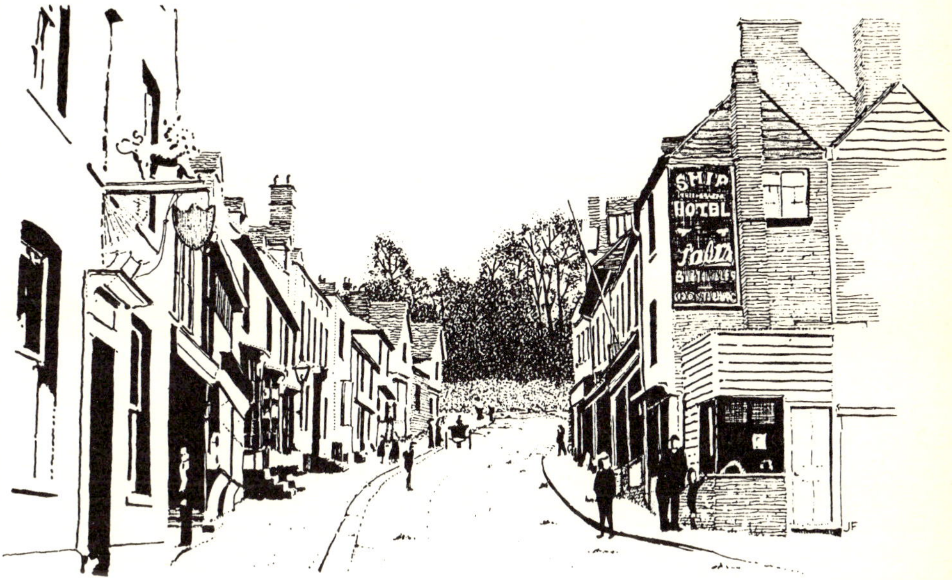

MARKET HILL, MALDON

"My last two miles or so to Maldon were again by pony and trap. The farmer's son driving. He left me outside the cottage, apologised again, and wished me well."

"I made my way indoors. It was two in the morning. Moira's mother greeted me, only to receive a shock on seeing the state I was in. I talked the mishap down, and asked to see Moira. The bloody mess was covered with a clean towel, and I went upstairs holding my hand behind my back."

"Moira looked awful, but raised a slight smile for me. Our meeting was but a few moments, for the midwife asked if I would go and fetch the doctor, because the situation was serious. I took a swig from a whisky bottle, and made my way up the High Street, and rattled on the doctor's front door."

"I'll be with you in a few seconds," was the reply from an upstairs window. With a lamp in one hand, and his bag in the other, we raced down the High Street, but loss of blood and weakness had overtaken me.

"Come, my lad. You should not let an old man out-pace you." I tried to explain my predicament.

"I'm sorry, Mr Summers, I will have to attend to you after I have delivered the baby." I thanked him, and explained that I was not seeking help for myself.

"The next hour was agony for me, both physically and mentally. I was given the task of maintaining the fire and providing a constant supply of hot water. The screams from Moira upstairs, and the torture of my wounds, drove me again and again to the bottle."

"As day dawned, I heard another cry. My heart leapt within me and my pain momentarily went, but it was another half-hour or more before I was permitted to enter the bedroom. I was then given but a glimpse of the child, a boy. I was able to smile at Moira and congratulate her with a kiss, and was then ushered downstairs out of the way.

"I sat with my head resting on my good arm, spread out across the table, happy but stupified with spirits, and with my other hand racked with pain. It was the doctor's voice that aroused me. "Now, young man, I will deal with you."

"He unravelled the towel and bandages from my hand. I cringed in the process. I heard him say, "Good God!", then he went and brought the midwife. He gave me laudanum to drink, to kill the pain. The midwife eventually laid across my arm, and the doctor, on the other side of the table, hacked and cut away the smashed bones and flesh."

Jimmie watched closely as Skip related the event. It was obvious that the old man must have re-lived those moments, many times, throughout the years.

"It was nine-thirty before I came to. I awoke to find myself lying on the sofa, my arm strapped to my shoulder. The room was clean and tidy again. The lady from next door provided me with a breakfast and sought to comfort me.

"At around eleven o'clock, I was in a fit condition to visit Moira. I sat down beside the bed. Her mother placed the little bairn on my good arm and left the room. Moira looked very weak, and from her weary smile I realised that all was not well. Holding the wee mite was a tremendous thrill for me, and Moira knew my feelings. We had never finally decided on a name for our firstborn. Moira laid her hand on the baby lying on my arm. I was aware that she did not appreciate that my other arm was out of use.

"What shall we call him?" I said.

"Let's call him Jamie, after my grandfather." Her voice was very quiet.

"Yes, darling, you will call him Jamie, but I will call him Jimmie." She raised a little laugh.

"You Sassenach! But promise me you will make a sea captain of him, on one of those large liners."

"Yes, dear. I promise you, I will train him, and we will be proud of him." She squeezed my arm gently and fell asleep. I sat silently watching her, and then Jamie. A great new future rose up before me. It was but temporary.

"Within the hour, I was racing around Maldon, trying to find Doctor Harris. Moira was worse, and Jamie was having difficulty breathing. I sat in suspense, awaiting the doctor's diagnosis. At last he came down and stood beside me. I dare not look up. His hand was on my shoulder, "Young man, life has dealt you a viscious blow. It grieves me to tell you, but the baby can live only an hour or two, and your wife may not even survive him. I only pray that, somewhere in that young life of yours, strength may be given for you to rise above the ordeal."

"Within the hour, a minister came into the house. Moira's mother insisted the circumstances demanded it. By this time, Mac had returned, and we stood around the crib and bed, Moira's mother and father, the midwife, the minister and myself. What he said, or did, I was oblivious to. My mother-in-law told me that Jamie died while he was praying, and that Moira died soon after."

For a while the old man neither opened his eyes nor spoke. The only noise that could be heard was the singing of the birds and the buzzing of the bees. Jimmie sat stunned by the revelation of how and where he began to fit into the story.

"Yew be Mr Brown?"

The voice startled them both. A lad of around sixteen years had found his way to where they were sitting.

"It all be round t'other side, sir. Mrs Deeks said to eat it before it gets cow'd. I'll collect the box abowt four," he said, and was away.

What had arrived came as a great surprise: a W.D. Haybox. Jimmie dragged it into the galley, and there spread the contents onto the table. There was roast pork and potatoes, green peas, Yorkshsire pudding, a can of thick brown gravy and, for sweet, a large gooseberry pie with custard. They sat, one on each side of the white boarded table.

"It's the first time I've seen a spread like this since before Nell passed away," said Skip, "I'm very grateful to you, Jimmie."

"Don't thank me, Skip, thank Mrs Deeks. I only asked for ham sandwiches, and this is what we receive."

Both men looked at their plates, piled high, like children at a birthday party waiting for the word 'go'.

Skip looked shyly at Jimmie, "What would Nell say now."

"God forbid that we should ever be so proud or ungrateful, Skip. Let us do the honours together."

"For what we are about to receive, Lord, make us truly grateful. Amen."

Jimmie noticed that Skip secretly wiped a tear from his eye before enjoying the spread. They ate their meal, and shared a bottle of beer. While Jimmie washed the pots, Skip had twenty minutes nap.

They took again to their seats under the shade of the awning.

"It's your turn to talk, Jimmie."

"Not so, Skip. I realized that it was extremely sad and emotional for you this morning, but please continue your story."

"If you insist, but there are parts of the story of which I am thoroughly ashamed."

"Moira and the babe were buried together the following week. After that, I lost myself along the sea walls. I watched the tide flow in. I watched the tide recede, to be absorbed in the mighty ocean. I would sit for hours, just thinking that mankind was like the tides. Youth flows on, gently at first, then, like a mighty rushing wave, man seeks to inundate all within or beyond his reach. Then, some mysterious power says, "No further", and he retreats to an ocean of obscurity.

"A week later, I was confined to bed, driven mad with my hand which had turned septic. I was prepared, and waited to die. Tetanus had taken over.

Nell travelled from Oxford, and she and my mother-in-law nursed me to health again. Six weeks or more later, Nell returned to her school, and I promised that I would return as soon as I could settle the business of boat and cottage. For a week, I went out on the boat with Mac, but I realised that I was of little help, and our relationship was far from mutual. The crunch came one morning, at breakfast. I had spent a sleepless night. I still suffered great pain from my hand. Mac had spent a fruitless night fishing, and the meal was taken in complete silence. I rose, turned to Mac and his wife, and said, "I have decided to sell the boat and cottage."

"I was prevented from finishing what I had to say. Mac got up from the table, and stood in front of me in an agressive mood. "You ungrateful sod! I saved your life, you killed my daughter, and now you will sell our house and my livelihood over my head."

"Wait, Mac, wait. Let me finish," I shouted. His wife tried to intervene, but he was raving mad.

"You are useless, an outcast of your own society who thinks that money can buy you just what you want. You've had all you wanted from Moira ..." He never finished. A red light flashed in my brain, and I hit him with all the power I could muster. He crashed to the floor, his head striking the table on the way down. But for me too, the pain was excruciating. I had used my right hand, and undone two months of Nature's healing.

"Mac at last rose from the floor, blood pouring from his head and mouth. "I'll give you four hours to leave Maldon. If you have not gone, I am determined to kill you."

"He left the room, accompanied by his wife. The lady from next door came to attend to me. My few possessions, mainly books brought home from India, were transferred to her house. I told her I would contact her in due course. I apologised to Moira's mother, and explained that, because of Mac's impetuosity, it would be necessary for me to reconsider the generous offer I had intended to make, but that for the meanwhile they could live in the cottage in peace, and Mac could fish to his heart's content. She put her arms around me, and kissed me."

"Please understand that nothing Mac said is true, I know you leave with a broken heart. I will always love you, as I loved Moira. Go, and God bless you."

"That afternoon, my hand heavily bandaged and strapped again to my shoulder, and a bag of food in my other hand, I trudged my way through a little village called Tiptree, on my way to Colchester. I slept the night in a haystack, and arrived in the town the following morning. I sought a doctor to dress my hand, then fixed up some lodgings. I had to share a room with an Irishman about my own age. "A very quiet man," said the landlady. It was Paddy. We had nothing in common, other than an interest in boats. He quickly made it plain to me that, provided I did not probe into his life, he would not probe into mine. The agreement suited me admirably. During the following days I was very grateful to him. Although I realised he was a tough, hard man, he certainly cared for me.

Chapter Twenty-four

A New Way of Life.

"It was, perhaps, a month later when Paddy came to me one morning. "Will you not help me to buy a boat, Todd?" I looked at him, surprised. "Sure, though I say's to meself, it's a lovely ship and it would serve us grand."

"You say us, Paddy. What would I be on a ship with a hand like this?"

"Goddam man! Nelson fought the French with one arm and one eye. I'll soon have you managing a bloody barge!" We walked down to the Hythe, to where it was berthed. I was somewhat disappointed; it was not exactly my idea of a fine ship. She lay there, in the mud, feeling sorry for herself. Paddy saw my dismay.

"Good heavens, man! I'll have her looking as though she has just left the stocks, in no time. Think of it. We can be independent, have a home of our own. If we haven't done sufficient freights in three years, you can lash me to the anchor and drop me in the North Sea."

"He raised my hopes. Somehow, I trusted him. He meant what he said. We shook, left-handed, on the quayside.

"I returned to Oxford, leaving Paddy to prepare the barge, while I arranged the payment. I arrived in time to be present at Nell's wedding. I stayed but a couple of weeks in the city. Although Nell seemed disappointed by my plans for the future, she wished me well. "Please keep in touch. The fact that I have married does not mean that we do not need each other," she said.

"Once more, back at Colchester, I soon saw that Paddy had achieved

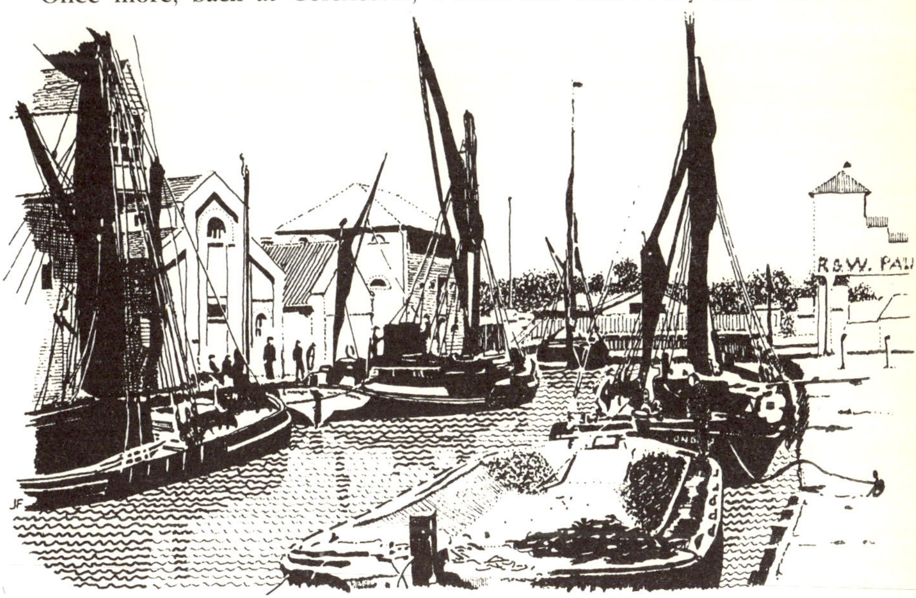

THE HYTHE, COLCHESTER

wonders. My solicitors had settled plans for payment, and the 'Linton' was formally handed over, eighty per cent mine and twenty per cent Paddy's. We decided to re-name her. It was more through Paddy's wit than any serious intention.
"It may well be the answer to our problems," he said, as we ate our breakfast in the lodgings for the last time. We both laughed! "'Maywell' it shall be," and that is what it remained.
"There was no doubt about it, Paddy was a born seaman, and a wizard with the sail. While I was getting my bearings, he had secured our first freight. The 'Linton' was built around 1860, perhaps not a true Thames barge, but qualified to do the same work. Within the next few years, I was to learn just what could be achieved with an eighty-foot craft, sailing into almost impossible berths, in and around the East Coast waterways.
"I also quickly learned that, while Paddy excelled in seamanship, he was hopeless where business and money were concerned. Whatever money we shared he drank away, and at last he asked me to keep control of the cash, to give him sufficient for baccy and a reasonable amount for beer, and to keep in safe custody whatever was due to him from trading.
"It was but a month or two before I had news from my solicitors that Mac and his wife had vacated the cottage at Maldon, and returned to Scotland, taking the boat with them. I was advised to take action against Mac, but I told them to sell the cottage and forget the boat.
"During the next eight years, we shipped everything from glass bottles to sheep. We sailed from Lincolnshire to the Isle of Wight. Although I was still a disillusioned man, the new way of life suited me.
"Paddy had made his home in the foc's'le, and I in the aft quarters. As far as the bargeing fraternity were concerned, we were considered oddities, although Paddy covered up for my rather reserved nature.
"During the middle-seventies, we were frozen in berth above the Pool. I took the opportunity to visit Nell in Oxford. Young William was somewhere around seven or eight years old. It was then I learned of her husband's failing health. Tuberculosis had got its grip. I felt extremely sorry for them. Richard, Nell's husband, was such a delightful man. I suggested they move to the East Coast, where the sea air might be beneficial to him, and I would be closer to hand.
"Nell, realising the outcome, decided on the move, and that is how we finished up at the 'Plovers', Burnham. The move took place in the Spring but, sad to say, Richard died in the Autumn. From then onwards, Burnham became our home port. Even Paddy had a permanent room with a family nearby, when ashore.
"During the late-seventies, the 'Maywell' began to show signs of her age, and we then condescended to ship horse dung, hay and straw. While we could not carry the large hay cargoes, like the 'Stakies', we could still make a living. It also enabled us to spend a little more time in Burnham. For me, it was to share in Nell's loneliness. I am not so sure about Paddy, although he was always ready to go ashore when the 'Maywell' brought up. Early one morning, during the summer of 1879, Paddy came into the galley. I had just prepared breakfast.
"Todd, we must have a serious talk. Last night, I lay in bed thinking, which

often happens when I'm unable to have my quota of beer. The good Mother told me that it was about time I returned to the Emerald Isles, and put right my wrongs. I may not be sure, but I felt she was giving us a word of warning, because if we sail this crate many more times up and down the Swin, it will drop to the bottom and leave us, like the Blessed Lord and Saint Peter, standing on the water, and I don't think I would have the faith to walk ashore, though I can't vouch for you."

"I take your point, Paddy. The warning must not be ignored. I cannot swim, and my faith would not keep me bouyant for more than five seconds."

"We made our plans. Paddy would return home for three or four months. The 'Maywell' would go into dock for a complete overhaul, and I would have a long, well-earned rest, and notify Paddy when we were ready to sail again. I contacted Tom King, and made the necessary arrangements. We decided to fit two more freights into Sutton's quay. On the first trip, I went to my solicitors and made arrangements for Paddy to be able to draw cash from a local bank during his stay in Ireland. That afternoon I paid him ten pounds. He wanted to rig himself up with new clothes. It was the first time we ever really quarrelled.

"You old skinflint," he called me, "after twelve years is that all I'm worth?"

"No, Paddy, you are worth a hell of a lot more."

"Then I want it," he yelled.

"You can have it when you get to Ireland, and not before."

"You don't trust me, after all these years, Todd, I'm ashamed of you."

"I do trust you, Paddy, but not with money. Prove to me how you are able to spend the ten pounds."

"It was some while later, he stormed off the ship. It must have been around midnight when I was disturbed by shouting, asking which was the 'Maywell'. I went on deck. Two policemen, dragging a body like a sack of coal, asked if I had a Paddy on board.

"Not at the moment," I shouted.

"Then take this one." They threw him by the arms and legs onto the piled dung. I asked that they help me to get him below.

"Leave him there for the night, skipper. That's all he's fit for."

"I turned his face away from the dung, and left him to sober up. While he snored away, I lay awake. A strange depression had come over me. At first light, I heard footsteps on deck. Paddy had come to. A short while afterwards, I heard them again. I put my head above deck, to see Paddy making his way from the 'Maywell', a bundle on his back. He had left me.

"I lay on my bunk feeling responsible. Unable to sleep, I took down the log book. I had not filled it in for about a week. I would now record Paddy's departure. As I made up the days, I then realised that Paddy had left me on Friday, 13th June. I knew now why I was depressed. The 13th June, 1866, somehow my life revolved around that date. Thirteen years had gone by, thirteen years of utter waste. I had a feeling of emptiness, and my stomach ached within me.

"Had Fate treated me better, I would now have Moira and Jimmie, a fine boy of thirteen, and who knows, a lovely daughter as well. But I had nothing, only misery. I wrote a letter to Nell, telling her that, by the time she received it, the 'Maywell' would be burned out, and I would be on my way back to

India. I would keep in touch, and wished her and William future happiness. From sheer exhaustion, I fell asleep."

Chapter Twenty-five

The Secret Unfolds

"The knock on the door annoyed me. Why should Charlie, the dung-loader, want me so early? I grunted for him to enter. I opened my eyes and was taken by surprise. One of the dockside urchins had dared to enter my cabin."

Jimmie felt like butting in. This was where he entered the story, but then he realised it would be prudent to let Skip tell the story in his own way.

"They were the curse of the docks. I know many were waifs and strays, hungry and homeless. They lived by begging and stealing, but this one had entered my sanctuary. I yelled at him. He was prepared for a getaway, but then, for reasons unknown, I demanded him to stay put."

The old man opened his eyes and looked straight at Jimmie.

"You may not believe what I am about to tell you. You can call it fantasy, if you like. I leave it for you to decide, but in those few moments, I had a vision. I have always belittled anyone who made such claims, but for me, this was absolutely real. I saw the boy, scruffy-looking and with tattered clothes, trembling like a leaf. Beside him stood a tall man, dressed in officer's uniform, his peaked cap held firmly in his raised hand. I saw Moira, radiant and smiling, looking me straight in the eyes, and in her charming Scottish lilt she said, "Todd, you promised me you were going to make Jamie into a ship's captain." The vision disappeared as quickly as it had come, and you stood there, in front of me. My reactions must have been somewhat confusing to you.

"Your only interest was where we took the dung to, but I was confronted with the decision of what to do next. If my recollections are correct, I asked you how old you were. I well remember the reply. It was as though I had been stabbed with a dagger. "I'm thirteen today, sir." I gasped. You were my boy, standing in front of me, an utter disgrace. I was still in a trance. Then I acted on impulse, and told you to start work. I soon realised that my reply had you confused. It seems remarkable to me that your concern as to where we were going was so great, and that Woodham Ferris should play such an important role in our lives.

"As you made your way from the cabin, I suddenly required to know your name. Your reply pressed the first dagger further into my heart. "Call me Jimmie, that's wot my movver calls me."

"While the words pained me at the time, they have, over the years, been secretly a source of inspiration to me. Jealously, I treasured them as the words of that little mite I held in my arms at Maldon.

"You will now understand why I was so overwhelmed at the time, and the very fact that you should drop to your knees and ask if you could help me, sealed for me your future."

There was a long pause. Jimmie watched, as his old skipper sought to mouth his next words.

"Yesterday, that vision came true. You stood before me as Captain Brown, and all I could do in return was to present myself deceitfully in the guise of a railway guard."

Jimmie watched in silence, and held the old man's hands, as Skip unashamedly cried.

Some minutes later he left, and went to the galley to make a pot of tea. He steeped Skip's mug with rum. They drank, and ate a large slice of fruit cake, supplied by Mrs Deeks. The lad turned up to collect the haybox, and shouted a cheery goodbye, as Jimmie put a half-crown in his hand.

Skip had now recovered from the emotional strain of his storytelling; the rum also taking good effect.

"That, Jimmie, brings you up to date. I trust I have not bored you."

"Not one bit, Skip. I admire and appreciate all you have told me. I feel my life story is almost complete, and I shall be indebted to you to the end of my days."

"I am also grateful to you, Jimmie, in the way you have fulfilled your role, unknowingly, but I am mystified as to why you say that your life story is almost complete."

"Because, Skip, I have yet to learn what happened to you between 1901 and 1922."

Skip looked surprised. "Is that necessary, Jimmie?"

"To me, yes. But I will not burden you any more. That will do for tomorrow. We have been sitting quite a lot today, if you feel fit enough, can I suggest we take a little walk around the fens?"

"That is a very good idea, Jimmie, but please, no somersaults!"

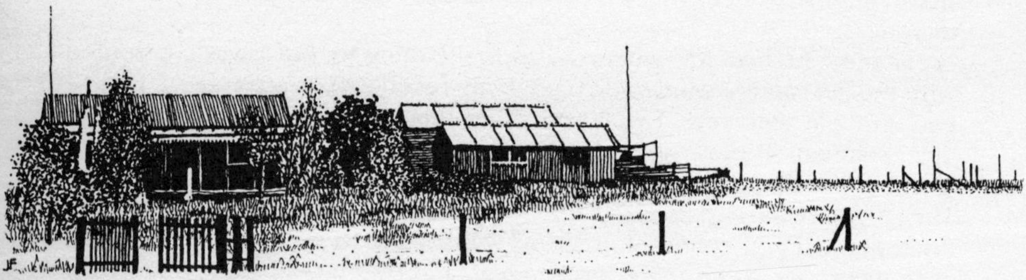

THE DRIVE, FENN CREEK

Chapter Twenty-six

The Loss of Paddy and the 'Maywell'

The next morning, they took their seats again. June was excelling itself with a spate of hot, dry weather.

"What I have to tell you today, Jimmie, may not be so exciting. It reveals the worst about me, and I trust you will accept it as the foolishness of an old man.

"First, let me say that Paddy returned and apologised to me the night before you first sailed with us.

"The fact that you eventually left the 'Maywell' to join the Merchant Navy gave me a sense of satisfaction and hope. Both Nell and Paddy followed your progress with interest. It was early in 1901 that we returned to Burnham to find Nell ill. She told me not to contact you concerning her illness because you were due to take some special exams. Sadly, she died within two days.

"The loss of my sister had a dour effect on me. I often feel that Paddy suffered me in silence. We continued with the freights, but I made little use of the cottage. I recall returning there, after an absence of three months, to find a letter from you, telling that you were awaiting your final results, but had taken an appointment whereby you would be in Australian waters for five years. I put it to one side, and told myself that I would attend to it later. For reasons unknown, I have never seen the letter since, and to my shame, I never did anything about it. The following week, we sailed up to Saltcotes Creek to collect a freight from the brickfields. Paddy and I took the opportunity to visit the Railway Hotel for a meal. We were pleasantly surprised, on our arrival, to find a crowd of people milling around the station

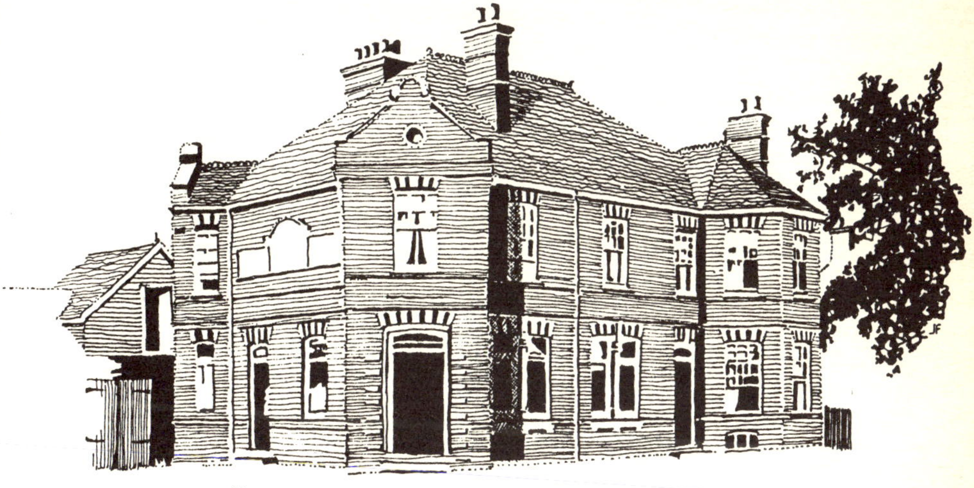

RAILWAY HOTEL, HULLBRIDGE ROAD

and hotel grounds, where long tables of food were displayed and drink seemed to abound. I asked an attendant the reason for such festivities.

"It's the last of the sales, sir." As nothing seemed obvious, I again enquired, "What is being sold?"

"Plots, sir." He could see my confusion. "It be Eyott's Farm. It's the last day. Help yourself to food, and you can drink what you like, it's all free. But don't nod your 'ead too often when the auctioneer gets on the table, or you'll go 'ome owning arf of Woodham!"

"Paddy and I enjoyed the spread, and we studied the proposed layout of roads and plotland. The agents, I remember, were Messrs Prothero and Morris, auctioneers from Cheapside, and they were in conjunction with Messrs Spurgeon and Son, of Maldon. I admired their regal taste for road names: Victoria, Albert, Louise, Alexandra, York and Connaught. With our local knowledge of the area, it was not difficult for Paddy and I to visualise the scene of the development.

"I would like to live there," said Paddy, pointing to some plots overlooking Fenn Creek and up to the mainstream.

"If I were to choose, it would be near the Fenn Bridge. The fens have a fascination for me."

"Then let's do just that," said Paddy, "the poor old 'Maywell' can't last much longer, and neither can you or I. Let's buy some plots, sell the 'Maywell' and settle down here. We can have a small craft and enjoy the river as well."

"I was inspired by the idea, as well as surprised by Paddy's sudden desire to become domesticated. I bought the plots on which we now sit, and four more for Paddy, bordering the river. Our future plans were to give up freighting in the late summer, load the 'Maywell' with all the necessary materials and equipment and build ourselves a dwelling place. In fact, I began to design a prefabricated bungalow, which would require little work to be done after erection.

"It was during June that we left the Hythe, Colchester, with a load of grain for Manningtree. We went down the Colne, on the ebb, and we were making way along the Wallett. The wind was in our favour, Paddy had given full sail and the old girl was doing us proud. We would round the Naze and bring up in the Stour for the night.

"Angry clouds, sweeping from off-shore, and the sound of distant thunder, raised my suspicions. Paddy was certain it would pass astern, but I disagreed, and suggested he took in some sail. His reaction was quite offensive.

"Todd Summers, you are losing your nerve! I know when to take the sail in by now," he shouted above the sudden rising storm. I clung to the wheel with all my might. I dare not lose her head. I yelled again for Paddy to take in. He looked to the sky.

"It will all be over in five minutes, Todd. Hold her there."

"A tremendous gust of wind heeled the 'Maywell' over onto her starboard beam. I could not believe it possible for her to right herself. Suddenly, Paddy raced around and began to take in sail. As the 'Maywell' wearily lifted herself upright, I sighed in relief. Our respite was momentary. A flash of lightning cracked down on the deck, followed by the crashing of the mast and rigging. The 'Maywell' wallowed in her plight.

"I rushed to Paddy's aid. He lay trapped between the foc's'le winch and the

main mast.
"Jump clear, Todd," he called, "I'm finished." I tried to raise his hopes.
"I'm sorry, Todd, I was a fool. Get clear while you can." Suddenly, the 'Maywell' lurched again on her starboard side, and began to sink. From the morass of sail and lines, I emerged to the surface to secure a hold onto a hatch cover. A fishing smack picked me up within the hour, and took me to Harwich. Paddy's body was never found.
"At the inquest on the loss of Paddy, I reported what had happened, but did not tell of the dispute between the two of us. Witnesses from the shore gave evidence, saying that we were running before the storm on full sail. This, I could not deny. The coroner, in his summing up, stated that while he did not attribute the loss of life and ship to me, he was mystified that two lifelong seamen, with our knowledge of the age and condition of our craft, should engage in the exploits of teenagers. "As the skipper of the 'Maywell', you must feel responsible. I can only express the court's sympathy for your lapse of judgement." I left that building a broken man, Jimmie."
"But it was not your fault, Skip. You must realise that."
"I was the skipper, and therefore responsible. Two days after the inquest, I returned to Maldon on the 'Waveney'. Distorted stories of the incident were already spreading throughout the bargeing fraternity. I had never really been accepted in their midst, although I blame my own aloofness for that, but I had provided just the right conditions for those who wished to degrade me."
"Skip, may I please intervene. Why do you punish yourself? In all my years with you, I realised that men chaffed you. There may have been one or two who resented you, but you are punishing yourself when you say you were not accepted."
Skip hesitated. "Do you really believe that, Jimmie."
"Yes, Skip. I do."
"Then that is a real comfort to me. Your words confirm what Nell once said to me."
"Can we carry on from Maldon, Skip?"
"Yes. It was around six in the morning when I left the 'Waveney', and walked up the hill. For a while, I stood looking at the cottage where Moira and Jaimie died. My spirits sunk lower than one could imagine possible. "You are useless, an outcast of your own society." The words of Mac, her father, rang through my mind. Thirty-five years later, I had proved his words true."
Jimmie wanted to interrupt, then decided against it.
"Why I did not walk straight back to the Blackwater, and end it all, I could never understand, until yesterday. Aimlessly I wandered through the town. What few people there were about had little time to even notice me. I took the road to Fambridge, I had not the courage to take the Mundon Road. I slept under a thick hedge during the day, and arrived at my cottage in Burnham after midnight."

Chapter Twenty-seven

Return from Death's Door

"It was not until the following evening that Mrs Stevens became aware of my presence. Because of her devotion to Nell, I let her into the cottage. I abruptly stopped her giving me the local account of what had happened to the 'Maywell', and explained what I required of her.

"As you know, she was a sensible woman and I knew that I could trust her. I needed food. I wanted to see Tom King, but I did not have the courage to leave the cottage. She played her part admirably for the next few weeks. Tom arrived the next evening. He did ask me for my version of the loss of the 'Maywell', and I felt he believed me. We then got down to the plans of converting a fishing smack into a habitable craft. I requested that on no account was he to divulge my name. "Tell your workmen what you like," I told him.

"It was mid-September before the work was completed. During this time I kept myself fit by walking during the midnight hours. Tom came for his final instructions. I told him of my plans to sail to Canvey Island, and sought his assistance in preparing my getaway. For three nights we transferred goods and chattels from the cottage to the smack, now moored on the fairway.

"On the last night, I told Tom that my agent would be taking over the premises within a few days. He would settle the remainder of the account. I thanked him for his help and his confidence. As I locked the door of 'Plovers' and handed him the key, even in the dark, he read my thoughts. "Just take the pleasant memories, Todd, leave the others behind." They were the words of a wise man, but I did not take his advice.

"He rowed me out to the smack, and helped me raise sail. We shook hands, "I trust you will find a good berth on Canvey, Todd. Goodbye, and God bless you."

"He pushed the dinghy away, and rowed back to shore. I slipped the buoy and sailed downstream, conscious that I was deceiving the man who had come to my rescue. The light of the moon assisted me in finding my way into the Roach. I dropped sail and threw over the anchor. The tide would be beginning to flow at four in the morning. It fitted nicely with my plans.

"Before I left the Roach, I changed into the railway guard's uniform. This I had bought in London on my return from visiting my solicitors to settle my affairs in Burnham. A swig from the bottle was all I needed to set me on my course.

"I passed Burnham town quay at four-thirty. As the sinking moon silhouetted the buildings, it made me feel sad and terribly lonely. I was closing yet another chapter in my morbid existence. I hardly used any sail, the flood would get me to my destination."

"But not to Canvey Island," put in Jimmie.

"I'm well aware of that, Jimmie, but if you want to hear the story of my

failings, you must not interrupt."
"I'm sorry, Skip, please continue."
"The sun rose, crimson red, reflecting in the high cloud. A depression was building up, and by the time I sailed past Fambridge it was raining.

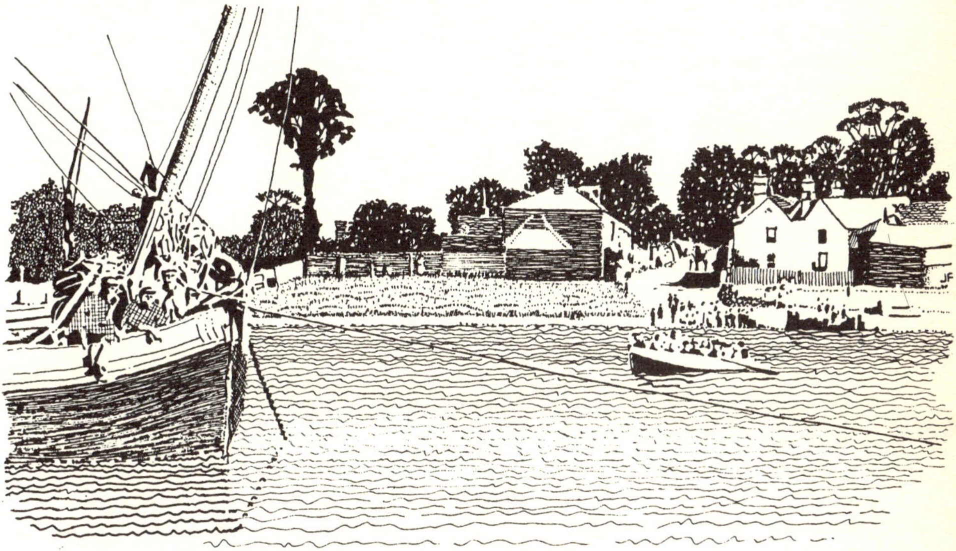

CHILDREN CROSSING RIVER AT HULLBRIDGE FERRY

Approaching Hullbridge Ferry came as a relief, there were no barges moored. I would soon be turning into Fenn Creek and safe from prying eyes. The rain came down in torrents. I was soaked to the skin. As I drifted past the ferry, the children going to Hullbridge school from Woodham Ferris stood forlornly awaiting their turn to cross. The pathetic look on their faces, as the rain swept down, made me feel really sorry for them. Those already on their way across waved at my unusual turnout. I felt that Tom Hitchins had no idea who had passed him. I turned into Fenn Creek, and waited for half-an-hour for sufficient water to get me past Eyott's Farm. By ten o'clock, I had nudged the smack into the Whalebone Creek, my journey's end."
"Throughout the day the rain never let up. I worked frantically to sheet up my possessions, stowed on the roof deck of my new home. I had eaten little during the day, so by evening I was weary and virtually at the end of my tether."
"During that night I awoke, sweating profusely, and had developed a dreadful throat. For the second time in my life I felt dreadfully ill. Throughout the next day, rain and wind did battle with the sheeting. I did my best to re-lash it, but finally gave up in despair. My temperature had weakened me. I crawled onto my makeshift bed, placed the rum bottle beside me, and decided to sweat it out."
"The second night, I had severe attacks of ague, and hallucinations. I did not even have the strength to pick up the rum bottle. I awoke from one trauma, shouting at Nell to leave me. She was dressed in her white wedding

dress, standing in the stern of the boat. I slept; I woke; then a few words kept haunting me: "The darkness falls at Thy behest." I could not dispel them, nor imagine what they meant."

"By a supreme effort, I grabbed the bottle, drained the last dregs, and laid back exhausted. For a short while I began to collect my thoughts again. The haunting words began to make sense. "The darkness falls at Thy behest." That was what I had been doing all my life, bringing darkness to everyone around me: my mother and father, Moira, Paddy and Tom King. I had deserted them. At my behest ... I had now brought myself to this little creek to live in my own dark world."

"I had even refused Nell's offer to take some part in my morbid existence. It was all at my 'behest', but now the Almighty had seen fit to bring it to a close. I would die in defeat."

Jimmie watched as Skip regained his composure, amazed at the depth of the man's thinking. Skip looked at Jimmie, and gave a wry smile.

"That should have been the end of the story, but it is to be continued, after a cup of tea."

"To wake and find oneself in a comfortable bed, with a large log fire burning in the hearth, was bewildering. A young lady walked into the room and looked rather surprised.

"Are you feeling better, Mr Clark?" she asked.

"I don't really know, ma'am. Should I be?" I suddenly panicked. "Where am I? Am I in hospital?" She put her hand on my forehead.

"Be calm, Mr Clark, you are quite safe, in Eyott's Farm. Try and go to sleep again." The next time I awoke, a doctor was examining me.

"It is nice to see you come back again, Mr Clark. You have had us on edge these last few days. If you can bear with me, I need a few questions answed." I nodded my approval.

"First let me tell you that you have been extremely ill. Fortunately, you have come through, and providing you are patient you will fully recover. Secondly, would Nell be your wife? You have mentioned her name a few times. So far, we have had no reply from your address."

"Nell is my sister, doctor. She died some months ago. I am a bachelor. I have no relations for you to contact."

"Thank you, Mr Clark. I will see you in a couple of days. You are in good hands." I questioned my host, later that day.

"How do you know I am Mr Clark, and what my address is?"

"Because it is stitched inside your uniform, sir. We gathered you come from near Cambridge."

"Yes, ma'am. I intend to settle down nearby."

"No further questions were asked that day, and I decided that Mr Clark would be my name forthwith. Strangely enough, the thought that my name could give away my identity had not occurred to me. The ruse of the uniform had played an essential part in my act of deception.

"My hosts were a young married couple, and their job was to oversee the occupation of the plotland by the purchasers, on behalf of landlords, during the break-up of the estate. Reg filled in my missing days for me. They had seen me sail up Fenn Creek and around the farm perimeter, then watched me moor in the Whalebone Creek. Because of the heavy rain, he had not bothered to check on me. He had seen me lash the tarpaulin over the smack, and assumed that I had returned to my home town. He said that a number of the newcomers were weekenders from London, and my activities did not appear unusual.

"It was during the morning of the third day that two boys came rushing to his door to say that strange things were happening on the boat in the creek. He took the man who worked with him and went to investigate. Everything seemed in order, so he told the lads to run off, but they insisted they had heard noises from inside. He then scrambled on board, lifted the tarpaulin and saw me laying in a dishevelled heap on the floor. He called Fred on board, and they decided I was dead and that they should send for the police. Then, I moved my arm. The shock made Fred step backwards and he fell into the creek."

Jimmie laughed.

"Have a good laugh, my boy, because there's nothing else in my story to amuse anyone."

Jimmie accepted the rebuff, "Please continue, Skip."

"Reg told me that, on further investigation, they concluded that I was in a coma, and needed a doctor rather than a policeman. Fred took the horse and raced to Wickford to get Doctor Marshall. Reg sent the boys home, and returned to Eyott's Farm to change his clothes. Later that day, they carried me on a home-made stretcher into the farm. For the next three days, Doctor Marshall rode twice a day to see me.

"For security reasons, he sailed my boat and moored it in front of the farm, without disturbing anything, he assured me. I expressed my thanks for all they had done, and hoped that I would not encumber them for much longer. That was not to be, for I remained at Eyott's Farm for another six months.

"It was after three months that I complained to Doctor Marshall about my slow progress. He gave a peculiar grunt, "Mr Clark, very few men who have suffered the degree of pneumonia that you had, live to tell the tale. What surprises me about you, is that you virtually stepped into your grave, and then apparently decided to step out again. Have you any particular reason for doing so, or could it be that the Almighty is not ready for you? If you will forgive me saying so, I find you a fascinating man.

"First, you arrive on the scene giving the impression that you are a railway guard taking an early retirement. From your physique, I would have concluded that you were a life-serving seaman, and by your education and bearing, a member of the gentry. I have a shrewd suspicion that one of those attributes does not apply to you. Would I be encroaching too much on your privacy if I asked whether my diagnosis is correct?"

"I was like a fish caught in a net, Jimmie. After all the medical skill he had bestowed on me, I could not bring myself to lie to him.

"Doctor Marshall," I said, "I thank you that you should be so interested in me. It would appear that your stethoscope conveys more information to you than just my heartbeat. But to answer your questions. With so much time at my disposal, I too have given serious consideration as to why I am not in my final resting place. In many respects, I wish I were.

"My last thoughts on the boat were that I had come to that situation in life from which man does not return, and I accepted it as fair recompense for the way I had conducted my life. So, I rule out your suggestion that I changed my mind.

"Your remark that the Almighty was not ready for me may have been said light-heartedly, but on reflection, and whilst I am loath to say so, you may be correct. Therefore it could possibly be that you have been instrumented by the Almighty to prolong my life, so that He can deal with me as I rightly deserve.

"With regard to my attributes, it would appear that I have fallen down in my act of deception. To answer your other question, I must crave your confidence in what I tell you." He assured me that whatever I told him would be confidential.

"You are absolutely right, doctor, I have been a seaman all my working life. My father was a gentleman of high rank in government circles. His son did not continue his example. Your diagnosis was correct: I am not a railway guard. I am not on the run, or wanted for crime. I just wish to settle down, on the fens, to do my natural history studies, uninterrupted by those who knew me. My name is not Mr Clark, but the fact that it was in the uniform means that it will be my pseudonym for the future. My real name is Tobias Summers, or Todd. I trust, doctor, that rather scanty information will suffice."

"Yes, Mr Clark, I will ask no more questions, and appreciate your intentions. I ask but one favour, that is, when you settle down on your new abode I may visit you, purely as a social caller." We both stood up and shook hands.

"Thank you, doctor, for all you have been to me over the last three months. Your favour is not only granted, but welcomed."

Once more, Skip's story was interrupted, as dinner was brought by the boy from the 'Whalebone', until the meal was consumed.

Chapter Twenty-eight

Eyotts and Plotland

Later that afternoon, Skip continued.

"My stay at Eyotts was longer than intended. My hosts insisted I remained until the Spring. I acepted their hospitality on the condition that I paid my way in full. I spent the Christmas on my own: they returned to Gloucester for a few days.

"By March, my health was back to normal. Reg had acquired a man to help to dig and form a ramp opposite my plot, so that we could pull the boat up on land. Having missed the Autumn Springs, a high March Spring would be needed. On the 20th March, 1902, I sailed the old smack up the Whalebone Creek on the crest of the tide. The water covered the fens from bank to bank, like an inland sea.

"To make life difficult, I required the boat to be pulled up stern first, which intrigued my helpers. I told them I wanted it pointing in the right direction for a quick getaway, which caused great amusement.

"With the help of four horses and tackle, the task was completed without any problem. The men received their pay and drank their bottles of beer around the old smack, and wished me the best of luck in my new home. One of the horsemen, I noticed, eyed me with suspicion. He tackled me before leaving. "Mr Clark, I reckon 'as 'ow I noo y'r brother; he were a skipper on an owd barge that used to come up to Eyotts. 'E 'as 'is 'and done up in a leather glove like yew. Todd Zummer they use' to call 'im and 'e were edicated."

"If ever my brain was required to work fast, it was then. I realised that his saying 'my brother' was just an attempt to catch me. I laughed aloud, "My good man, if you could have seen me navigating this monstrosity up the Crouch, you would hardly credit me as a skipper of a barge. I have no brother, therefore you must be implying that I am Todd Whatever-his-name-was. You must remember, there are dozens of men like me around, with their hands shot off because of the war, and even a railway supervisor is expected to have the vocabulary befitting his task, but please do not feel embarrassed for misjudging me."

"He looked at me very sheepishly, "I do beg yur pardon, sur, and I will tell my pals at the 'bone I were dreadfully mistaken."

"Don't you worry, my man, we all make mistakes."

"Crafty old blighter," thought Jimmie of his shipmate.

"When the team had left, I sat down on a box and wiped my brow. Reg moved over and placed another box opposite me and sat down too. "I admire the calm way you answered the horseman, Mr Clark." I sensed a note of suspicion in his voice for he had been calling me Nobby for many months.

"Do you challenge my answer to him," I said. I realised I had spoken sharply; it showed a sign of weakness. "I have no need to, Mr Clark. The horseman's questions confirmed my suspicions. He was right, but he had no grounds on which to confirm his theory." I felt like the 'Maywell', when she dropped the wind from her mainsail.

"Perhaps you will be good enough to explain yourself, before I make any further comments." I was playing for time.

"Mr Clark, it has never been my principle to tread on a man when he is down, and you are the last person on earth I could do it to. I never had any reason to disbelieve you, until you told me the number of the plots you would be occupying, and they did not tally with the Mr Clark on my schedule. I realised how ill you had been and thought it was a lapse of memory on your part. I checked with my office in Maldon. They informed me that a Mr Tobias Summers was the rightful owner of the plots in question, and that he was a barge skipper from Burnham-on-Crouch. They advised me not to take any action until you actually occupied the site." I sat like a schoolboy in front of his headmaster, awaiting punishment for playing truant.

"So, what are you going to do?" I asked. He smiled and took my hand.

"Nothing whatsoever. I will just keep calling you Nobby Clark. Only Mary and I know your secret; not even Dr Marshall knows that." A feeling of satisfaction crept over me at his last remark. I was at least one up on him there."

Skip looked at Jimmie. "Tell me, what is it about people that make them tolerate people like me?"

Jimmie shook his head. "I think your sister could have answered that question better than me, Skip."

"I was very sorry when Reg and his wife eventually left Eyotts. They had stood by me in my hour of need, shielded and protected me from all the enquirers. They fascinated me with the stories of malpractice by the purchasers of plotland: fencing in land that did not belong to them; moving boundaries overnight; enclosing roads; and assaulting one another. Some even walked their boundaries carrying twelve-bore guns. It was more like the Gold Rush than a quiet country backwater. Strangely enough, while all the fighting went on, many people never claimed their rights of possession, due to the fact that they were too drunk at the time of paying their deposit to even know what they had signed for."

"Over the next few years, Eyotts Farm had many changes. I lived a life of complete solitude, and it was some years before little weekend huts began to spring up in the most unforeseen places. By then the hedge had grown around me, and I learned from hearsay during my visits to the 'Whalebone' that I was known locally as the 'Hermit of Woodham Fenn."

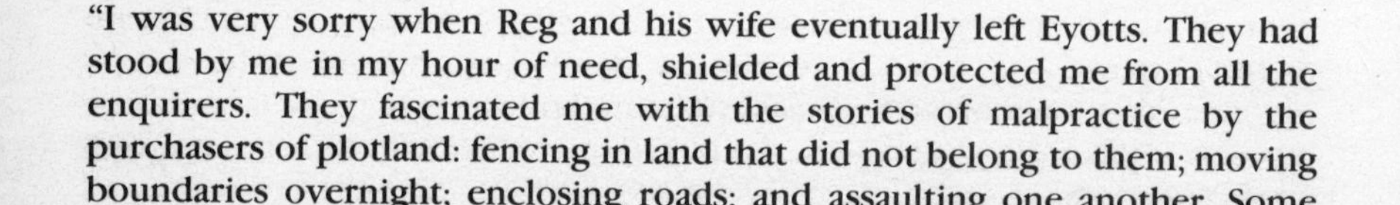

PROPERTIES NEAR FENN CREEK

"For years, I studied every square yard of the fens. I investigated the change of seasonal habitat, the action of meadow land taking over saltings and marsh. I searched the creeks and riverbeds, and studied the peatlayers for evidence of bygone settlements. I am now confident, from what I have found and read, that this quiet backwater contains the secrets and the history of mankind, going back over many thousands of years.

"People arriving in this scattered village assume they are the first humans to live here. Far from it, Jimmie. We are but intruders on the past.

"I think I must have known every bird and beast in the area, and they knew me. I have reset many a broken wing or leg for their families. Once, I even nursed a young vixen back to health. I thought, for a while, she had become domesticated, but when fully recovered she killed a couple of my chickens and proudly presented me with the remains. I turned her out of the compound, but she did not really leave me until the next mating season. I feel certain she must have brought all her litters along to tell them of her gratitude towards me, because I have never lost a chicken by foxes since, and that was in 1906.

"For years, I did battle with the bird-catchers. They were a cruel lot, and abused me terribly at times. They would harness-up decoy birds with horse-hair threads, and tie them onto a seeding thistle, then set up nets. The fluttering decoy would attract its fellows of the species: finches; linnets; and even sparrows. With a clap of the catcher's hand from the right direction, the birds would fly into the nets. They were then caught and dipped into yellow dye and sold as canaries in the London markets. Skylarks were lured by the use of rotating mirrors, and pheasants and partridges were caught by using green peas with a short length of horse-hair threaded through. I have found many a bird choking to death, and usually it was only mercy to kill them. So you see, Jimmie, while I was not very popular among the bargeing fraternity, I was likewise very unpopular amongst the country people.

"I knew little of the war, except to see the aeroplanes, both British and German, and also one of their Zeppelins. Dr Marshall kept me up to date on his occasional visits. While I managed reasonably well, I did suffer at times from periods of deep depression.

"It came to a climax in 1918. For a whole week, I did little but drink spirits, and storm around my garden. After a night of utter torment, I released my fury on the galley door. I took the axe and began to smash it down, shouting at the top of my voice. Having expended all my strength, I laid across the table, exhausted, my head buried in my hands.

"I am not certain how long I laid in that position, I only know someone was holding my hands. "How often do you have turns like that, Mr Summers?" It was Dr Marshall. I completely broke down before him. "If the Almighty has any mercy at all, why does He let me continue living?" I cried.

"He made me swallow some tablets which had a dramatic effect on me. Gradually, he got me to talk. I told him about Moira, my father and mother, how I had deserted you, and he listened patiently. He even made me a cup of tea, and joined me himself. I don't know how long he stayed, but when I awoke it was to find that I had almost slept the clock around. My poor old nanny goat was bursting its bag with milk.

"Dr Marshall had left a letter on the table, with some tablets. "Please come to my surgery, in Wickford. The walk will do you good." I did that walk every month for a year. He had saved my life again. He was convinced that you would return to me, after the War. I must admit that, by 1921 I had given up hope. That, Jimmie, finishes my account of myself."

"Thank you, Skip, I appreciate all you have suffered, both physically and mentally. To re-tell your story has caused you much pain. We are together again now. Shall we take the advice of Tom King - leave the bad behind and carry on with the good?"

"Yes, Jimmie. With you at hand, I'm sure I can." They shook hands.

"Do you know, Jimmie, I am beginning to think the Almighty played some part in our coming together again."

"I am inclined to agree with you, Skip."

The next day, Jimmie and Skip viewed the plots of land originally purchased for Paddy.

"They are still in my name, and they are yours for the asking," said Skip.

Chapter Twenty-nine

Jimmie Moves to Woodham

It was mid-August when the people of the village watched, yet again, a large steam traction engine pulling a passenger coach of the Great Eastern Railway, on a purpose built limber, from the station goodsyard, along the Hullbridge Road, up the baked mud track of Victoria Road, along Louise Road, up the hill over York Road, then across the fields to Connaught Road. The boys, away from school, followed and milled around, watching the spectacle, while men with large sections of wood were prepared to place them in position to prevent the coach slipping, or even tipping, in the deep ruts.

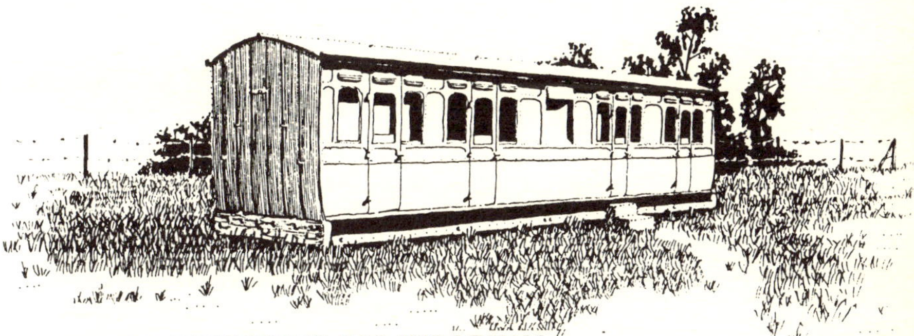

JIMMIE'S FIRST HOUSE IN S. WOODHAM

It was all part of Jimmie's country estate. Plans to build a small bungalow alongside would come later. From Enfield, Jimmie and Emily moved to Brentwood (that was to be their town residence), an easier journey to their new country dwelling at South Woodham. By the following summer, Jimmie had purchased a twenty-foot motor launch with sail, and the bungalow was fit for habitation. Skip still lived his reserved way of life, although he spent many afternoons and evenings talking to Emily and Jimmie, and had an occasional trip on 'Maywell III'.

Mid-October, 1923, was warm and bright. The pressure of work on the bungalow and garden had eased up. Soon, Jimmie and his sister would return to Brentwood for the winter, and it suddenly occurred to him that he had now been in the area for nearly fifteen months without finding time to visit Hullbridge. He walked over to Skip, to ask if he too would care to visit one of their old haunts.

"No Jimmie, I feel it's more than my bones will allow. You remember me to anyone who may have known me, and have a good day."

A good half-hour's stroll along the fen creek bank and mainstream brought Jimmie to the ferry. It took another ten or fifteen minutes before Tom Hitching, the ferryman, realised he had a customer waiting to cross. His eventual arrival on the Woodham bank gave him an unexpected surprise.

"Jimmie, boy! What the devil are you doing here, standing like a forlorn mariner? Get in and take a seat."
They shook hands, Jimmie sat down, and Tom pulled away.
"How much is this trip going to cost me?"
Tom laughed. "Usually threepence, but for a man of your status, two and six! And if old Todd had been with you, I should have charged a guinea."
"I can see you still drive a hard bargain, Tom."
The old ferryman pulled skillfully on the oars, gave a hearty cough and spat a wad of baccy into the tide.
"He was rather a queer stick, your skipper, but with due respect, he was superior to the general run of bargemen. I doubt whether he did anyone any harm, and it was a pity they did not accept him. There, I expect he's been dead a few years now." Tom hitched his boat to the old quay post. "Right, Jimmie, let's get into the bar and share a drink."
"Yes, Tom, Skip was a queer one, and still is. I tried to get him to come with me this morning, but he sends his best regards."
"You surprise me, Jimmie. I was told, years ago, that he had gone to Canvey Island to die."
"I was told the same story, then found him disguised as a railway guard, living on a boat on the Woodham fens. It has been his home since the turn of the century."
"Well darn me, Jimmie. That rings a bell with me. I must have seen him sail within a few feet of me, as I rowed the youngsters over to school. The kids waved and shouted, but he took no notice. The crafty blighter did not want me to recognise him. I can remember the boat was loaded sky-high, and it was teeming with rain. Anyway, its nice to hear that he is still hale and hearty."
Ducking their heads, they stepped into the heavily timbered bar. Four men sat talking. They all seemed very young to Jimmie.
"Meet a man who sailed barges up the Crouch before you lot knew which end to find the Mizzen. Today, he is Captain Jimmie Brown, hero and survivor of the 'Cannondore'".
They all stood up. "Pleased to meet you, captain," they said in unison.
"I am surprised that newspapers have now reached Hullbridge," laughed Jimmie.
"Not only do we get them, but some of us can read them as well," returned Tom.
"Fill the glasses, Mary. This round's on the house, but charge them double for the next."
"Not so," butted in Jimmie, "that will be my privilege."
The news of Jimmie's arrival soon spread around the little cottages clustered nearby. Three elderly gentlemen arrived who knew the 'Maywell' and Jimmie, and for the next few hours they talked freely and drank to each others' health. Their war service, ships and barges dominated the conversation. At two o'clock, Tom called "Time". Jimmie thanked all for the reception he had been given and raised a toast for all men at sea.
The scream of "Help!" brought the jovial scene to a sudden halt. All eyes turned to a frantic woman standing in the doorway.
"A horse and cart and two men are being washed down the river!" she cried.
Men left the bar within seconds and raced to the water's edge. The ebb had

been running for half-an-hour and was gaining momentum. In the centre of the river, some two hundred yards downstream, the men could see the tumbril almost submerged. The horse, still in the shafts, was thrashing its forelegs frantically to keep its head above water, but the driver and mate were not to be seen. Men raced to the Brickfield Wharf to collect a dinghy, in the hope of cutting off the beleaguered animal. Another took his bicycle and headed towards Rayleigh, some three miles away, for the police, while Tom, with Jimmie and a young lad and his bike, rowed to the Woodham bank. The lad was then sent off to cycle onto Woodham village, a mile away, to fetch the local policeman and other helpers. Meanwhile, men in a rowing boat searched the area. Standing on the Woodham Wharf, Tom and Jimmie discussed the possibilities of what could have happened. Perhaps the men had jumped clear, got ashore, and made their way to Marsh or Peatlands Farm for help. Or was the lady mistaken in seeing two men? Could the drivers be having forty winks after their lunch break? Maybe their horse had strayed or bolted. All were possibilities. They walked the banks nearby, but found no clues.

On the Hullbridge bank, it could be seen that the horse had succeeded in crossing the outgoing tide, and the cart had come to rest in the mud nearby the Brickfield Wharf. Men were already standing to their waists in water, trying to release the animal.

News travelled quickly and, within the hour, people were gathered on both banks, trying to solve the mystery of the missing men. Tom had returned to the Hullbridge causeway to row the children from school back to Woodham, accompanied by their schoolmaster.

As Jimmie lifted some of the smaller children from the boat, he could sense their fear and concern. Many had fathers and elder brothers who drove the tumbril carts that distributed the stones from the wharf to the surrounding road works. So far, it had not been confirmed who had or may have been drowned.

With the receding tide, more and more mud and seaweed-covered banks became exposed, and organised searches were being made. Men and women followed the tide.

The first alarm was raised by two fourteen-year-old boys who, against instructions from the schoolmaster, had wandered along the east Woodham bank saltings. The glint of a brass buckle on the belt of one man, covered by seaweed on the bank, was enough. It was another hour before the second man was found, further downstream. The infestation of crabs was proved by the mutilation of the bodies in such a short space of time.

It was later confirmed that the two men were Thomas Deeks, landlord of the Whalebone Inn and also a haulage contractor, and Sidney Osborne of the Fenn Cottages. Both men left a widow and four children.

Later that evening, Jimmie made his way to Skip and conveyed the sad news. Sidney Osborne had lived but three hundred yards along the creek from the boat.

The whole village mourned the tragedy, but what made it harder to bear was the fact that, had the men stayed on the cart, the horse would most probably have taken them safely to shore.

Early the following morning, horsemen endeavoured to get the horse over the ford to return it to the Whalebone stables. Once again, the children were on their way to school and, it being low tide, a pony and cart was their means of transport. They were told to stand well to one side, and be quiet. The animal was led down the Hullbridge causeway, with a sack covering her head. Slowly, she made her way over the slippery stones, led by two men who held the halter and stroked and carressed her. They stopped at the water's edge. The horse's feet touched the flowing tide, and suddenly she gave a strange whinney that frightened the young children. Then she raised herself onto her hind legs, turned, then dragging the men over the stones, shook the sack from her head. She raced up the causeway, and galloped some two miles in the Rayleigh direction, before being recaptured.

One of the outcomes of this tragedy was the local demand for a bridge, to put an end to the dangerous practice of ferrying the children to and fro to school. Eventually, the message got through to the authorities, although it was another five years before a primary school was erected in South Woodham.

Just before Christmas, 1924, Jimmie visited Skip. The idea was to encourage him to come to Brentwood for the festive season. He had refused in 1923, but this time Jimmie's hopes were high.

He arrived at the boat to find his shipmate ill. "I'll be alright in a few days. Don't bother me. Just get me some food and drink."

From the boat, Jimmie made his way to the local Post Office to get a telegraph message to Dr Frew of Wickford, who arrived later on his motor bike.

"We must get you to hospital, Mr Clark."

"No, thank you, doctor. Just let me die here."

"My job is not to let you die, but to get you better. I shall arrange for an ambulance to collect you."

"Then let it take me to Jimmie's house in Brentwood."

Jimmie gave his approval.

Very well, Mr Clark. I will visit you there."

Skip's stay at Brentwood lasted eight weeks, but with Emily's care and attention, and the comfort of a nice home, he made a full recovery.

Once fit, Skip's only desire was to get back to his beloved fens.

Chapter Thirty

To Burnham: Mr King's and the Storm

During the early summer of 1925, Skip enjoyed some short trips on the 'Maywell III', down to Fambridge and up to Battlesbridge. The sight of a passing barge on its way to or from the mills gave Skip and Jimmie nostalgic moments.

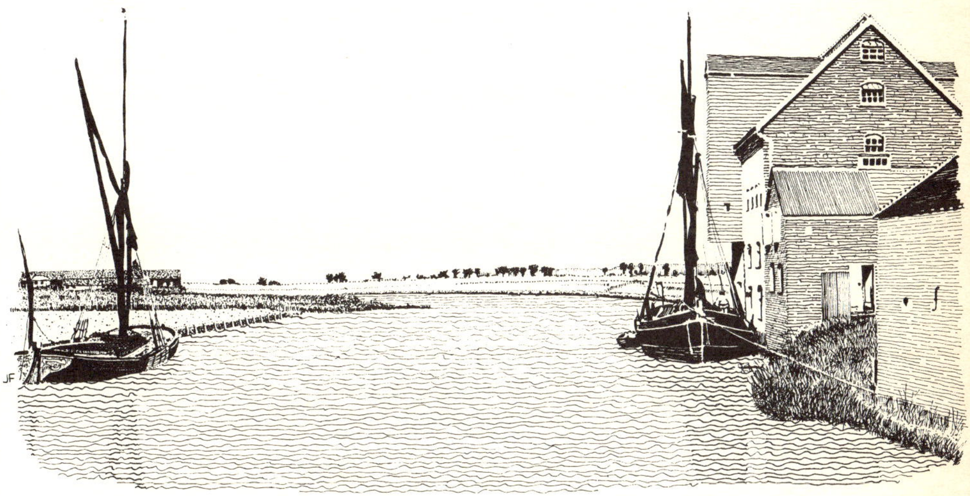

BARGES AT BATTLESBRIDGE

In mid-July, it was necessary to take 'Maywell III' to Burnham for engine maintenance. To Jimmie's surprise, Skip suggested that he should accompany him.

"If it's only to see Tom King, it will be worth it," he said.

They left the creek at eight in the morning, on the ebb. As they passed the Hullbridge ferry, they were intrigued by the to-ing and fro-ing of men working on the shafts in preparation for tunneling under the river. A large gantry had been erected to drive steel piling into the marshland. Men pushed little steel tip-up trolleys, loaded with mud, along lines on the river bank. The normally quiet area, graced only by the barges, was now a place of industrial activity.

Already, gangs of men, starting from different points, had been digging a trench some four feet wide and seven feet deep to take the large twenty-eight inch cast iron pipes that would convey the water. They had made their way through villages and farms, up hills and across valleys. The twenty-five mile track had brought upheaval in its path. Every bit of earth had been dug by hand or the pickaxe, whilst horses and men manouvered the one-ton pipes into position, all to get the much needed drinking water from Langford,

near Maldon, to Southend-on-Sea.
Skip and Jimmie arrived at Burnham soon after ten o'clock. Jimmie left Skip to have a few minutes sleep whilst he sorted out the whereabouts of Tom King. This being achieved, Skip was taken to spend the day with him, while Jimmie and the mechanics overhauled the engine.
It was four o'clock when Tom King, plus one or two old timers who had gathered, shook hands and waved the Woodham pair goodbye. The wind being south-easterly, and there being a flowing tide, Jimmie hoisted sail. Skip held the tiller. It was a repeat in miniature of fifty years sailing out of Burnham on the tide for the two veteran seamen.
As they brought up to the fen jetty early that evening, Jimmie helped his shipmate from the boat to shore. They walked up the slope to the bungalow to enjoy a good meal prepared by Emily. Drinking coffee afterwards, Emily was aware that Skip's eyes were closing.
"Would you care to stay here the night?" she asked.
"No, thank you, dear, but I must be on my way. It's been a long day."
The walk across the fields would take but ten minutes. The evening had turned extremely humid and storm clouds were building up fast to the south-east.
"You don't have to escort me, Jimmie," said Skip, pointing with his stick. "I know which direction to take. I can make the cabin before that storm breaks, but I can envisage you getting a wet shirt before you get back."
"Thank you for your consideration, Skip, but after such a wonderful day, it would complete it for me to know you were safely in your cabin."
Little was said as they plodded the sun-baked ground. Skip needed all his breath to complete the walk. Stopping at the gap in the hedge, Skip put his hand on Jimmie's shoulder.
"Thank you, my boy, for all you have made possible today. Meeting Tom King has enabled me to clear up another problem from my past. I have always felt guilty about the fact that I knowingly deceived him. I now have but one other person to whom I must make amends, but that's a spot of rain, so off you go, and goodnight."
Jimmie headed back home as quickly as possible. There was a crack of lightening, then a roaring sound, as a cyclonic wind lifted dust and hay in a vortex before him. The crash of thunder seemed to shake the very earth beneath his feet. He dug his stick hard on the ground and pushed himself forward. Hailstones began to sting his face, as they ricocheted from the hard ground. For the last hundred yards, Jimmie crunched and slithered over the rolling stones of ice. His arrival back at his bungalow was greeted with relief by Emily.
"Skip said I would have a wet shirt and he was certainly right."
For the next three hours Jimmie sat smoking his pipe, watching the storm edge its way along the Crouch valley. It was three o'clock before he went to bed. The storm had passed, but heavy rain continued. It was eight-thirty the next morning when Emily awoke him, and it was still raining. Their journey back to Brentwood was cancelled. After breakfast, Jimmie donned his wellingtons and oilskins and crossed the fields to see how Skip had fared.
"I expect he'll tell me he never heard a sound, when I get there," he thought.
The fact that Skip had not opened up the galley did not surprise him. After

such a night, no one could be blamed for over-sleeping. He knocked with his stick on the door of the corridor leading from the galley to the boat, and shouted, "Ahoy, Skip."

He heard the reply of a tired man. "Come in, Jimmie."

He passed through what Skip called his rest and study quarters to the sleeping quarters, in the bows. The old chap lay, half asleep.

"Have you had breakfast yet?" asked Jimmie.

"Not yet, but I could do with a drink of tea. Then come and sit down here, I have something to tell you."

Tea made, then drunk, Jimmie made himself comfortable on a low stool beside Skip.

"I did not have a very good night, and feel the effects this morning."

"I don't think you have any reason to excuse yourself, Skip. Half the country will be feeling the same."

"I very much doubt if there are many who would have had the same experience as I have had during the last twelve hours. I was not expecting you today. I take it you have cancelled your trip. In that case, I can tell you what happened while it is fresh in my mind. Do you recall what I was telling you when the rain started last night, Jimmie?"

"Yes, Skip, that there was someone with whom you wanted to make amends. Do I assume that I am the person in question, because I am at a loss as to what it could be about."

"Good gracious, no. We have made our peace long ago." He paused. "When I told you my life story, I left one important issue out. I felt at the time it did not really concern you, or that it would benefit you. But of late, I have reconsidered my thoughts, and decided you should know all. Hopefully, you may use my experience as a warning to my fellow men."

Jimmie detected a slight break of voice as Skip spoke, and studied him.

"Please don't look at me with suspicion, Jimmie. I am completely compos mentis. I have yet to explain what happened."

"I'm sorry Skip. Please continue."

"Hold my hand, Jimmie. I need your strength to help me tell my story."

Jimmie laid his left hand on Skip's right. He could feel it trembling.

"You may recall me telling you, when we were re-united, that I was brought up in a strict Non-conformist family. With Nell, I enjoyed our way of life and had a great appreciation of the Christian faith, as taught me.

"After Moira and the baby died, and my fight with her father, you will recall I headed for Colchester. Plodding my way over Tiptree Common, my hand was driving me almost insane. My feet were blistered and sore and I stopped and sat on a log. Then, on the spur of the moment, I stood, raised my face and shook my clenched fist to the sky and, in defiance, cursed God at the top of my voice. In my temper, I said that, from that moment of time, I would renounce all I ever believed about Him, and would never, never forgive Him for what He had done to me.

"It was some years later that I confessed to Nell what I had done. She was shocked, and pleaded for the rest of her life for me to change my way of thinking. Last night, things came to a climax. I did not bother to go to bed, I just sat in my chair thinking: thinking that, after confessing the error of my ways to Tom King, he had forgiven me, and I felt better. I had told him

I saw no reason why he should forgive me. He said it made him feel better as well, if he did.

"I sat watching the storm, then it occurred to me that, if I forgave God for what He had done to me, I would feel better in mind and soul.

"Suddenly, I heard someone calling outside, "Todd, what about me?" I ignored it at first. Nobody could be outside on a night like this, and only you knew me as Todd, and it was not your voice. But I heard it again, at least twice, "Todd, what about me?"

"Good gracious," I thought, "it's Emily. Jimmie has not arrived back at the cottage." I went to the door and opened it. The wind and rain rushed in. I shouted, "Come in, Emily, come in," but I saw nor heard nobody. I waited, then with extreme effort managed to close the door against the storm. I returned to my chair, mystified. I took a swig of rum and continued to watch the storm illuminate the fens. Then, I had a strange feeling that I was not alone. Surely no one came in when I had the door open. So convinced was I that someone was present, that I walked into the galley to satisfy my curiosity. There was not a soul to be seen. Satisfied, I sat in my chair and dozed off.

"I expect it was a clap of thunder that woke me. Somehow, I had a strange feeling that someone was holding my hand. I remained sitting with my eyes closed, not the slightest bit afraid. It felt comforting. "Todd, you cannot forgive God, you must ask Him to forgive you. Please, Todd, before it's too late." It was Nell's voice. I wanted her to stay. I opened my eyes, but she was gone. Suddenly, I became afraid and trembled. I was alone. A flash of lightening and a crash of thunder shook the boat. I gave vent to my feelings. I shouted through the roof of the cabin, to God, at the top of my voice.

"I have sailed the seven seas, in tempest and in storm. You are not going to scare me into submission now, by claps of thunder and strange voices in the night." I took the rum bottle and raised it to my lips, but did not drink. I decided I would sort out this phenomenon with a clear head, so instead, I made a cup of tea. I waited until I felt composed. There must be a logical answer to the circumstances I had experienced.

"It had been sparked off by me telling you that there was still one to whom I must make amends. That meant forgiving, which was something I found difficult to do. I was then ready to bargain with God. I would forgive Him, and enjoy freedom from my lifetime of remorse. The voice outside may have been a figment of my imagination, but it was real enough to make me open the door. As for the holding of my hand, and the message from Nell, I had, and still have, no explanation, yet I knew from experience that, when it came to debate, she was usually right. I decided I would give her message serious thought.

"The storm gradually moved away and, as the rain came down, it had a calming effect on me. I looked at the clock. It was three in the morning."

Jimmie felt the old man's thumb grip his finger.

"I knew there and then that Todd Summers was about to make the greatest decision of his life. Without any feeling of emotion, I rose from my chair, came into my sleeping quarters and got down on my rickety knees, and said something like, "Almighty and Omnipotent God, I have done battle with You for the greater part of my life. I once loved You, then I hated You.

I once owned You, then disowned You. I once praised You, then cursed You. I once honoured You, then brought dishonour to Your name. I now realise that, while I forsook You, You have never forsaken me. You gave me Nell as a guiding angel for the loss of Moira, and Jimmie for the loss of the baby. You have brought me through illness and shipwreck to this moment of time. I humbly confess defeat. You are more than Conqueror. For the sake of your Son, please forgive me for what I have been to you, and my fellow men. Amen." I don't know how long I remained in that position, Jimmie, but at last I got into bed knowing my life-long battle was over, and that I was at peace with God."

There were a few moments silence.

"Thank you, Jimmie, for listening so patiently. Please would you make me another cup of tea?"

Picking up the two mugs, Jimmie thoughtfully made his way towards the galley. A muffled call caused him to return quickly to find that Skip had slumped forward onto the bed.

He dropped to his knees and lifted his old shipmate gently back onto a pillow. His breathing was very heavy and slow. Jimmie waited a few minutes until it became steadier.

"Will you be alright while I run to the Post Office and get a message off to the doctor?" asked Jimmie.

The reply was very quiet. Skip opened his eyes, "No, Jimmie. I only want a doctor to keep me alive. I don't need one to help me die. Just stay with me, I am on course for running into harbour. You have been a good shipmate, Jimmie, from the very first day I met you."

Jimmie felt the thumb of Skip's mangled hand lose its grip from around his forefinger, then watched his arm drop mechanically to the floor. Skip was dead.

Carefully, Jimmie laid the skipper's gnarled hand over his chest, pulled the blanket up and left him in peace with the world and in peace with his Maker.

Chapter Thirty-one

Jimmie's Final Duty

Later that day, Skip's body was removed to the local mortuary at Hillview Works, Wickford Road. The cremation took place the following week. Jimmie, Emily, Steve Donaghue and a Mr Carter, from Skip's solicitors, were present.

That afternoon, the disposal of Skip's estate was discussed at Jimmie's bungalow. Steve Donaghue had already taken care of the goat and chickens, and it was agreed that he should keep them. Skip's diddy-box, with contents, were for Jimmie's good pleasure. His books, the papers he had written on Natural History and Ornithology, plus monies and land, were all donated to charities. That evening, as Mr Carter and Jimmie walked to the station, the solicitor asked whether Jimmie was satisfied with the outcome of the Will. Jimmie stopped in his tracks.

"Sir, if you are inferring that I was expecting financial gain, I can soon put you right. The alteration to Mr Summers' Will in 1923 was with my full approval, as you are well aware. Other than his books, his estate was left to me if I were still living. I made it plain on my return to England that I only wanted the person, not the pence. Therefore I am satisfied with the execution of the Will, sir."

"I meant no offence, Mr Brown, by my question. You only confirmed to me the man your friend described, and I truly sympathise with you on your loss."

Ten days after the cremation, Jimmie sat with Emily, enjoying afternoon tea on their verandah.

"Conditions this evening should be ideal," he said. "I will go and see if I can find some thrift, then all will be ready."

At seven o'clock exactly, Jimmie made his way to the jetty. Under his arm, he carried a shallow whicker basket, about fifteen inches in diameter. In the centre, lay Skip's tarred bowler, and beneath that lay his ashes with a lock of Moira's hair that Jimmie had found in the diddy-box. The whole was surrounded by thrift and sea lavender. He took his place in the dinghy and placed the floral tribute in the stern. Emily gave a wave.

The mission on which he was now embarking would be his benefactor's last wish, one which came as a pleasant surprise. He pulled away from the jetty. It was a neep tide, so would not be hard to row against. He turned the sharp bend in the river and headed for the mainstream, some three-quarters of a mile away.

The evening was calm and still. The only sound he could hear was the plying of the oars into the water. It was just as Skip would have wished. The sudden scrambling of a cow onto the bank on the Battlesbridge side attracted Jimmie's attention. Soon there were six cows abreast. They lowered their heads almost to the ground, as in deep meditation. Some three hundred feet along the Woodham bank, ten cows and two calves of Farmer Lewin's herd stood like sentinels. They were lowing quietly, as though trying to tell

Jimmie they understood.
A little further, sheep chewing cud on the saltings rose slowly to their feet to face the lonely oarsman in silent reverence. Jimmie raised his head in wonder. There, behind the sheep on the sea wall, some ten to fifteen rabbits sat on their haunches, their forepaws held closely together, as though in the spirit of prayer. Even the sea birds, flying overhead, changed their course and glided silently down, almost onto the floral tribute, as though paying their respects to the one who, over the years, tended and nurtured their sick and wounded.
From the time of Skip's death in the cabin, Jimmie had shown no signs of visible emotion. He was not a hard-hearted man. He had told himself he accepted the fact of death. Skip had certainly experienced a hard and difficult life, but he had died a contented man, therefore he saw no reason to shed tears.
He rested a while upon the oars. The scene he was now witnessing on this quiet summer's day, he realised, could be repeated any evening, but tonight it was as though it was the final rehearsal.

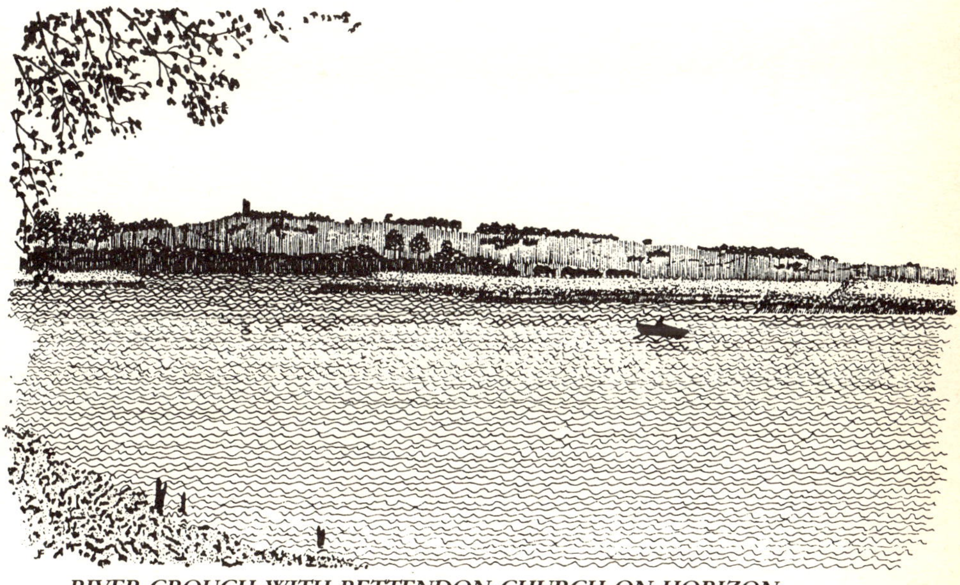

RIVER CROUCH WITH RETTENDON CHURCH ON HORIZON

He searched his thoughts. Skip, who had sailed the old 'Maywell' up this very river as far back as 1870, who had traded with the few locals, and had then decided to settle down as a hermit and naturalist on the fen in 1901, was now departing the area, almost unknown and certainly unmourned, except by Steven, Emily and himself. It seemed, in some ways, a little ungracious.
But now it appeared that the very creation on which he had devoted his life was reverently paying its respects.
He was well aware that Skip, throughout his life, had shown little devotion to his fellow man, and during the last couple of weeks, he had come to

understand a little of the man's mental conflict. It was apparent that, other than Moira and Aunt Nell, he alone was the only person to whom Skip had expressed any form of love or appreciation.
With the sun dropping in the western sky, silhouetting Rettendon church on the high ground, the flowing tide reached its peak, then stayed in its motion, before receding. Not a human being or boat was in sight, and it seemed an idyllic moment for quiet reflection. Around him lay the saltings, clothed in thrift and sea lavender. The silent sheep and cows, even the rabbits, looked on. No better setting could be provided for Jimmie to relieve his pent-up emotions. He looked at the hard-topped bowler. "I am well aware that you are not under there, Skip, I am well aware that you are not in the ashes, but where I believe you to be, I will surely follow."
The words came from a broken-hearted man. For a few moments, his thoughts returned to the night when, in the little crutched bedroom in Burnham, he had cried for joy because he was the happiest boy to leave the London slums.
Tonight he was unable to prevent himself crying again, because of the man who had meant everything to him. Tears dropped unchecked into the cupped hands supporting his bowed head. Slowly, the tide turned, and Jimmie felt the boat being caught up with the ebb. He slipped the oars into the rowlocks and pulled away into the mainstream, past the Hullbridge causeway and up level with Brickfield Wharf.
The barge, 'Athena' was berthed alongside, but no sign of life appeared on deck. Jimmie stowed the oars and drifted with the tide. Taking the basket, he lowered it reverently onto the water, and stood silently watching as the swirling river carried its burden to the open sea.
A lone seagull swooped low over the last tribute, then downstream like an escort to the unknown.

For some fourteen years, Jimmie and Emily shared their days between Brentwood and the now-called South Woodham. They watched as the village slowly developed, and poultry farms grew to cover every available free space. By the late 'thirties', eleven small shops dotted the village, plying for trade from the five to six hundred residents. Five churches now catered for their spiritual needs, but two pubs still allayed their thirst. Two cobblers repaired their soles and two garages replaced the blacksmith. A number of village builders sought to expand and maintain the ever-increasing array of huts and houses built in the most outlandish places.
By 1928, a three-class primary school had been erected in the Hullbridge Road. The eleven to fourteen-year-olds took the train to Battlesbridge, and then walked the mile or so to Rettendon school. It was disputed by parents as to whether this journey was more hazardous than that to Hullbridge. Because of the length of the 8.40 train, which was a through train to Liverpool Street, the children would get into the rear coaches and then jump from the compartment onto the railway track at Battlesbridge. After that, they had to negotiate the turnpike crossing, which was becoming notorious for accidents.
In South Woodham, a Women's Institute Hall and Smallholders' Hall, the pride of the Essex villages, competed to provide entertainment. Gradually,

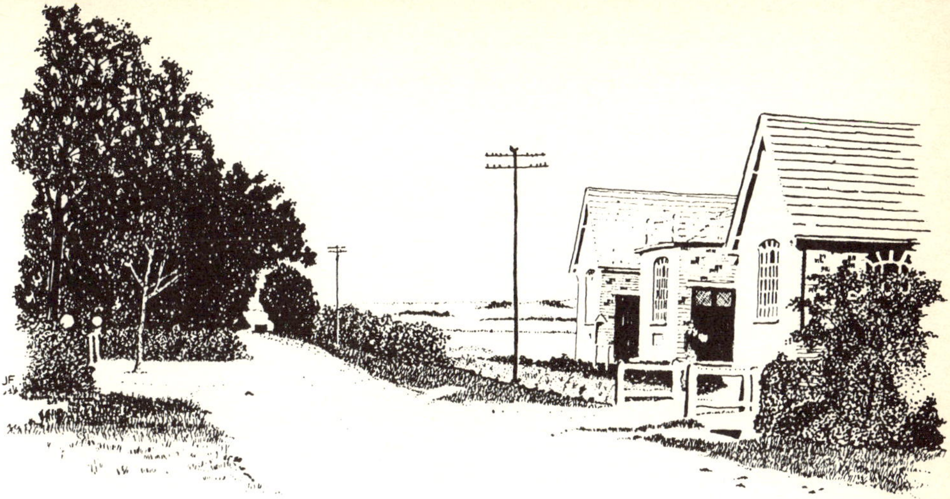

THE SMALLHOLDERS HALL, HULLBRIDGE ROAD

motor cars replaced the horse and trap, and by the early 'thirties, electricity replaced the paraffin lamp and the candle.

While the river still ebbed and flowed, it carried or provided a different way of life. The barges gradually decreased, until it became a rare occasion to see the red sails floating over the green fields. Small pleasure yachts, motor boats, even speed boats came - the quiet river had turned into a rush of man against the tide.

The little rutted track called Hullbridge Road became surfaced. Ditches were piped, and concrete kerbs replaced grass verges. Then the poultry farms decreased, and local farmers did not bother to plough. Aeroplanes buzzed overhead, and on a summer's night, Jimmie and Emily would watch as countless searchlights stabbed the sky, seeking to pin-point the impendent invader. This was but a rehearsal for war.

Over the years, they observed the independent attitude that had grown between the parent village of Woodham Ferrers and its offshoot, South Woodham. This had now become self-contained. Its train service and limited bus service, along with the advent of motor cars, more bicycles, and local businesses, had changed the days when residents of the area were dependent on the village on the hill for their existence.

The annual August bank holiday carnival and fete brought the divided villages together, not exactly as the return of a long lost son, but more in a spirit of competitiveness, and in the desire to get even over their petty differences. This often became apparent in the judging of sports and exhibits.

August bank holiday Monday, 1939, was marred by the rumblings and movements of troops and tanks on the Continent. The whole country was living on borrowed time, and already many local lads had been called into the militia.

Jimmie decided he would take a walk along the sea wall to the Hullbridge ferry, cross over for a drink, then make his way home. He had lost the desire to visit the local fete.

He sat for a rest on the round brick tunnel shaft, smoking his pipe. Youngsters were swimming and paddling. Men were sailing their little pleasure boats, the sails fluttering in the breeze. The whole atmosphere gave relief from the present political situation. Dick Hymas was having a heyday, rowing hikers and cyclists to and fro. The scene was all so different, thought Jimmie. Even the old Anchor Inn, which had been devastated by fire in 1936, had been replaced by a fine new building facing the river. But new polished counters and comfortable furnishings had no real attraction for him. When the opportunity arose he walked to the water's edge and shook hands with Dick.

"Can I take you over now, Jimmie? I'm sure there will be someone who will give you a welcome in our new pub."

"No, Dick, it's not for me. Will you please remember me to any I knew," he said, handing Dick a pound note. "Share a drink with any I know, for old time's sake."

They shook hands again. Jimmie took one last glance up and down the river, and made his way along the Hullbridge Road.

To passers-by, he was but an old man. No-one would ever know his love of the river that had for him been a lifetime's experience. He would, with Skip, soon pass into obscurity, and men would know of neither their coming nor going.

Eventually, Jimmie and Emily moved to Walton-on-the-Naze, on the Essex coast. Jimmie grieved at the appalling loss of life caused by a war, unexperienced in kind before. The beastly atrocities, the helplessness of women and children against a wicked tyrant were too awful to bear. Emily died, and life became lonelier.

The war ended, and once more Jimmie could sleep in peace and watch the children play on the sands. August, 1947, saw an endless stream of visitors and Sunday School treats. It was a bumper year. He took his deck chair to his favourite spot, and settled down. A group of children burrowed deep into the sand nearby. 'South Woodham S.S.' was the notice pinned on their banner.

"Where do you come from?" Jimmie asked, expecting 'South Woodham' in reply.

"We come from Wapping, Mister."

It sparked off a lifetime's memories as he watched the children enjoy their day. With his newspaper laid across his face, he dropped off again to sleep.

"Come on, Jimmie, they have all gone home. Now it's your turn."

The deck chair collector always left him until last. He lifted the paper, and tapped him on the head.

"Wakey! Wakey!"

For Jimmie, the collector's action meant nothing. For the collector, it meant a shock.

Jimmie Brown, ex-slum boy, ex-barge boy, ex-sea captain, now eighty-one years of age, was dead.

Epilogue

August 1947

"Where is South Woodham Ferrers?"
The enquirer was a lad of some fifteen years old.
"I'm not sure, David," was his mother's reply, "but I've a feeling it's near Chelmsford, in Essex. What makes you ask that question?"
"Father said I can accompany him tomorrow. He has a special task to execute, and requires my help. There must be water there, as it necessitates taking the dinghy."
Father and son arrived at their destination at about seven-fifteen the next evening, having followed a detailed map. The last mile had required travelling down a narrow lane and over a level crossing, then finally surmounting a large hump in the road. They found themselves on a stoney beach, confronted by a tidal river some four to six hundred feet wide.
Getting from the car, they spread the map on the bonnet to clarify their position. Pointing across the river, father suggested, "that would be the village of Hullbridge. That is the Anchor Inn, facing us. The old planking and posts must be an old wharf, but I cannot see the brickfields."
Looking further afield, he saw the flint tower that was marked, and another wharf edge out into the river and, a little further downstream, another wooden jetty.
"It would appear, David, that the brickfields have disappeared, but this is definitely our appointed place of mission."
David could wait no longer.
"Father, will you please tell me why we have come to this desolate spot? Why all the secrecy? Are you seeking to dispose of me?"
"No, David, nothing like that. Solicitors get some extraordinary duties to perform throughout their careers, and this evening's task is a first one off for me."
"That may be so, father, but may I also tell you that solicitors have a happy knack of talking without telling you anything. So what are we here for?"
"Yes, David, you are quite right, I appreciate your comments. In the box on the rear seat of the car we have the ashes of a certain Jimmie Brown, who died recently. He requested that they be committed secretly, and without fuss, to the waters of the River Crouch, near the brick wharf, at the ebbing of the tide, as near as reasonable to eight in the evening. That precisely is our task, and now we must wait until the tide turns, which should be at seven-fifty, according to the River Authority."
They untied the dinghy and settled it in the water, placed the box in the stern, then waited at the water's edge.
Their journey from London had been hampered by violent storms, and secretly David's father did not fancy being on the river under such conditions. Fortunately, the rain had eased as they approached South Woodham, and the evening sun cast long shadows through the breaks in the clouds.

Slowly, the flowing tide eased, and man and boy watched the ceaseless miracle of the changing tide.

"This is the moment, David. You are oarsman."

With a push of the oar they headed downstream. As they approached the old wharf, David stayed the oars and held the dinghy against the tide. From the box, his father removed a small whicker basket, made by the deceased especially for the occasion. It contained the white cap of a captain of the Merchant Navy and a crumpled water colour of a barge. Beneath, lay his ashes, and on top, an illuminated card, beautifully written in Old English. 'Today I follow the course set out before me by my beloved Skipper, Benefactor and Friend. Jimmie.'

Reverently, the basket was raised and placed on the water. From a piece of paper, the words were read aloud. "These last earthly remains of the said Jimmie Brown we commit to the waters of his beloved river, to be carried by their endless ebb and flow to the oceans, and resting places of the countless number of his fellow seafarers. Amen."

As David's father rowed back, his only remark was that, to his knowledge, not a living soul had witnessed what they had done.

"Apparently, that is how he wanted it."

"The only living thing I saw was a seagull escorting it downstream," said David.

They reloaded the dinghy onto the car and took one last look at the river. Dusk was falling fast, and they were wanting to get away from the solitary spot.

As they waited at the gates of the level crossing in the village, David asked, "What do you know about Jimmie Brown and his skipper, father?"

"Virtually nothing David. He was a client of the firm and I was given the task to do because I had a boat. Of the Skipper I know nothing at all. But who knows, perhaps one day someone will put pen to paper and write about them."

The gates swung back and as they drove on they both said,
"Goodbye, South Woodham Ferrers."

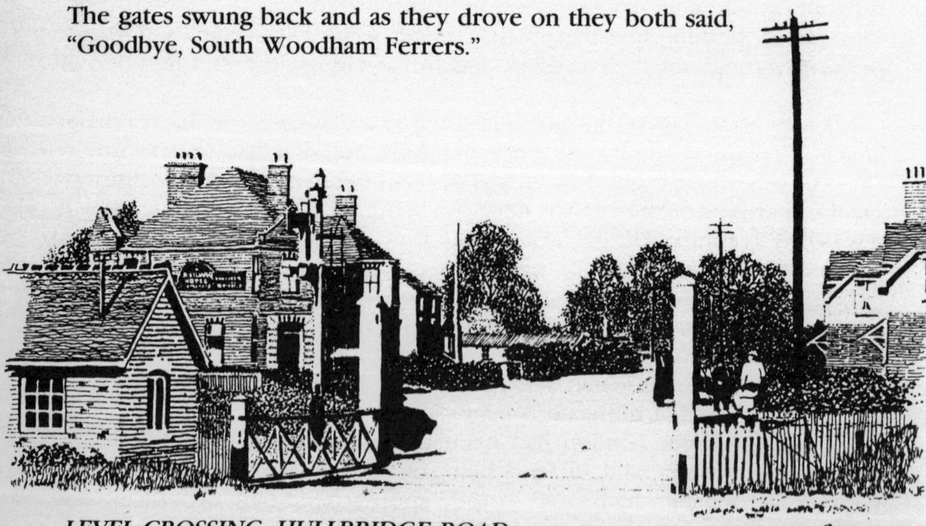

LEVEL CROSSING, HULLBRIDGE ROAD

The Personalised Consultation in Aromatherapy

of related interest

Integrating Clinical Aromatherapy in Palliative Care
Carol Rose
Foreword by Rhiannon Lewis
ISBN 978 1 83997 160 0
eISBN 978 1 83997 161 7

Aroma, Aromatherapy and Trauma
Helen Nagle-Smith
ISBN 978 1 80501 279 5
eISBN 978 1 80501 280 1

Working with Unusual Essential Oils
Helen Nagle-Smith
Foreword by Jennifer Peace Rhind
ISBN 978 1 80501 179 8
eISBN 978 1 80501 180 4

Aromatherapy and Women's Mental Health
An Evidence-Based Guide to Support Emotional Wellbeing
Pam Conrad PGd, BSN, RN, CCAP
ISBN 978 1 83997 624 7
eISBN 978 1 83997 625 4

The Personalised Consultation in Aromatherapy

A PRACTITIONER GUIDE

Annie Prince

Foreword by Rhiannon Lewis

Illustrations by T.M. Prince

SINGING DRAGON

LONDON AND PHILADELPHIA

First published in Great Britain in 2025 by Singing Dragon,
an imprint of Jessica Kingsley Publishers
Part of John Murray Press

1

The Presence 5 practices on pp.32–33 from Zulman, D.M., Haverfield, M.C., Shaw, J.G. *et al.* 2020 "Practices to Foster Physician Presence and Connection With Patients in the Clinical Encounter" has been reproduced with kind permission from Dr Zulman and JAMA.

The CARE Measure Report on pp.34–35 has been reproduced with kind permission from Dr Stewart Mercer © Dr Stewart Mercer 2004.

The extracts from *Hydrosols: The Next Aromatherapy* (2001) beginning p.122 have been reproduced with kind permission from Suzanne Catty.

A CIP catalogue record for this title is available from the
British Library and the Library of Congress

ISBN 978 1 80501 146 0
eISBN 978 1 80501 147 7

Printed and bound in Great Britain by CPI Group (UK)

Jessica Kingsley Publishers' policy is to use papers that are natural, renewable and recyclable products and made from wood grown in sustainable forests. The logging and manufacturing processes are expected to conform to the environmental regulations of the country of origin.

Singing Dragon
Carmelite House
50 Victoria Embankment
London EC4Y 0DZ

www.singingdragon.com

John Murray Press
Part of Hodder & Stoughton Limited
An Hachette UK Company

The authorised representative in the EEA is Hachette Ireland,
8 Castlecourt Centre, Dublin 15, D15 XTP3, Ireland (email: info@hbgi.ie)

For Ted

My Anam Cara

"In this love you are understood as you are without mask or pretension"

JOHN O'DONOHUE

Contents

Foreword

The therapeutic encounter in complementary therapies is built on a foundation of core qualities that ensure the safety and effectiveness of the treatment itself. They provide the space and opportunity for expression, transformation and deep healing that, in the context of an aromatherapy session, are further enhanced and facilitated by essential oils coupled with therapeutic touch techniques. These core qualities foster a positive healing environment and contribute to the overall success of the aromatic intervention.

This text details and develops the core elements of the personalised aromatherapy treatment and is written by an experienced aromatherapist who has honed her own approach through intensive studies coupled with life experience delivering care in the sacred space of the therapy room and bedside. Annie Prince has trod the privileged aromatic path over many years in the company of clients and has witnessed the transformative power of aromatic interventions when all the core qualities are aligned within the therapeutic space. She has understood the importance of marrying the intangible with the intelligible and uses these insights to weave an aromatic synergy of client-focused care.

This book is therefore about presence, connection, empathy and meaningful encounters for priming and delivering safe, effective care. It is about communication, respect, intentional practice and the importance of being fully present and focused on the needs of the Other. It is about helping the client to reconnect with themselves and with nature to find solace and space for resilience and restoration. It is also about the sanctity, stillness, space and beauty of the therapeutic encounter, the importance of a heart-centred approach and the requirement of active, compassionate listening. In an age of virtual connections, it reminds us of the privilege and necessity of the face-to-face therapeutic encounter as central to true transformation.

All these core foundational qualities need to be cultivated by the

aromatherapist and implemented in every therapeutic interaction. They require awareness, sensitivity and practice to open the doors and opportunities for healing. Teaching others about the therapeutic encounter requires insight and sensitivity grounded through longstanding experience of care delivery. These skills are, like this book, honed over time and cannot be rushed.

Most therapists setting out on their aromatherapy journey require guidance, coaching and encouragement, with clear examples of good practice of the art of aromatherapy. This sensitive aspect of aromatherapy can often be overlooked or skimmed over in the rush to acquire knowledge and tangible skills through online learning or through fast-track aromatherapy education. Yet becoming an aromatherapist is more than simply the acquisition of knowledge and skills; it demands that we are able to truly meet the person in the privileged therapeutic space in such a way that there are no limits to their healing potential.

For experienced therapists, there is also a need for reflective practice to recalibrate, remember and realign with the true power of an effective aromatherapy intervention. This book is therefore for all aromatherapists no matter how far along they are on their aromatic path.

Lastly, this book is also about authenticity, kindness, sensitivity and grace – all qualities that for me epitomise the author herself who has journeyed for so many years in the field of healing minds, bodies and souls. This personal text reflects her own journey and the insights she has wisely gathered into her aromatic basket along the way. Each insight shared is a wise gift, a precious jewel and a tool for reflection and healing. Annie Prince has also done what many authors have not achieved – she has nurtured, harvested and distilled down her life experiences and learnings into this succinct text that you hold in your hands. Nothing is superfluous. Every word and phrase are to be savoured and reflected upon. I am honoured to write this foreword.

Rhiannon Lewis, clinical aromatherapist, director of Essential Oil Resource Consultants and host of the International Clinical Aromatherapy Network

Acknowledgements

It gives me great pleasure to acknowledge the following people who have had an influence on this book and on my life.

The former may never have seen the light of day were it not for the prompting and encouragement from Rhiannon Lewis, who said to me one day, "I think you have a book in you." Rhiannon has this amazing ability to see potential and to push people out of their comfort zones. As a guiding light in the world of clinical aromatherapy I am fortunate to have studied with her on several occasions including in her beautiful Provencal home, an experience I shall never forget. I continue to learn indirectly from her through the portals of the Botanica Conference Series, the Essence of Clinical Aromatherapy (ECA) Seminars and the International Clinical Aromatherapy Network (ICAN) platform, all of which are spearheaded and directed by her. So thank you Rhiannon for your tireless work for our profession, your support and your knowledge. You are an aromatherapy rock star.

It is fitting, too, to acknowledge my earliest teachers on this healing path: Barbara Allpress and Sharon Erdrich who introduced me to the art and science of aromatherapy, and to the wonderful Dr Sridhar Maddela who made the study of anatomy and physiology so engaging.

I honour, too, all the authors from many disciplines referenced in this text. Thank you for the wisdom I have gained from you. Special mention must be made of Peter Holmes, Gabriel Mojay, Felicity Warner and Robbi Zeck. Your work has been an inspiration to me when working with the emotions.

Special mention to Suzanne Catty for her generosity in permitting me to include her research on the benefits of hydrosols. Thank you.

I am indebted, too, to the work of Doctors Abraham Verghese, Bernard Lown, Robin Youngson and Lissa Rankin whose belief in taking the time to get to know the patient as a fellow unique human being,

treating them with respect and compassion, has become a cornerstone of my practice. I salute your work.

To Candace Pert, your book *The Molecules of Emotion* has become my bible. To Sherry Turkle and Johann Hari, who eloquently document the importance of connection in our modern world and the need to reclaim conversation, I love your books.

I must mention also Carole Guyett and Vivienne Campbell, who through their herbal teachings changed how I view the natural world and deepened my connection to the plants.

I honour the work of John O'Donohue whose exquisite writings uplift the spirit and help me find beauty in our tortured world.

I honour the memory of my mother, Mary, one of the best teachers I ever met. I remember how you took an interest in each student, encouraging them to take pride in their appearance, to believe in their abilities and self worth. As a home science teacher the work that your falsely labelled "less able students" produced for your Xmas display was tantamount to entering a deluxe delicatessen. You were a strong, independent, resilient woman ahead of your time and you walked through the world with grace. I carry your values in my heart as well as your love of gardening and cooking.

To my dear father, Jim, one of nature's gentlemen, who never failed to believe in me, you taught me the value of Irish hospitality. I can still hear, ringing in my ears, your words "you are heartily welcome" whenever a guest crossed the threshold of our home. Home was a sacred place.

To my children, Sean, Mark, Beth, Jo, Amy, Patrick and Ruth, you are a complete joy. Fiercely intelligent and quick witted, it's impossible to get a word in edgeways when you are all together, but that's what I love about you. You are thinkers and you challenge my thinking and keep me on my toes. Most of all you are good, caring people, and for that I am most proud.

For my six grandsons, Thomas, Jacob, Lucas, Jesse, Jack and Carlos, you give me hope for the future. Your innocence, sense of wonder and connection with nature as young children is heartwarming. Spending time with you is a treasured gift. You help me to slow down, to be in the moment, to be kind and patient. You make me a better mother.

To Sarah Hamlin, Claire Robinson and all of the editing and production team at Singing Dragon, thank you for your dedication and the opportunity to publish with you. Special thanks to Carole McMurray for her unfailing encouragement and for being such a pleasure to deal with.

Thank you to photo lithographer Peter Deutschle of Spectragraphics, who prepared Terry's drawings for prepress.

To the clients who have shared their stories and trusted me with their healing journey I can only say a profound thank you. It is a privilege, a responsibility and a humbling experience to have worked with you.

And last but not least to Ted (Terry Prince), my lovely man, thank you for your beautiful drawings. Melding our passions of art and aromatics in this written text has been very special to me.

Annie

Introduction: A "Scentimental" Journey

My earliest scent memory is of freshly cut grass in the field opposite our house in Clontarf, Dublin, Ireland. I would have been about three years old. Instantly I am transported back to the land of my birth, from which I would be uprooted at the age of six when my father moved to England in search of work. I remember distinctly how I hated this move, even down to the accents. Everything was foreign to me; I didn't belong there and my sense of self was shattered. It was the most traumatic event of my life and gave me a deep appreciation of the plight of the emigrant.

For the next dozen or so years the memory that predominates is the anticipation and joy of returning to Ireland for six weeks every summer to spend time with my mother's family in Mayo and Galway, and the scents that fuel this are the smell of the sea when we boarded the Liverpool to Dublin ferry and the fragrance of newly mown hay on a summer's day on my uncles' farms...

At the age of 18 I attended University College Dublin to study modern languages and during this time spent a while in France and Spain as an au pair. I remember the vibrancy of life in Madrid, the Rastro market, the Prado museum, the smell of paella, gazpacho and tortilla, all of which I learned to make, and in particular the smell of 4711 Eau de Cologne by Muelhens: a citrusy fragrance with a blend of a dozen or so essential oils, refreshing, uplifting and used in the children's grooming.

Looking after four children under eight in France was good training for the large brood I would subsequently have. The very strong scent memory I have is of the pine trees in the mountains of Barcelonnette and the Cote d'Azur and of course the staples of French life, exquisite food, baguettes, croissants, divine cheeses, wine and herbs. That's when I fell in love with France and returned as an English assistant to the Lycée de Jeunes Filles in Albi, spending a year immersed in Gallic culture,

sadly spending too much time hanging out with other English speakers instead of living with a family to become fluent.

I also at one point spent time on my own spiritual quest working with the sick in Lourdes, a place of pilgrimage for Roman Catholics. I remember the smell of the baths deemed to have miraculous healing waters, the damp misty air over the hills, the aromas of the local patisserie and the fragrance of frankincense in the thurible as it swung backwards and forwards during the religious ceremonies. Little did I know what an important part *Boswellia sacra* (Frankincense) would play later on in my life. This experience gave me an insight into the suffering of others and the myriad ways we seek comfort.

After qualifying as a teacher I spent three years as a new bride teaching in Nassau, the Bahamas, where the smells were of the sea, sand, sunscreen, chalk in stifling hot classrooms, gin happy hours, mojitos, pina coladas and conch salad saturated in lime juice. My two eldest boys were born there, an interesting experience in itself, being turfed out in 24 hours regardless of the duration or difficulty of the labour and having only a copy of Dr Spock's *Baby and Childcare* book for guidance! Then of course there followed the wonderful baby smells of newborn skin, baby baths and talcum powder. Experiencing the expat culture of Nassau gave me an appreciation of different ethnicities, and teaching fuelled my interest in the diversity of human beings and the human condition. I have always loved people's stories, which would serve me well in later life as an aromatherapist specialising in dealing with those suffering from mental, emotional stress.

Making the decision to come and live in New Zealand, an emigrant once again, was not easy at the time but one I certainly don't regret. The next 12 years saw me step back from the educational world to bring up my family of seven beautiful children. Pregnancy was a time of great joy for me; a ferocious maternal instinct was at play. I was never healthier and craved a raw food diet. I learned a lot about nutrition and my experiences leave me well placed to work with pregnant women.

During this time my interest in natural medicines was awakened, namely in homeopathy, herbs, flower essences and essential oils. Arnica was a well-used remedy with my fearless brood, who had a third of an acre of garden with tall trees and all sorts of hazardous rope bridges and so on to explore. An interest too in self-development, life purpose, personality types and mental, emotional, physical, spiritual connection was fuelled by my avid love of reading. Studying the enneagram (a model

of the human psyche taught as nine interconnected personality types) and reading John O'Donohue's works had a profound influence on my thinking and interaction with others.

A love of nature and gardening has always been central to my life. The aromas of the New Zealand bush are earthy and unique from our native trees such as *Leptospermum scoparium* (Manuka), *Kunzea ericodes* (Kanuka) and the majestic *Agathis australis* (Kauri), to name a few. To me there is a sacredness and tranquillity in this forest space respected and well understood by the local Maori. It was to provide a stunning backdrop for my treatments a few years later after qualifying as an aromatherapist.

In 1990 another milestone and traumatic event took place in my life when my mother died in the west of Ireland and four months later my father. It was a catalyst for change and I felt a deep connection to my roots, resulting in the creation of Ballyglass House, my artisan bakery, named after a favourite uncle and aunt's house in County Mayo where I spent many a happy holiday and weekend escaping university life. The initial idea was to make Irish soda bread, not commercially produced in New Zealand, but the business soon expanded to 12 breads, a porter cake, whiskey cake and my mother's famous Irish plum pudding which took ten hours to make. She was a home science teacher and her spirit filled that business.

So for ten years the aromas that filled the commercial kitchen in our home were those of yeast rising, freshly baked bread, dried fruits soaked in Guinness and whiskey and the smell of newly minted labels, boxes and ribbons, as everything had to be beautifully presented. I have a strong sense of the aesthetic. We supplied the top restaurants in Auckland and sent our puddings to Air New Zealand first class, David Jones in Australia and Huka Lodge in Taupo, a favourite of the late Queen Elizabeth II. Our products were all handmade, high quality and we appeared on television, in *Cuisine* magazine and won two major food awards including the Massey University Enterprise award. My mother would have been proud.

However, the glory was not to last as my health deteriorated, resulting ironically in a coeliac diagnosis! All that making and eating delicious home-made breads was nearly killing me. And so I stopped, returned to teaching for a while and pondered the future.

My overwhelming desire was to do something that nurtured people. Enter the Abbaye Notre-Dame de Sénanque in Gordes where the scent of the lavender fields imprinted itself on my psyche and never left. I had

found my new path; came home to study for the Diploma in Aromatherapy and 16 years later I am still studying. I think I have a slightly obsessive-compulsive nature. Whatever interests me is what I study ad nauseam. Running my artisan bakery, it was all about entrepreneurship, marketing, packaging, bread making, health requirements, nutrition. Teaching is all about logic, lesson planning, learning styles, enjoyment, connection. Now my bedside table is stacked with books on essential oils, anatomy and physiology, the mind–body connection, biophilia, human connection and such like.

Much self-directed study followed the diploma, along with classes in Australia and Provence with the incomparable Rhiannon Lewis, of Essential Oil Resource Consultants, delving deeper into the chemistry of essential oils and the multiple interfaces of application. I was asked to return to Wellpark College of Natural Therapies to teach the Diploma of Aromatherapy, which I did for two years, rewriting it, incorporating the knowledge I had gained overseas.

As you can imagine the scents that filled, and continue to fill, this part of my life were exquisite, taken from the multitude of essential oils from leaves, flowers, fruits, resins, seeds, woods. Of course *Lavandula angustifolia* (Lavender true) figured strongly but also favourites such as *Picea mariana* (Black spruce), *Cistus ladaniferus* (Rock rose), *Citrus medica* (Lime), *Boswellia sacra* (Frankincense) and *Rosa damascena* (Damask rose), to name but a few. A whole new world opened up to me in the shape of anatomy, physiology, chemistry, botany and the magical world of perfume.

In 2010, while meandering around the elegant and expensive Place des Vosges, in the heart of the Marais district in Paris, I suddenly found myself outside an aromatherapist's dream: no. 18, Christian Louis, Maître Parfumeur. An Aladdin's cave with a vast array of shimmering bottles beckoned, holding their secrets from the natural world. In the midst of this glorious sanctuary of scent was Christian Louis himself, bursting with energy and passion, brandishing testers, accosting everyone who walked through the door, engaging each one in conversation, scrutinising, interpreting each character through a suggested personalised scent. His desire was to offer "mille et un senteurs" (a thousand and one perfumes) to the world.

For him perfume was an emotional language of truth, to reflect the memories, passions, inspirations, interactions of everyday life. His extraordinary creations paid homage to people as diverse as the Dalai Lama, Carla Bruni and Mozart or celebrated the likes of the abolition of slavery or his beloved Bayonne Rugby Club.

"Bleu Mogador" reflected "the charm of Morrocan Islam" with its bouquet of rose, patchouli, heather, osmanthus flowers and spices.

"Eau de Curé", named after the ancient Gallet parish priest from the walled city of Clairence, exuded aromas of bread, incense, myrrh, orange flower, honey and musk.

"Eau de Tobago" for men, with blond tobacco, leather, tangerine, cedarwood, nutmeg and musk, was described as "perfume of a Caribbean adventurer".

"Hegoak for Women and Men" had exotic and enigmatic descriptions such as: "Head notes, first world blond tobacco, heather, mandarin, black pepper; Heart notes, second world lily, green leaves of the violet plum; Base notes, symbolist binary." What's all that about?

Children were not forgotten in this aromatic world: "Potxolo Parfum Enfant", with berries, citrus, sandalwood and musk, was "reminiscent of acid drop sweets".

Not all was fanciful or weird. "Eaux d'Euskadi" for women was one of my favourites, evoking the green countryside of the Basque region. It was floral and green with hyacinth, mayflower, juniper, dogrose, grapefruit, green tea, lemon, pimento and black pepper. And so Euskadi became my Parisian scent. What memories does this little bottle hold for me? The long awaited moment at Gare du Nord to hug my eldest sons after three years and to meet my beautiful new Iranian daughter in law; the joy of Paris, its art, its history, its culture, its way of being, the joy of sharing it all with my *anam cara* (the Gaelic term for "soul friend", reflecting a deep and lasting bond between two people).

And what about the exquisite musky heady scent of the VIP perfume "Magdalena" with notes of damask rose, violet, iris root, arabian myrrh, olibanum, patchouli and vetiver, described as "suggesting memories of an encounter"? Its perfume resides in a cemetery in Kilconly, Co. Galway, in a porcelain box with two letters, photographs of my children and grandchildren and laid to rest at the graveside of my dear parents who had passed away 20 years before, without me. "Magdalena" therefore will forever remind me of that sunny autumn day, Wednesday 29 September 2010, when I went to pay homage to the people who gave me life and every pore oozed with grief suppressed for two decades in the cells of my being.

I treasure these scents and the memories they hold for me. I treasure the world of aromatherapy.

And so here I am today working in my own business, treating clients, making products and teaching small groups about the real meaning and power of aromatherapy. Teaching runs in my genes. There are a lot of us in my extended family.

My greatest love and passion is conducting aromatherapy massage treatments as it combines so many skills and embodies deep human connection in a unique way, resulting in profound health benefits.

You might wonder why I have bothered to tell you about my "scentimental" journey to becoming a clinical aromatherapist. Well, I have a belief that age and life experience are great assets when it comes to treating clients. As this book will illustrate, it requires great listening skills, knowledge and empathy to be a successful therapist. I would hope that the many diverse experiences, joys, sorrows and challenges that have filled my life have made me a better person, a little wiser, more compassionate and understanding, better prepared to deal with the emotional/mental stresses endured by so many in today's world.

This book is intended as a practitioner guide for serious aromatherapists. Its central tenet is the importance of the therapeutic relationship and the personalised conversation, at the heart of, and crucial to, the success of any treatment. It incorporates also the fundamentals you need to know to practise well and includes my own massage sequences for the head, hands and feet, invaluable for those not trained in massage but keen to incorporate a simple form of aromatic touch into their practice. They are structured in a way that is easy to learn and are extremely effective in inducing a state of deep relaxation and stress release.

I hope you find this book helpful and that it will shine a light on this most exquisite and powerful modality.

Sláinte, Annie

CHAPTER 1

The Need for Resilience in a Post Pandemic World and the Place of Aromatherapy

"A sad soul can kill you quicker, far quicker than a germ"

JOHN STEINBECK[1]

2023 and the world is in crisis. Geopolitical unrest abounds; climate change threatens our very survival and Covid 19 has ripped through the world leaving a trail of death, fear, anxiety and exhaustion. It changed life as we knew it. The world stopped and social isolation compounded our misery.[2]

Loneliness became a serious issue. Loneliness kills and is comparable in its detrimental effects to obesity or smoking cigarettes. More than 58% of Americans, for example, are considered lonely and a report in October 2022 referred to their "battered psyche". Several governments have appointed ministers for loneliness, such is the state of disconnection in our technology dominated world.[3]

Harvard professor Robert Putnam has been studying and documenting the decline of the collective structure and community involvement for decades, leading to social isolation and the shutting of ourselves away in our homes. His book *Bowling Alone: The Collapse and Revival of American Community* is sobering reading.[4]

When asked by social scientists how many close friends they could turn to in a crisis, the answer from the majority of Americans in 2004 was, frighteningly, none.[5]

The biologist E.O. Wilson believed "People must belong to a tribe". Through extensive research on the effects of social isolation and loneliness, psychologist John Cacioppo and colleagues have discovered what

Johann Hari describes in his book *Lost Connections*: "we have become the first humans to ever dismantle our tribes. As a result, we have been left alone on a savanna we do not understand, puzzled by our own sadness."[6]

Beloved author, theologian, poet and philosopher John O'Donohue in his book *Eternal Echoes: Exploring Our Hunger to Belong* states "something within us cries out for belonging" and when we are "cut off from others we atrophy and turn in on ourselves".[7] He suggests that a sense of belonging evokes understanding and the eternal values of truth, goodness, justice, beauty and love. He believes "we have unlearned the grace of presence and belonging" in modern culture and have instead "a gaping emptiness".[8]

Dr Vivek Murthy, Surgeon General of the United States, in his equally sobering book *Together: The Healing Power of Human Connection in a Sometimes Lonely World*, describes the epidemic of loneliness as a public health concern running "like a dark thread" through many issues such as violence, anxiety, depression and addiction.

He calls it the "great masquerader", appearing in various states of anguish such as anger, sadness, fear and despair and resulting in feelings of shame, self doubt, low self esteem and a belief that we are unworthy of being loved.[9] He says "the ability to talk to one another is broken" and "to be a healer you have to learn to listen, to learn, and to love".[10]

Lissa Rankin MD sums it up succinctly when she says, "Loneliness poisons the body."[11]

Add to this the pace of twenty-first-century life and the pressure to succeed, along with the major life traumas of abuse, divorce, bereavement, serious health issues, poverty, unemployment, homelessness and cost of living, endured by so many, then it is hardly surprising that these stresses chip away at our fortitude, undermining our resilience and giving rise to anxiety and depression.

According to the World Health Organization (WHO) more than 280 million people suffer from depression worldwide.[12] In my own country the 2017/2018 New Zealand Public Health Survey revealed that one in six adult New Zealanders would be diagnosed with a mental disorder at some point in their lives.[13] This includes depression, bipolar and anxiety disorders. Shockingly, we have one of the highest youth (15 to 24 years) suicide rates in the developed world.[14]

Taking all of this into account, the need for resilience is indisputable; that ability to adapt when faced with adversity, to mentally and emotionally bounce back from difficult life events.[15] Trauma specialist Bessel van der Kolk describes it simply as "the capacity to face reality".[16]

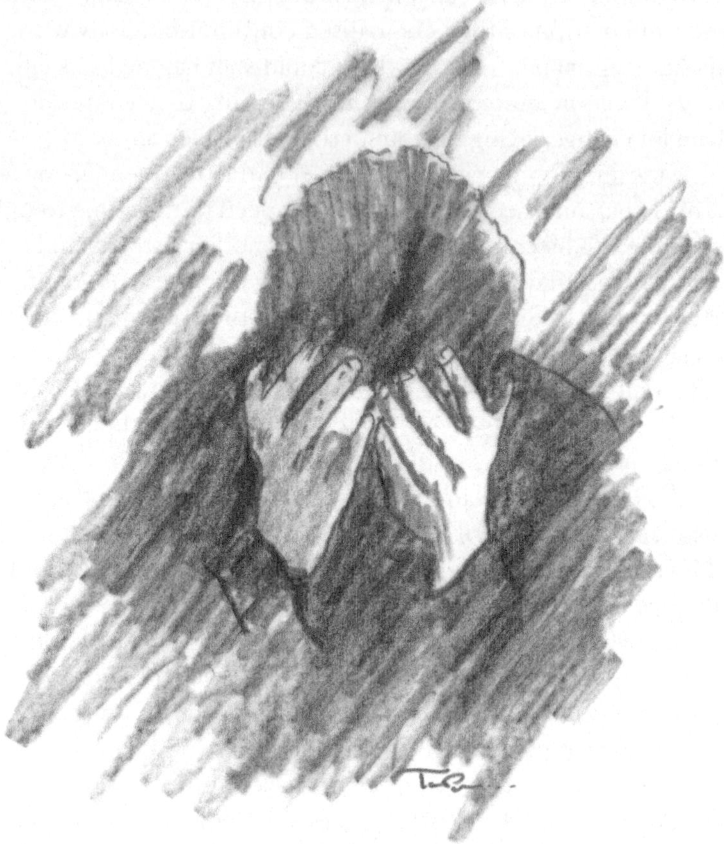

Anguish by T.M. Prince

We have a greater capacity to flourish and to be resilient when the five pillars of holistic wellbeing, mental, emotional, physical, spiritual and social, are in homeostasis.[17]

Where, then, does aromatherapy sit in this complex world and what part can it play in nurturing our resilience?

The answer lies in the fact that aromatherapy is a modality which treats the whole person, addressing just that, the five aspects of wellbeing. We don't shy away from delving into the emotional, mental world of our clients. How could we, with aromas having open access along the olfactory route to the limbic system, seat of memories and emotions? Like it or not, aroma triggers psychological and physiological reactions in the body. "With Aromatherapy, individual human life plays a role; the life story of a woman or a man receives recognition and respect."[18]

The uniqueness and beauty of an aromatherapy massage treatment is the combination of the personalised consultation, body work and bespoke essential oils, each of which could stand alone in its efficacy. The result can be quite profound in the ability to activate the reset button for change, laying the foundation for resilience.

The most important aspect and driver of the treatment, in my opinion, is the personalised consultation. We need to take time to talk to one another, to listen to and validate one another's stories, to honour one another as unique human beings trying to make sense of life. In a world fractured by disconnection from self, others and nature, we need to reclaim conversation.

The renowned cardiologist Professor Bernard Lown believed that the majority of ailments presented to doctors are functional, resulting from the ups and downs of life and often stemming from "an aching heart".[19] How on earth can we ascertain what's troubling people, and subsequently help them, if we don't take time to talk to them?

Lissa Rankin MD poses the challenging question "Without the healing power of listening, loving touch, nurturing care and healing intention, what are we offering patients beyond straight technology?"[20]

The purpose of this book is to delve a little deeper into the therapeutic encounter and the personalised consultation in the context of an aromatherapy massage treatment, and to show how we enlist the power of the mind through talk and access the emotions through bodywork, creating what Pert describes as a "loop of healing".[21] Add to that the use of essential oils tailored to the client's needs and we have a singularly unique and powerful modality to help nurture resilience and build connection in our stressful world.

My hope also is that these words may be a helpful guide to students of aromatherapy to consider how they conduct their clinical treatments and to illustrate for all healthcare practitioners the importance of keeping the client's needs front and centre through taking the time to have a deeply personal conversation.

> There is nothing magical about clinical aromatherapy just as there is nothing magical about essential oils. They work because our sense of smell is our most powerful sense and because our olfactory system is so closely tied to many other important systems in the human body.[22]

During Covid 19, essential oils were powerful tools to help manage stress, insomnia, fatigue, lack of focus and depression.

CHAPTER 2

The Importance of Conversation and Human Connection

> *"Face to face conversation is the most human – and humanizing – thing we do. Fully present to one another, we learn to listen. It's where we develop the capacity for empathy. It's where we experience the joy of being heard, of being understood. And conversation advances self reflection"*
>
> SHERRY TURKLE[1]

When I was teaching the Diploma of Aromatherapy, the students, during their clinicals, were forbidden to hand out intake forms for clients to fill in. Instead they had to engage in a conversation in order to build up trust, empathy and respect and to learn how to monitor body language. They had no shortage of willing participants who thrived in this atmosphere of care and attention.

I feel deeply passionate about this practice, born out of my own experience over the years of always being given a form to fill in, in any healthcare situation, and feeling a profound sense of disconnection between myself and the person to whom I was about to entrust an aspect of my wellbeing.

I vowed as a therapist that I would never do that. The idea that I would say to a client "sit over there and pour your heart and soul on to that piece of paper" for me, a stranger whom you don't even know if you will like, let alone trust or respect, is anathema to me. Why would I do that? Form filling is tedious, loathsome and certainly not conducive to opening one's heart, risking vulnerability. We're human beings. We connect through speech. When did we become so disconnected from one another?

I am a companion on this person's journey and I want to be there from the moment they arrive to the moment they leave. When they have shown sufficient faith in me to come and unburden themselves, surely I need to respect them as a unique human being by giving them my undivided attention in a face to face conversation.

We are a social species. We are wired to connect. According to Maslow's Hierarchy of Needs, love and belonging, the desire for connection and being part of a group, along with food, water and safety, are our most important needs for a fulfilling life.[2]

Maslow's Hierarchy of Needs

Self actualisation

Desire to become the best that one can be.

Esteem

Respect, self esteem, status, recognition, strength, freedom.

Love and belonging

Friendship, intimacy, belonging, sense of connection.

Safety needs

Personal security, employment, resources, health, property.

Physiological needs

Air, water, food, shelter, sleep, clothing, reproduction.

Brené Brown defined connection "as the energy that exists between people when they feel seen, heard and valued; when they can give and receive without judgment; and when they derive sustenance and strength from the relationship".[3]

The 80 year long, and ongoing, Harvard Study of Adult Development, the world's longest study on happiness, revealed the perhaps not surprising truth that the greatest predictor of happiness is the quality of our relationships.

It bears witness to the importance of human connections. Those who are more connected to family, friends and community are happier, healthier and live longer than those who feel less connected to others. The massive global experiment of isolation during the pandemic made it clear that the physical presence of another human being cannot be duplicated by a machine.[4]

Scientist Matthew Lieberman affirms our need to connect as fundamental to our species and states that social pain is as real as physical pain.[5] Sadly, although we are living in a time of great digital connectivity, we are lonelier and more disconnected than ever before. In the words of Johann Hari, "Loneliness hangs over our culture today like a thick smog."[6] Worryingly, it has a profound impact on our mental and physical health, raising levels of the stress hormone cortisol, which can compromise our immune system, causing vascular problems, inflammation, heart disease and an increase in anxiety and depression.[7] Research has shown it is even a predictor of premature death![8]

In her groundbreaking, thought provoking book *Reclaiming Conversation* Sherry Turkle shares her thirty years of research studying the effect of technology on our relationships.[9] She is by no means anti-technology but she is most definitely pro conversation. Without conversation her studies show that "we are less empathic, less connected, less creative and fulfilled".[10] I found it quite disturbing that so many of the students she interviewed were terrified of face to face conversation or even speaking on the phone. Both practices they said left them feeling too vulnerable. Texting and email were their preferred means of communication and many had to be taught how to have a conversation! In the past twenty years a 40% decline in the markers for empathy was seen in college students, linked to the presence of digital communication.

Turkle goes on to say that even a silent phone disconnects us. Its mere presence keeps conversations light, for fear of interruption, and blocks empathic connection.[11] Her views are supported by the research from Yale by Dr Joy Hirsch reported in Neuroscience News:

> Neural signaling during online exchanges was substantially suppressed compared to activity observed in those having face-to-face conversations, researchers found.
>
> The findings were published Oct. 25 in the journal *Imaging Neuroscience*.
>
> "In this study we find that the social systems of the human brain are more active during real live in-person encounters than on Zoom," said Hirsch, the Elizabeth Mears and House Jameson Professor of Psychiatry, professor of comparative medicine and neuroscience, and senior author of the study.
>
> "Zoom appears to be an impoverished social communication system relative to in-person conditions."
>
> Social interactions are the cornerstone of all human societies,

> and our brains are finely tuned to process dynamic facial cues (a primary source of social information) during real in-person encounters, researchers say.[12]

Kevin Kelly goes even further to declare, "Smartphones are the new sugar and fat. They are so potent they can undo us if we don't limit them."[13]

The good news is that Turkle believes we are resilient and that conversation cures. "Speaking and listening with attention are skills. They can be taught."[14]

The great Jewish thinker of the twentieth century, Rabbi Lord Jonathan Sacks, talks about the underrated art of listening and describes it as one of the greatest gifts we can give to another human being in distress. His words are worth repeating:

> It is an act of focused attention. It means being genuinely open to another person, prepared to enter their world, their perspective, their pain. It does not mean that we have a solution to their problem. There are some problems that cannot be solved. They can only be lived through, so that time itself heals the rupture or loss. When we listen, we share the burden so that its weight can be borne. There are times when friendship calls simply for a human presence, a listening ear and an understanding heart, so that soul can unburden itself to soul.[15]

He recounts the story of Viktor Frankl, holocaust survivor and renowned psychiatrist, who spoke on the phone in the middle of the night to a woman contemplating suicide, giving her numerous reasons to live. She did indeed choose to live, but when asked why, she replied that his willingness to listen to her trauma in the middle of the night indicated a world worth living in.

All of this brings me to the importance of the personalised consultation, which is at the core of the therapeutic relationship.

Andrea Pennington MD describes "positive relationships as one of the top ten traits of resilience".[16] Relationships where we feel empathically connected, heard, understood, supported, mirroring back our strengths to encourage resilience.

This relationship between therapist and client, doctor and patient, has been shown over decades of research to be central to the success of any treatment. Often it is the only meaningful relationship where the individual can reveal themselves in all of their totality, in a safe,

nurturing, respectful, non-judgemental and confidential space.[17] Its importance is poignantly and powerfully illustrated by Lissa Rankin MD in her book *Mind over Medicine* where she shares her journey as a physician. She describes herself as an unlikely candidate to research mind, body, spirit medicine having been brought up in a strict methodist home with a rigidly sceptical physician father.

Suffering multiple health issues in her twenties and thirties she eventually succumbed to burnout and had a suicidal breakdown. After years of long shifts, churning out forty patients a day at seven and a half minute intervals, she became completely disillusioned. This was not the kind of medicine she signed up for. She wanted to be a healer, a compassionate listener bringing comfort to her patients. Every day was "chipping away at her integrity" which Harvard doctors now call "moral injury".[18]

She left to get herself well and to delve into why we get sick when the mind is unhealthy and we are disconnected spiritually. She returned to a holistic practice, choosing to spend an hour listening to her patients' stories. She saw that her patients were sick because "They were gut wrenchingly lonely or miserable in their bad relationships, stressed about work, freaked out about their finances, profoundly depressed or suffering from a huge load of unhealed trauma."[19]

She began to see remarkable healing in her patients from longstanding illnesses. She said she hadn't done anything other than "ask good questions and listen with love".[20] She asked questions that dug deep into their personal lives. When she questioned "What's missing from your life?" most of them wept and there was an outpouring of what needed to change.

She healed from her own trauma by working in a fulfilling and heart-centred way and pursued her research into radical remissions. The life changing "aha" moment in her career was a letter from a patient who had wanted to talk to her about an intimate problem but reneged because she saw "her eyes were blank" and she "never let go of the door handle".[21] I can't think of a more powerful symbol for disconnection in the therapeutic relationship than fingers on the door knob ready to usher you out.

She now jokes that she "practises love with a little medicine on the side".[22] She argues that the mind has the power to alter the body's physiology through positive belief, nurturing care from the right healthcare provider, wise life choices in relationships, work, finances, and a fulfilling creative happy life.[23]

Bessel van der Kolk agrees that "feeling listened to and understood changes our physiology; being able to articulate a complex feeling, and having our feelings recognised, lights up our limbic brain and creates an 'aha' moment." He goes on to say, "Silence reinforces the godforsaken isolation of trauma." While it keeps us "dumbfounded, the path out of it is paved with words".[24]

In today's stressful and often lonely world I believe the personalised consultation in aromatherapy, and indeed in any form of healthcare practice, is crucial to alleviating this sense of aloneness that so many feel and most importantly to contributing to successful treatments.

CHAPTER 3

What Do We Mean By the Personalised Consultation?

"The essence of medicine is addressing a human being;
A human being is more than a heart, a lung, an organ that is dysfunctional
A human being is a mind, a soul, a presence"

DR BERNARD LOWN[1]

These insightful and beautiful words from Professor Bernard Lown, renowned medical pioneer in cardiology and Nobel Laureate, speak to the heart of the personalised consultation, which is to find and connect with that unique "presence" for the betterment of the client/patient.

In his inspiring book *The Lost Art of Healing* he stresses the importance of getting to know the patient behind the symptoms and "not concerning oneself with fragmented body parts".[2]

He regards talk as one of the "underrated tools of the physician's armamentarium"[3] and laments the lost art of listening being taken over by technological procedures, thus changing the doctor/patient relationship.[4] He believed that healing began with listening first and foremost to the patient's story and that information gathering was not just about the disease but grasping what was "agitating a patient's mind".[5] What a wonderful phrase: "what is agitating a patient's mind".

His very readable book recounts many of his patients' stories. As an acute observer of body language, if a patient was not responding to treatment he would ask, "What is going on in your life, what are you not telling me?" Invariably there would be a mental or emotional issue which, when resolved, enabled the patient to focus on healing.

In an interview, "The Inner Landscape of Beauty", John O'Donohue expands this view by saying "Our biography is not our identity" and quotes the fourteenth-century German mystic Meister Eckhart as saying, "There's a place in the soul that neither time nor space, nor no created thing can touch," meaning a place where we have never been wounded, where there is still a sureness, a seamlessness, a confidence and a tranquillity. O'Donohue goes on to say that the intention of prayer, spirituality and love is to visit that "inner sanctuary" or, as Dr Lown says, to find that "presence".[6]

For O'Donohue, "Presence is the way a person's individuality comes toward you. Presence is the soul texture of the person."[7]

For me this is the sacred essence of the therapeutic encounter, the purpose of the consultation, to navigate towards that "inner sanctuary", that place of healing, to find and connect with that "presence" through the deeply personal conversation.

A similarly inspiring doctor is Abraham Verghese, Professor of Medicine at Stanford Medical School, who believes in the old fashioned thorough examination from head to toe, while getting to know the patient's life story.

He of course embraces the advances in modern medicine, but teaches his students that just as important is the doctor/patient relationship. In fact he refers to the **sanctity** of that relationship.

He describes a ritual whereby, before engaging with a patient, he washes his hands and reminds himself that he is about to enter a sacred space to listen to a stranger who has come to tell his story. He quietly offers a little prayer that he may be of service.[8]

My reaction is always thank God you are teaching these future doctors and what a gift you are to the healthcare profession.

He regards the first moments of the doctor/patient encounter as critical. Why then would those first moments be "sit over there in isolation and put your heart and soul on to that piece of paper" or, worse, online?

Verghese and researchers identified five evidence-based practices to deepen the therapeutic relationship and personalised consultation. They are known as the Presence 5 practices.[9]

- **Prepare with intention**: Familiarise yourself with the patient you are about to meet; create a ritual to focus your attention before a visit.

- **Listen intently and completely**: Sit down, lean forward and position yourself to listen; don't interrupt; your patient is your most valuable source of information.
- **Agree on what matters most**: Find out what your patient cares about and incorporate these priorities into the visit agenda.
- **Connect with the patient's story**: Consider the circumstances that influence your patient's health; acknowledge your patient's efforts, and celebrate successes.
- **Explore emotional cues**: Tune in, notice, name and validate your patient's emotions to become a trusted partner.

All of these aspects, in my opinion, are, or should be, part of the personalised aromatherapy consultation and, in an ideal world, part of every healthcare practice.

Dr Robin Youngson, author of *A Time to Care*, makes the powerful observation that "our compassionate caring is the most powerful thing that can elicit the healing response".[10]

These inspirational doctors embrace the art and science of medicine when "body and spirit are probed"[11] and stress the importance of getting to know the patient's life story through conversation and focused attention.

Professor Verghese, on being interviewed about transforming medical education, talks about the ubiquity of smartphones and screens taking us away from being truly present with the other. He reminds us that "one of the timeless principles in medicine is that it is always about the human being, an individual person at a particular point in life".[12]

Lown believes "patients crave caring which is dispensed largely with words".[13]

The Consultation and Relational Empathy (CARE) Measure is a consultation process measure developed by Dr Stewart Mercer and colleagues in the Departments of General Practice at Glasgow University and Edinburgh University. It serves as both a teaching and assessing tool for the quality of consultations in the context of the therapeutic relationship and is a great guide to empathic practice.[14]

CARE Measure Report

CARE Patient Feedback Measure for

*** Type name of Practitioner here ***

Please write today's date here:

☐☐ / ☐☐ / ☐☐
D D M M Y Y

Please rate the following statements about today's consultation.
Please mark the box like this ☑ with a ball point pen. If you change your mind just cross out your old response and make your new choice. Please answer every statement.

How good was the practitioner at...	Poor	Fair	Good	Very Good	Excellent	Does not apply
1 **Making you feel at ease** (introducing him/herself, explaining his/her position, being friendly and warm towards you, treating you with respect; not cold or abrupt)	☐	☐	☐	☐	☐	☐
2 **Letting you tell your "story"** (giving you time to fully describe your condition in your own words; not interrupting, rushing or diverting you)	☐	☐	☐	☐	☐	☐
3 **Really listening** (paying close attention to what you were saying; not looking at the notes or computer as you were talking)	☐	☐	☐	☐	☐	☐
4 **Being interested in you as a whole person** (asking/knowing relevant details about your life, your situation; not treating you as "just a number")	☐	☐	☐	☐	☐	☐
5 **Fully understanding your concerns** (communicating that he/she had accurately understood your concerns and anxieties; not overlooking or dismissing anything)	☐	☐	☐	☐	☐	☐
6 **Showing care and compassion** (seeming genuinely concerned, connecting with you on a human level; not being indifferent or "detached")	☐	☐	☐	☐	☐	☐

7	**Being positive** (having a positive approach and a positive attitude; being honest but not negative about your problems)	☐	☐	☐	☐	☐	☐
8	**Explaining things clearly** (fully answering your questions; explaining clearly, giving you adequate information; not being vague)	☐	☐	☐	☐	☐	☐
9	**Helping you to take control** (exploring with you what you can do to improve your health yourself; encouraging rather than "lecturing" you)	☐	☐	☐	☐	☐	☐
10	**Making a plan of action with you** (discussing the options, involving you in decisions as much as you want to be involved; not ignoring your views)	☐	☐	☐	☐	☐	☐

Comments: If you would like to add further comments on this consultation, please do so here.

CHAPTER 4

The Personalised Consultation in Aromatherapy and Its Core Role in an Aromatherapy Massage Treatment

"Give sorrow words: the grief that does not speak
Whispers the o'er-fraught heart and bids it break"

SHAKESPEARE, *MACBETH* ACT IV SC. 3

The following four aspects of an aromatherapy massage treatment are inextricably linked, but at the very heart, driving everything, is the personalised consultation to find and connect with the client's unique "presence" and to tailor the treatment to their needs.

1. **The preparation**
2. **The personalised consultation**
3. **The massage**
4. **The essential oils**

Underpinning all four is the power of **intent** to nurture the client, to endeavour to return them to a degree of homeostasis. Practitioner intent and focus cannot be underestimated.

Cutting edge research conducted at Princeton, Massachusetts Institute of Technology (MIT), Stanford and many other prestigious universities reveals that the universe is connected by a vast quantum energy field; thought has its own palpable energy, and the power of intention can profoundly affect all aspects of our lives.[1]

Cleve Backster discovered telepathic communication between all

living things.[2] Physicist Fritz-Albert Popp further developed this work through his discovery of biophotons, minute particles of light emitted by all living things and used for communication. He found that our thoughts and intentions could augment or diminish something else's light.

The Love Study, conducted by Radin, Schlitz and Stone, was the first major scientific demonstration of how intention physically affects the recipient, almost like a minuscule electric shock. For the most powerful effect the healer or sender needs to become "ordered" mentally and emotionally, focused, motivated and empathetic. People appeared to receive healing deep in their bodies by being "retuned" to the more coherent energy of the healer's intention.[3]

In a number of studies on healing, the electroencephalogram (EEG) waves of the recipient synchronised with those of the healer during moments when healing energy was sent. Similarly, brain mapping showed evidence of brain wave synchrony.[4]

The HeartMath Institute (HMI) was established three decades ago to research energy field environments, the human heart, emotions and stress. Studies conducted by the HMI have revealed the heart as a multifaceted source of intelligence sending signals to the brain and all parts of the body. The powerful electromagnetic field generated by the heart can be detected up to five feet (1.5 m) away from the body and produce measurable effects in others.

Our thoughts and emotions emit energetic fields which affect our environments, thus influencing our relationships. Attitudes of appreciation, love and compassion change our energetic fields, facilitating a state of coherence between mind, body and emotions.

Scientific evidence has shown that positive emotional states directly affect the autonomic nervous system (ANS) that regulates our physiology, creating a cascade of positive effects throughout the body. Stressful emotions make our heart rhythm jagged and erratic. Positive emotions even out our heart rate variability sending coherent signals to the brain that bring all our systems into alignment, creating clear thinking, emotional stability and effective decision making.

The importance of intent on our part as therapists is therefore clear. We need to be working from a place of heart centred coherence which will be felt by those close to us. The HMI has simple techniques we can use to bring about a state of coherence such as:

- Imagine that you are breathing in and out deeply through the heart.

- Picture someone, something or some place that you love.
- Breathe in a feeling of gratitude, love and compassion. (www.heartmath.org)

Positive emotions increase our coherence level and signal to the brain that all is well. This simple technique can be used anywhere anytime for a few minutes, to reduce stress and improve our interactions with others. It is part of my preparation with intent before giving any treatment.

In the words of Dr Pénoël, "Even the most biological and purest essential oils can never replace the warmth of light from the small flame that shines in the depths of the heart."[5]

Focused intention and compassion are therefore the ground rules for the treatment.

1. The preparation

For me the aromatherapy treatment, incorporating the in depth consultation and massage, is a ritual. And the ritual is the same whether I am treating a friend, a client or a family member. It begins a good hour beforehand when I prepare myself and the sacred spaces.

I ensure that the rooms are warm, the flowers are fresh, candles are lit, towels are wrapped around hot water bottles, fresh linen drapes the heated massage table and carrier oils are warmed gently. Next I visit the herb garden to choose the botanicals for a fresh herbal tea while tuning in to the person coming and what it is they may need from our plant allies. They are already front and centre in my focus. I don't like to be disturbed during this time.

Creating a beautiful, peaceful, **safe**, welcoming space for my clients is very important to me. I have a strong sense of the aesthetic and believe that beauty is healing and we need to be deliberate in creating the conditions for deep connection.[6] I am lucky, I look out on a forest garden. No Nature deficit syndrome here. I have nature on my side creating a beautiful environment to help induce a state of relaxation and reflection.

Renowned theologian, poet and philosopher John O'Donohue believes that beauty enables the heart and restores us to our higher selves with a greater sense of grace and elegance. He reminds us of Pascal's words that we should always keep something beautiful in our hearts to endure great bleakness, and that the root of the word "beauty" is the Greek word meaning "calling".[7]

Bessel van der Kolk stresses the need to feel safe with other people and considers it "the single most important aspect of mental health". When the message we receive from a therapist is "you're safe with me" we relax. For many this feeling of safety can come initially from someone else who is calm and confident.[8] We create this feeling of safety by our attention to detail in making the environment as pleasurable, beautiful and welcoming as possible and of course by our focused attention and caring interactions.

There are no time pieces, or, God forbid, technological devices, in my treatment rooms. Nothing that would say, "I only care about you for a limited time." There is nothing worse than a clock watcher. I've experienced it myself where I felt the practitioner focus was partly on me and partly on the next client's arrival.

"When we bring an attitude of business and hurry, we shut out caring and compassion."[9] If you must time watch, please be discreet. This may sound trite but actually it's the little things that make a difference. Attention to detail shows that we care. I want my client to know that at that moment in time they are the most important person in the world and they have my complete undivided attention and unqualified time.

Florence Nightingale, in her holistic approach to nursing, believed the cure is in the caring and that relaxation and the creation of healing environments for body, mind and spirit were a vital part of healing.[10]

Last, and most important, I prepare myself.

I "tune in" to ask for guidance in order that I may:

- Listen well.
- Ask the right questions.
- Give the right answers.
- Choose the right oils.
- Give a wonderful treatment.
- Bless the fellow human being coming in good faith to share their story.
- Focus on heart centred breathing.

The "tuning in" can be whatever is meaningful to you: your God, your higher power, the angels, the plant devas. It doesn't really matter. What is important is taking the time to be quiet and centred, to go over client notes if applicable, to set the intention to be fully present and of service, to work from a heart focused place of compassion and empathy.

John O'Donohue talks about "The Inestimable Power of Intention" and describes a blessing as a "powerful and positive intention" which "can transform situations and people". He describes it as an invisible form of grace which creates a "sheltering wall of rest and peace around a person".[11] We can learn much from the Celtic tradition of blessings marking milestones and thresholds signalling the start of a transformational journey. Preparing for the arrival of a client is, for me, preparing for a transformational journey, not to be taken lightly and requiring my full attention and respect.

2. The personalised consultation

"Just listen to your patient: he is telling you the diagnosis"

SIR WILLIAM OSLER[12]

Sir William Osler, often called the Father of Modern Medicine, was a nineteenth-century physician and one of the founding professors of Johns Hopkins Hospital. A wonderful diagnostician, his greatest influence was to insist that students learn from seeing and talking to patients.

After greeting my client I usher them into my consultation room where a tray prepared with a linen cloth, sprig of flowers and fresh herbal tea awaits them. A warm rug for the knees, assurance of confidentiality and consent for the treatment set the scene. Straight away the client feels cared for and starts to relax. Simple measures which carry the message of compassion and kindness.

John O'Donohue has some beautiful words about the importance of kindness, how "something deep in the human soul seems to depend on the presence of kindness; something instinctive in us expects it, and once we sense it we are able to trust and open ourselves."[13] When someone is kind to us we feel understood and seen. In the loveliest of words he describes how "kindness has gracious eyes; it is not small or competitive...it also suggests that your vulnerability, though somehow exposed, is not taken advantage of; rather it has become an occasion for dignity and empathy". When we show compassion or kindness to another "we are setting blessing in train".[14]

We sit face to face, no barriers. This is a level playing field marked by equality and mutual respect, and we have to earn that respect.[15]

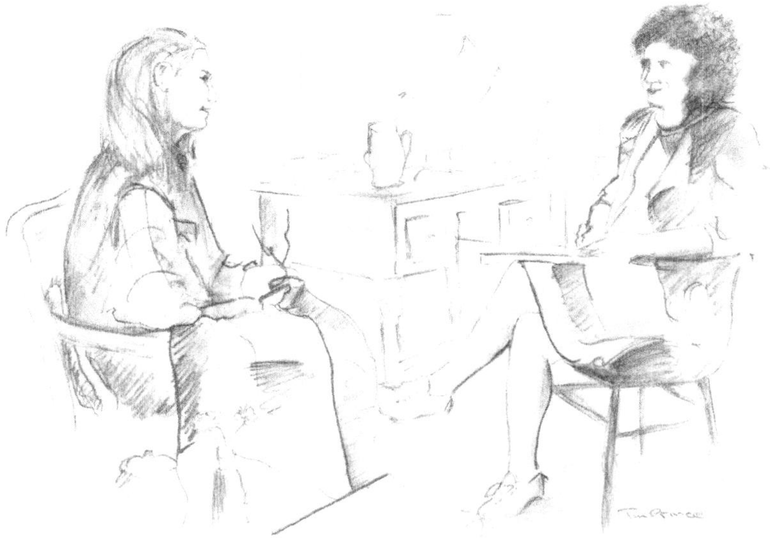

Connection by T.M. Prince

All the while I am observant of body language; this nonverbal way in which we reveal our "mental state and attitudes".[16] Is their handshake feeble or strong; how is their gait, are they trudging along with the weight of the world on their shoulders or are they upright and confident; do they have colour in their cheeks; are their eyes bright and lively or sunken and lifeless; do they look happy or sad, angry, nervous, depressed or exhausted; is their voice timid, unsure or loud, even overbearing; is there an unshed tear waiting to fall?

The consultation/conversation is the means by which I get a snapshot of the client, mentally, physically, emotionally and spiritually. The client information form is the basis for this conversation and is filled in manually (print, not digital) by me.

As previously stated, I feel very strongly about not leaving this task up to the client. It is so important to build up trust, respect and empathy by engaging in a face to face conversation, maintaining eye contact, monitoring body language, following the thread of the conversation which may lead to questions that are not written down but are crucial to understanding the client's situation.

Murtagh describes the role of listening with every fibre of our being and all of our senses to "the sounds and to the silences", to the messages

encoded in the words, [17] and Thich Nhat Hahn describes deep listening as "the kind of listening that can help relieve the suffering of another person".[18]

The reason I use pen and paper to take notes harks back to Turkle's research about screens and smartphones, even when closed, blocking empathic connection. She references studies that show that "open screens degrade the performance of everyone who can see them".[19]

Interestingly Carol Steiker, a professor at Harvard Law School, insists that her students take notes by hand and is convinced it forces them to be better listeners. "They can't write fast enough to do a transcript, so they have to figure out what is important."[20]

Note taking is part of how we learn to think. In the consultation process it focuses my complete concentration on the client's words.

My client information form is carefully structured to cover personal details, health history, lifestyle, relationships and, finally, emotional state. It allows the conversation to flow easily, building connection, before delving into the more "nitty gritty" emotional, mental issues. The last question, and arguably the most important, is a series of words describing emotions. The client is asked to circle the ones that they have predominantly felt over recent months. This is often the key to unlocking the floodgates of emotion, to tapping into underlying issues in the subconscious. At this stage, trust has been established and it is not uncommon for tears to flow, a healthy release in itself. Tears are the language of the soul. They are not a sign of weakness, instead they speak to deep grief, sadness, joy or pain.

Through unhurried conversation in a safe nurturing environment with no time constraints, the client feels valued and develops greater self awareness, achieving clarity around mental, emotional and spiritual issues.

To repeat the words of Pert, we enlist the power of the mind through talk and access the emotions through bodywork, thus creating "a loop of healing".[21]

The bond that is built up between therapist and client provides a secure anchor of support, a safe place. In our time poor, technology driven, often lonely lifestyle, this connection and "time out" is of great benefit.

Annie Prince Aromatherapy Client Information Form

The following detailed consultation is strictly confidential and its purpose is to ensure the efficacy and safety of the treatment. It forms the basis for our conversation and is filled in by the practitioner.

Are you happy with that?

Date: .... Name: ....

Address: ....

Phone No.: .... Mobile No.: ....

Email Address: ....

D.O.B.: .... Doctor: ....

Occupation: ....

Single/partner? ....

Do you have children? ....

Emergency contact number: ....

Have you had an aromatherapy massage before? ....

What is the reason for your visit? ....

....

Medical history:

Do you have any issues with the following?

Muscle/Joint pain		Pregnant/Menstrual problems	
Heart problems		Diabetes	
High/Low blood pressure		Digestive problems	
Blood clots		Respiratory problems	
Headaches/Migraines		Epilepsy	

Do you have any allergies/sensitivities?

....

....

Do you have any skin problems?

....

....

Are you currently taking any medication or herbal supplements?

....

....

Have you had any surgery in the last 2 years?

....

....

Family medical history: Any chronic illnesses?

....

....

Is your oral health good ? ....

Diet: Good/average/bad? ....

Exercise: Often/sometimes/never? ....

Alcohol intake? ....

Water intake? ....

Tea/coffee? ....

Do you smoke? ....

What do you do to relax?

....

....

Do you sleep well? ....

What is your memory like? ....

Do you suffer or have you ever suffered from depression? ....

Are you happy in your job/family/relationship? ....

Rate your stress levels 1 to 10 (1 being very low): ....

How would you rate your self esteem 1 to 10?......................

How would you rate your confidence 1 to 10? ....

How would you rate your happiness level 1 to 10?......................

How would you rate your energy levels 1 to 10? ....

Are there any scents you particularly like or dislike?

....

....

....

....

Below, please circle the words describing your predominant feelings over the past few months. Do not analyse them. There is no judgement attached to them. They are not right or wrong but feelings we can all have at times in our lives. It does not matter how many or how few, and please feel free to add your own.

Anxious Fearful Relaxed Depressed Despairing Happy Joyful

Sad Resentful Envious Contented Optimistic Pessimistic Tired

Enthusiastic Positive Ambitious Intolerant Critical Compassionate

Loving Generous Overburdened Fragile Worried Vulnerable

Grief Hopeful Hopeless

I have answered all the questions to the best of my knowledge. I understand that this treatment is not a substitute for medical examinations and/or diagnosis and it is recommended I see my physician for any physical ailment that I may have. I have stated all of my known medical conditions and take it upon myself to keep the therapist updated on my physical health. I am happy to receive this aromatherapy treatment.

Signature: .... Date: ....

Practitioner Form

Name: .... Date: ....

Clinical observations

....

....

....

....

Summary of presenting conditions

....

....

....

....

Therapeutic intent

....

....

....

....

Oils selected and why

....

....

....

....

....

....

At the completion of the consultation, bespoke essential oils are chosen to reflect the needs of the client:

- an essential oil for inhalation: one drop in a bowl of hot water placed under the massage table
- three essential oils for the massage blend diluted in a carrier oil at around 2%
- *Rosa damascena* (Damask rose), diluted at 3% in Jojoba for the facial treatment.

Inhaling the rose oil always results in a deep intake of breath and a sighing expiration as if the last vestiges of tension were leaving the body. Rose has such an affinity with the heart, but more about that later.

3. The massage

> *"The most natural way that we humans calm down our distress is by being touched, hugged and rocked"*
>
> BESSEL VAN DER KOLK[22]

> *"Your body does not lie. Your body tells you, if you attend to it, how your life is and whether you are living from your soul or from the labyrinths of your negativity"*
>
> JOHN O'DONOHUE[23]

The relatively new science of psychoneuroimmunology (PNI) explores the mind/body connection with the premise that homeostasis involves the interaction between behaviour and the nervous, endocrine and immune systems.

Physical disease is regarded as a powerful expression of a patient's emotional themes and life story. High stress has a mind/body connection.[24]

Trauma expert van der Kolk, in his book *The Body Keeps the Score*, states that when our emotional and rational brains are in conflict a tug of war ensues which for the most part is played out in "the theatre of visceral experience – your gut, your heart, your lungs – and will lead to both physical discomfort and psychological misery".[25]

He believes that to resolve traumatic stress we must restore the proper balance between the rational and emotional brains. He puts self awareness at the core of recovery and talks about conducting "limbic system therapy" to restore the emotional brain to a quiet state in which it can "take care of the housekeeping of the body", ensuring eating, sleeping, connection with intimate partners, protection of children and defence against danger.[26]

Recovery from trauma involves reconnecting with our fellow human beings in a safe space through compassionate conversation and recalibrating the ANS through breathwork, movement and touch.

Sometimes described as the mother of psychoneuroimmunology, Candace Pert in her fascinating book *The Molecules of Emotion* states, "The body and mind are not separate, and we cannot treat one without the other."[27] Furthermore she showed through her research how "the emotions travel between the two realms of mind and body as the peptides and receptors in the physical realm and as the feelings we experience and call emotions in the nonmaterial realm".[28]

She believed that the biochemicals of emotion run every system of the body. In her view the body is the subconscious mind storing deeper, older messages that cannot be healed by talk alone and need to be accessed by the touch therapies such as massage.[29]

Massage is regarded as one of the truly holistic health maintenance therapies because it promotes the flow of blood and lymph, improves nervous conductivity, soothes tension, increases vital energy and promotes a sense of emotional wellbeing. By inducing a state of relaxation we can ease muscle tension, which often relates not only to physical pain but to psychological tension and repressed emotions.

> Feeling worthless? Get a massage, a spinal adjustment, or a lot of good hugging, and see what happens. Your mind, your feelings are in your body and it is there in your somatic experience that feeling is healed.[30]

Aromatherapy massage combines the physiological effects of massage with the therapeutic holistic effects of bespoke essential oils chosen for the client after a comprehensive consultation.

The full body aromatherapy treatment, which I personally perform, is head to toe, deeply relaxing to the central nervous system, nurturing not painful, incorporating different techniques drawn from Swedish massage, holistic pulsing, acupressure points, reflexology and lymphatic drainage.

Something which I always do for first time clients is to give them permission not to talk to me during the massage! Unless there is any emotional release or they need to communicate about an aspect of their physical comfort, I encourage them to be silent to allow themselves to completely relax, reassuring them that while I am focused on the treatment and their needs I am fully present to support them in any way. It's surprising how many people appreciate the removal of any obligation to make conversation during the massage. The same applies of course to the therapist!

During the treatment, intent and focus are very much to the fore, working with the oils while being acutely aware of the life story I have just heard and the needs of the person before me. Acutely aware too of the privilege it is to touch another human being. I am reminded of the profound words of Tracy Walton: "By touching a body we touch everything that has happened to it... We reach across the isolation of the human experience and hold another person's legend."[31]

A privilege indeed and a responsibility. We need to know what that "legend" is so that we can truly connect with the client and be prepared for any emotional release during the treatment. Hence the importance of the personalised consultation to get to know the client's story.

To complete the treatment I spritz the aura with an aromatic mist to cleanse and protect energetically.

The aromatherapy massage treatment is a three part affair. It involves the client/therapist relationship, therapeutic touch and the inclusion of bespoke essential oils, all of which are interconnected.

How can we possibly put a treatment like this into a randomised control trial or distil it down into a petri dish? We can't, because of the complexity of the human being, the complexity of the essential oil chemistry, the unique touch and the complexity of the therapist at the centre bringing them all together. This is the art of aromatherapy.

Aromatherapy is an art and a science. Researching the pharmacological effects of individual molecules and essential oils is much easier than documenting and researching the art of aromatherapy, which encapsulates the whole treatment. That by no means belittles, or invalidates, the profound, almost indefinable results we can see in our clients as the result of an aromatherapy massage treatment.

The transformation is often remarkable. The eyes are the storytellers, they have more life. There is colour in the cheeks, the shoulders have dropped, the body is relaxed, movement is slow, the breath is calm, the voice is quiet. The tyranny of the intellect has been stifled. There is

often a sense of euphoria or bliss. It is like watching the parasympathetic nervous system kick in, in slow motion.

That's our "petri dish", our "randomised control trial" right there in the flesh and blood of the human being we have just treated. We need time to be fully present, for focused observation to monitor these changes. Having a "hand on the door knob" is anathema to the whole treatment.

For serious deep seated issues of course this treatment is only the first step on the road to recovery, but it can be a very important one in activating the reset button for change, in laying the foundation for resilience.

4. The essential oils

> *"Smells don't care what the mind or heart wants. Scents will find their way around the darkness of closed eyes, slipping past barricades of thought"*
>
> ERICA BAUERMEISTER[32]

These brilliant words by Bauermeister sum up magnificently for me the power and immediacy of olfaction. The effect is instantaneous, we can't "unsmell" an aroma.

Essential oils (EOs) distilled from various parts of aromatic plants or cold pressed from the rinds of fruit contain a complex cocktail of chemical components which contribute to their beauty and power, their "breathtaking versatility of application".[33]

In 2020 Dr Lizarraga-Valderrama published her review paper "Effects of essential oils on central nervous system: focus on mental health" in *Phytotherapy Research*.

> A large body of research confirms the multiple benefits that EOs have on the mental health of humans including anxiolytic/antidepressant effects, cognitive processing enhancement, attention enhancement, psychostimulant effects and memory improvement. Moreover, varying animal models have been used to elucidate the diverse molecular pathways involved in the therapeutic effects of EOs such as HPA axis, sympathetic nervous system, cAMP response element-binding protein (CREB) signaling pathway and neurotransmitter systems including serotonergic, DAnergic and GABAergic pathways.[34]

The aromatic molecules use the olfactory highway as an open route to convey their messages to the brain's limbic system, the seat of memories and emotions. The chemical messengers impact structures such as the amygdala, hippocampus and hypothalamus, thereby producing an emotional response and the release of neurochemicals which, in turn, influence various bodily systems including the nervous, endocrine and immune.

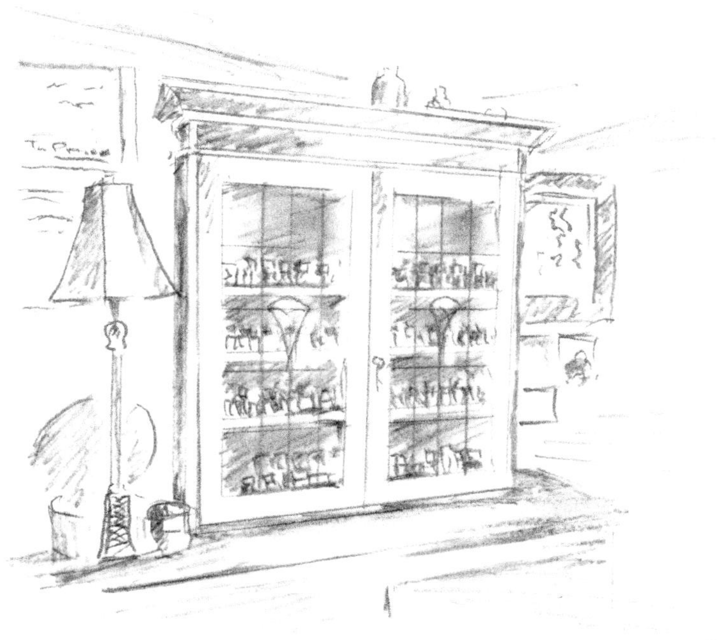

The Oil Cupboard by T.M. Prince

They thus work on many levels, mental, emotional, physical, spiritual – the pillars of holistic health, the bedrock of resilience. Fragrance influences how we think, feel and behave. Essential oils chosen specifically for the client's needs after the personalised consultation complete the holistic treatment and add a deeper level to the benefits of the massage.

Essential oils "possess properties which can affect the mind and emotions, to sedate, calm, uplift. They also have effects on bodily systems, they evoke memories, change perception, calm agitation, relieve stress, activate cognitive responses and affect intercommunication."[35]

The ability of odours to trigger involuntary autobiographical

memories, known as "the Proust effect", was demonstrated in the author's famous tome *À la Recherche du temps perdu.*[36] His protagonist upon eating a tea soaked madeleine was instantly transported back to his childhood and his aunt's kitchen where on a Sunday morning he would enjoy a similar treat. The memory was infused with a deep emotional resonance.

An important part of the personalised consultation therefore is ascertaining the client's particular aroma likes and dislikes. A strong preference either way can determine the choice of oils. Not all memories are happy ones.

To summarise

The **personalised consultation** is at the very heart of all aspects of an aromatherapy massage treatment for the following reasons:

- The purpose of the **preparation** and creation of the sacred spaces is to provide a **safe**, beautiful, nurturing environment conducive to having open, honest dialogue; to show by our attention to detail that we care.
- The **consultation** is the means by which we get to know the client as a living breathing fellow human being, in all their mental, emotional, spiritual, physical glory, negotiating the rigours of life and trying to make sense of it all. It's profound. It's nonjudgemental. It's a privilege and it is deeply moving.
- The **massage** is the follow up to the very personal consultation. It's the powerful but gentle way to aid release physically and emotionally. It's the means to bring about a degree of homeostasis and deep relaxation; to silence the inner critic, the mental tyrant; to just pour love into this precious human being. And don't we all need that?
- The bespoke and precious **essential oils**, nature's gifts, the tools of our trade, are chosen as a result of getting to know the "essence" of the person before us. In an almost inexplicable way they weave their magic into the psyche, bringing their innumerable gifts to body, mind and soul.

It's timely to note at this point that the quality of the essential oils is paramount for their therapeutic effect. Adulteration is rampant in the world of aromatherapy because essential oils are expensive to produce and are big business globally.

I always say to students that if you can't buy direct from distillers make sure your supplier does. A gas chromatography/mass spectrometry analysis of the chemical constituents is helpful (GCMS combines two analytical tools to identify and measure the concentration of chemical components in essential oils), and the botanical as well as common names, place of origin, part of plant used, method of distillation, organic or wild crafted, instructions for use and expiry indication is information that should be available.

It's timely too to mention our respect for endangered species and to be mindful of the oils we use, choosing alternatives to threatened species. Dr Kelly Ablard and the Airmid Institute do phenomenal work in this regard. Do check out their website (www.airmidinstitute.org) if you are unsure of a plant's status or if you would like to support their conservation work.

To survive the stresses of modern life we need to be resilient. While there are many effective ways to deal with stress and trauma including lifestyle changes, cognitive behavioural therapy, eye movement desensitisation and reprocessing, emotional freedom tapping, medication and psychedelic assisted psychotherapy, I believe that aromatherapeutic massage is in a league of its own.

It marries talk therapy with bodywork, "the gateway to the mind",[37] along with the use of essential oils whose aromatic molecules have a direct pathway to convey their information to the limbic system. There, their olfactory messages trigger the release of neurochemicals which affect mood and behaviour, and their energetic signatures in a mysterious way reach into the crevices of the human psyche.

It requires skill and training in the art and science of aromatherapy, bodywork, anatomy and physiology, conversational and listening skills, along with a deep connection to, and knowledge of, these extraordinary plant extracts, to effectively nurture resilience using the aromatherapy massage treatment plan.

When conducted in an unhurried, heart centred, focused way it is a deeply moving experience for both the therapist and the client.

It's a joy in my life, a privilege, a responsibility, my raison d'être.

CHAPTER 5

For Further Reflection: Nature Deficit Syndrome, Biophilia and the Case for Essential Oils

"Can you see any plants right now? If not you might want to fix that"

RUSSELL MCCLENDON[1]

Nature deficit syndrome is a thing. From being a race of hunter gatherers immersed in nature, living and working in the safety of groups, 55% of us are now urban dwellers and by 2050 the United Nations expects two thirds of humanity to be city dwellers.[2]

Living in a city environment poses well known risk factors for mental and physical health. Sedentary lifestyles, air, noise and light pollution linked to stress and fatigue, disrupted circadian rhythms giving rise to poor sleep, cognitive impairment and mood disorders, all can have a serious impact on our health.[3] Not to mention the effects of solitary living and loneliness, as previously discussed.

Thanks to a growing body of scientific research, however, spending time in nature has been shown to have a profoundly positive impact on our psychological and physical wellbeing. This is related to the term "biophilia", first coined in the 1960s by Erich Fromm and introduced into the world of biological sciences by E.O. Wilson. It means love of life and refers to our deep innate connection to the natural world and all living things.[4]

Much research has been done in Japan on the benefits of *shinrin yoku* or "forest bathing". Spending time in Nature has been shown to lower stress levels, pulse rate and blood pressure, improve sleep, reduce pain levels, improve cognitive performance, reduce negative emotions, improve mood and boost the immune system by enhancing the activity

of natural killer (NK) cells and the expression of anticancer proteins. The benefits can be felt for weeks afterwards. This is partly due to the effect of wood essential oils called phytoncides released into the forest air with antibacterial and antifungal properties which, when inhaled, increase NK activity.[5]

Furthermore, two theoretical frameworks on the psychological benefits of nature have been proposed by Kaplan and Kaplan. Attention restoration theory (ART) focuses on cognitive restoration. Nature captures our involuntary attention, allowing our voluntary attention processes to recover. Stress recovery theory (SRT) relates to the stress reducing capacity of natural environments which promotes positive emotions as well as decreasing arousal and negative emotions such as fear.[6]

Biologist Clemens Arvay talks about the inherent benefits of getting away from civilisation to where the inhabitants of the natural world are not interested in our pay cheque or bills; they do not criticise or judge us. We are free to just be ourselves.[7] So if we mock the tree huggers we may need to reconsider that behaviour!

The interesting thing is that we can reap some of the benefits of being in nature simply by observing plants or natural environments. Surgical patients in hospitals who looked out on natural scenery as opposed to brick walls have been shown to recover more quickly and need less analgesia.[8] Doctors in the UK can prescribe a green prescription in the form of looking after a potted plant to patients who are anxious or depressed.

All of which brings me to the case for essential oils. Here we have nature in a bottle. In an instant the inhalation of these highly concentrated aromatic essences can transport us from our grim concrete jungles to the lavender fields of Provence, the conifers of the Taiga and Boreal forests, the citrus groves of the Iberian Peninsula, the heady frankincense laden air of the deserts of Oman and Somalia, the cistus hillsides of Crete, the rose fields of Turkey and Iran, the herb gardens of Europe, the wild helichrysum of Corsica or the eucalypt forests of the Antipodes.

> Odors have a power of persuasion stronger than that of words, appearances, emotions, or will. The persuasive power of an odor cannot be fended off, it enters into us like breath into our lungs, it fills us up, imbues us totally. There is no remedy for it.[9]

One of the great advantages of essential oils is the ease with which we

can reap their benefits. It lies in the methods of application: roller balls, aromasticks, smelling salts, creams, spritzers or simply inhaling from the bottle or a cotton wool ball. One sniff can interrupt the cascade of stress hormones and help change our perspective.

Aside from their pharmacological effects on our physiology, it is their ability to lift the spirit, to calm, to energise, to reconnect us to the "green" world and to temper the emotions which elevates them to the subtle, energetic and spiritual domain. Which brings me to the next chapter.

> Smell is the primordial sense, more powerful, more primitive, more intimately tied to our memories and emotions than any other. A scent can trigger spiritual, emotional or physical peace and stimulate healing and wellness.[10]

CHAPTER 6

Subtle Aromatherapy and Aromatic Allies

"If you are a rational person with faith in the orderly progress of established science, you will believe hardly a word in this book, which deals with unknown forces in the vegetable world, human communication with plants, psychic powers, radionic pesticides and such 'nonsense'. If, on the other hand, you are irked by the strait jacket of materialism, you may find this one of the most encouraging books you have ever read"[1]

The fascinating book *The Secret Life of Plants* documents the groundbreaking work of Cleve Backster, a lie detection specialist, who demonstrated that plants respond to human emotions, thoughts, intentions and prayers.

The initially sceptical research chemist Marcel Vogel, after conducting his own experiments, declared that "man can and does communicate with plant life. Plants are living objects, sensitive, rooted in space... There is no doubt in my mind that they are extremely sensitive instruments for measuring man's emotions. They radiate energy, forces that are beneficial to man."[2]

There's a lot more to plants therefore than meets the eye. Indigenous cultures around the globe have recognised the spirit in all living things and understood the interconnectedness of people with the natural world. Stephen Buhner says it's not necessary to have a degree in chemistry to understand the medicine of plants. There is a deep intuitive feeling connected to it; an element of the invisible.[3]

Albert Einstein said, "The intuitive mind is a sacred gift and the rational mind is a faithful servant. We have created a society that honours the servant and has forgotten the gift."[4]

Subtle aromatherapy makes use of the vibrational, energetic qualities

of the essential oils "to affect the subtle body, the psyche and indeed the soul".[5]

Dr Florian Birkmeyer calls essential oils "Molecules of connectedness, The medicine of the soul".[6] They can touch us on a deep level causing subtle shifts in consciousness and emotional release. Felicity Warner, soul midwife and spiritual and holistic therapist for the dying, in her book *Sacred Oils* describes them as "sacred tools of consciousness" which have "energy signatures that resonate with the human soul and spirit".[7]

Marguerite Maury stressed the importance of tailoring the treatment to the individual's needs.[8] There are certain essential oils, however, which I find indispensable allies when dealing with mental, emotional and spiritual distress. These are usually chosen for their subtle, energetic and vibrational qualities rather than for their chemistry, although I am always cognisant of the chemical components from a safety point of view as well as their physiological effect.

The oils are chosen with a nod to the Doctrine of Signatures, Traditional Chinese Medicine (TCM) and my own personal experience and observations from working with them. I am indebted, in particular, to the work of Peter Holmes, Gabriel Mojay, Robbi Zeck and Felicity Warner who have so often been my companions on the healing road.[9]

What do we mean by the Doctrine of Signatures?

The Doctrine of Signatures proposes that the healing properties of plants are reflected in their physical features and habitat.[10] It provides us with tangible images to describe the subtle healing properties of particular plants and essential oils. It can be explained in terms of the following:

- the aroma of the essential oil
- the anatomy of the plant
- the habitat of the plant
- the part of the plant used.

The unique aroma of each essential oil reveals an aspect of its character and healing potential which often evokes powerful memories and emotions.

The shape, texture and colour of plants often reflect their subtle action. The vertical shape of a sturdy tree reaching upwards imparts a sense of direction and purpose, for example *Cedrus atlantica* (Atlas cedar) and *Cupressus sempervirens* (Cypress). The hard, tough texture of wood

suggests the ability of essential oils such as *Santalum spicatum* (Australian sandalwood) and *Cedrus atlantica* (Atlas cedar) to give us strength, endurance, equilibrium and a sense of groundedness and stability. In contrast, the soft delicate petals of *Rosa damascena* (Damask rose) and *Anthemis nobilis* (Roman chamomile) reflect the gentle comforting effect on the emotions.

The violet coloured flowers of *Lavandula angustifolia* (Lavender true) embody its calm, cool nature and mirror its affinity to the spiritual realm in the colour of the third eye chakra.

Root oils tend to be stabilising, strengthening, grounding, for example *Vetiveria zizanoides* (Vetiver) and *Angelica archangelica* (Angelica). If you have ever seen the long, matted, dreadlock like roots of the grass vetiver, you can imagine how nothing is moving where it is planted and indeed it is used to stabilise land.

Flowers produce seeds and scent for pollination and often have an affinity with the reproductive system. Highly scented flowers indicate a spiritually evolved plant and are a sign of intense astral activity. They deal with matters of the heart physically and emotionally and are supportive of the heart chakra, for example *Rosa damascena* (Damask rose) and *Jasminum officinale* (Jasmine).

Essential oils produced in the leaves of trees represent the "lungs" of the plant and have a great affinity with the respiratory system. In fact a diagram of the trachea, lungs, bronchi and bronchioles looks for all the world like an upside down tree with its trunk, branches, twigs and canopy of leaves, for example *Eucalyptus radiata* (Narrow-leaved peppermint eucalyptus) and *Cinnamomum camphora* ct cineole (Ravintsara).

The resins of *Commiphora myrrha* (Myrrh) and *Boswellia carterii* (Frankincense) have powerful wound healing properties, as demonstrated in their sealing of the cuts in the trees. They have a soothing, elevating action on the soul. As ancient essences, often used in religious rituals, they are healing also for deep emotional wounds of the spirit.

Seeds represent new life, creativity, moving forward, for example *Coriandrum sativum* (Coriander) and *Elettaria cardamomum* (Cardamom).

Jacquelin Guiteau is a Haitian spiritual teacher and herbalist who has studied western and eastern mysticism since the age of fourteen. After the devastating Haiti earthquake of 2010 he founded the Naturopathic Earthquake Survivor Relief Clinic with Julia Graves. He says, "[T]he Doctrine of Signatures is how the medicinal plants introduce their healing powers to the healer."[11] To Paracelsus, signatures are the knowledge of the inner essence based on outer characteristics.[12]

I am by no means an expert on TCM but I find the concepts of the Five Elements and yin and yang extremely helpful for understanding the energetics of the human body and the essential oils. For further study of TCM I highly recommend reading *Aromatherapy for Healing the Spirit* by Gabriel Mojay and *Aromatica* by Peter Holmes.[13]

Rather than document detailed essential oil monographs, listing chemical constituents and generalised actions, which are readily available in many aromatherapy texts, I would instead like to help you get to know some of the oils on a subtle level, to bring them alive through story and my own journey with them to the point where they have indeed become aromatic allies.

You may not like my choices, you might actually strongly dislike them, and that's OK. Working with essential oils is highly personal.

What I would suggest, if at all possible, is getting to know the plants first, sitting quietly with them, communicating, listening to their messages, being aware of how they make you feel, silencing the left brain for a while and allowing your intuition and your heart to speak to you. Subsequently you can work with the essential oils in the same way, simply through inhalation: direct from the bottle, a drop on a tissue, in an aromastick or diluted in a rollerball. When working emotionally or spiritually, low doses are called for; often one drop suffices.

Lavandula angustifolia (Lavender true)

If I told you that lavender completely changed my life, you probably wouldn't believe me, but it's true. In 2007 I was at a crossroads in my life, in between careers and on a journey back to health after a coeliac diagnosis. My unchanging mantra was: "I want to do something that nurtures people."

Enter the Abbaye Notre-Dame de Sénanque, that wonderful twelfth-century Cistercian monastery near Gordes in Provence. As soon as I rounded the bend of the winding road down into the valley and saw this magnificent edifice and the lavender fields surrounding it, I stopped in my tracks. I knew in that moment that somehow my life had changed and I would return.

Smelling the Lavender essential oil and sampling the beautiful products the monks had crafted from it triggered something in my soul. My fate was sealed. I returned to New Zealand to study aromatherapy

and haven't stopped studying since. I can't imagine a more nurturing profession. The mantra worked.

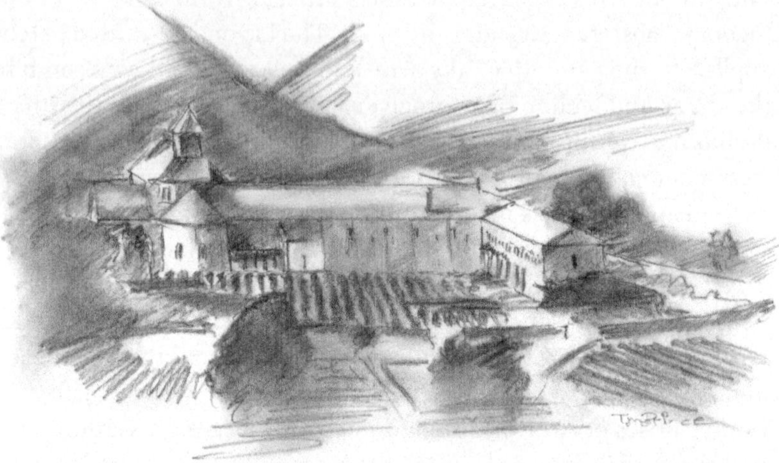

Abbaye Notre-Dame de Sénanque by T.M. Prince

I've always loved lavender, mind you, and have to have it in my garden. For me it's a symbol of home, of nurture, of love, of peace, of a wild cottage garden, of grace. It is a love token reminiscent of my teaching days when I would find a sprig on my windscreen to say, "I'm thinking of you."

It's the first scent I introduce to the grandchildren. Rubbing the flower heads between my fingers, the little faces of the infants are irresistibly drawn to the molecules of relaxation. As they get older a drop on their pillow at night is always expected at Grandma's "house of peace and calm" and they sleep, well, like babies.

Lavender is often referred to as "the Swiss army knife of essential oils", which sounds slightly ferocious. It refers of course to its amazing versatility as a skin healer, analgesic, antimicrobial, sleep aid, anxiolytic, anti-inflammatory, antispasmodic and mood enhancer. "A high quality essential oil of true lavender is an irreplaceable gift of Nature because it provides so many benefits."[14]

The main chemical components, the monoterpenol linalool and the ester linalyl acetate, contribute to the calming action on the central nervous system. High altitude French lavender has a high ester content increasing its sedative effects. I say to students that if you can only have one essential oil make it this one because it can do virtually everything.

Dr Lori Shook and Dr John Daniel of Kentucky Children's Hospital use an aroma patch with a drop each of *Lavandula angustifolia* (Lavender true) and *Anthemis nobilis* (Roman chamomile) essential oils, to help mitigate the stress endured by babies suffering from drug withdrawal (neonatal abstinence syndrome; NAS). The Lavender-scented patch is applied to the palm of a Zaky arm, a floppy green pillow resembling the shape and feeling of a caregiver's arm, placed beside the infant. Preliminary results show that the babies receiving the aromatherapy treatment spend 6.4 fewer days in the neonatal intensive care unit (NICU) and need less medication![15] Truly inspiring, compassionate care for these innocent children and another example of this gift from nature.

Despite its gentleness there is a strength and resilience in lavender as a result of growing in extreme conditions from blistering heat in summer to freezing cold in winter. When I visited the artisan distillery Verdon Roses et Arômes situated near the Gorges du Verdon, while studying with Rhiannon Lewis in Provence, it had a profound effect on me, not just witnessing where this hardy little plant grows so high up in the mountains but also seeing the work that goes into hand harvesting and distilling this aromatic so that we can reap the benefits. My respect knew no bounds both for the plant and the distillers.

I sensed in that moment the importance of knowing where and how the plant is grown; how and by whom it is harvested, distilled, packaged and how it is used and treated by the recipient. Everything and everyone carries an energy which can impact our precious oils. Support our ethical artisan distillers. Please.

Lavandula angustifolia (Lavender true) is cooling, calming, restorative, indicated for volatile emotions, fear, panic and nervous tension. Often called the "Grandmother" oil it is nurturing for self neglect. I have read that lavender enhances any blend and honours the higher spiritual realms.[16]

I use Lavender for the caregivers, the busy mamas, those on the treadmill of life who need to be stopped. I use it myself at night when the mind won't be still. A drop on the temple usually suffices. I dilute a drop in a carrier oil for the grandchildren's bush baths (our outdoor bath situated in the midst of a native forest) and subsequent massage. They have grown up with this ritual and respect the sacredness of the treatment room. No playing in there. The little four-year-old said to me one day, "You're a very good massager." The mantra came true.

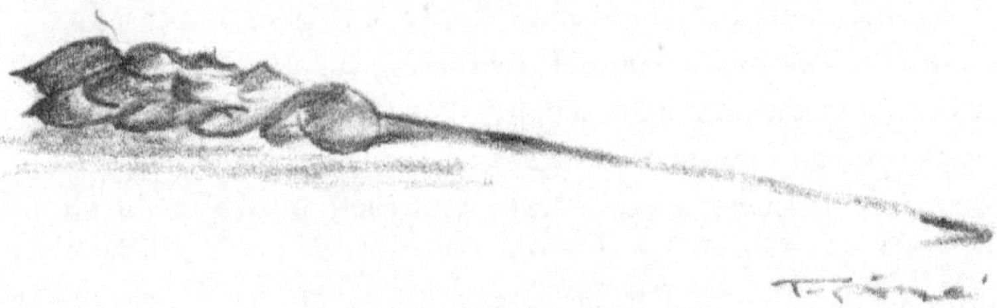

The Gift by T.M. Prince

Salvia rosmarinus ct cineole (Rosemary)

Salvia rosmarinus ct cineole (Rosemary) has been my companion while writing this book because it is good for the brain. Dr Mark Moss, in his research, showed that the inhalation of *Salvia rosmarinus* ct cineole (Rosemary) enhanced cognitive function and memory, due perhaps to the presence of 1,8 cineole which impedes the breakdown of acetylcholine necessary for synaptic communication.[17] Anyway I need all the help I can get, especially when it comes to keeping the ageing brain sharp!

Rosemary has long been known as the herb of remembrance and is a tonic for the body's yang energy, promoting circulation and energising the heart qi. Wonderful for sluggishness, mental fatigue and congestion, Rosemary is one of the best oils for boosting self confidence and is an "age old remedy for apathy and gloom".[18]

With its strong, invigorating, stimulating aroma I like to use it with the person who is world weary, lacking motivation and full of self doubt. I also find it useful for students studying for exams to reduce their fears and to help bring about mental clarity and focus.

Cistus ladaniferus (Rock rose)

I don't think I could live without *Cistus ladaniferus* (Rock rose). One of the ancient spiritual essences, it is sometimes called the "phoenix plant" as the seeds regenerate in the heat of burned earth after fire. The plant produces a sticky resin to protect itself. I love the analogy of rising from the ashes of fire. Who amongst us hasn't had to rise from the ashes of trauma at some time in our life? The oil is a tremendous tissue healer, haemostatic and wonderful for trauma on all levels. When we are shaken to the core it restores equilibrium. The aroma is deep, intense, long lasting. One drop diluted is all that is needed to address emotional shock.

I remember the young man, tense, exhausted, depressed, eyes sunken, cowed by the state of the world's inequalities and injustices; plans in disarray because of a pandemic. One drop of *Cistus ladaniferus* (Rock rose) on a cotton ball, one intake of breath, was all it took to fire the parasympathetic nervous system into action. Deep sighs, shoulders dropped, the body slumped in the chair, the eyes closed, a calm settled around and within him. It was extraordinary. The light in the eyes came back, the mind became quiet, the spirit was uplifted. No, I couldn't live without cistus.

Helichrysum italicum (Everlasting, also called Immortelle)

A wound healer on all levels physical and emotional, *Helichrysum italicum* (Everlasting) has been hailed as "liquid stitching" such is its ability to heal wounds and regenerate cells.[19] Regarded as one of the most powerful aromatic essences, *Helichrysum italicum* (Everlasting) works with deep knots in the psyche, longstanding anger and resentment often stemming from childhood trauma. Described as "honey for the psyche" it restores compassion for self and others.[20]

Often called the arnica of essential oils, Immortelle has anticoagulant activity and an ability to dissolve clots and treat bruising. It's not difficult to see the analogy between that and emotional blockages. It works well over the solar plexus to dissolve tension and depression from long held frustration.[21]

I remember the client who for years carried rejection and a profound lack of self worth and held it all in the solar plexus area, the seat of our personal power and where I like to think we digest life's experiences. Initially she found it almost unbearable to be touched there. Immortelle helped heal her. It took time but it worked. Her body released the deep seated, false, belief that she was "not enough", and gentle anointing of the solar plexus chakra became a comfort, not a threat.

Agonis fragrans or *Taxandria fragrans* (Fragonia)

Agonis fragrans (Fragonia) is a relatively new and unique West Australian oil grown and distilled by the Paperbark Company. Chemically one of the most balanced essential oils, not only in the molecular groups but within the individual components, the oil is valued for its ability to harmonise and rebalance. Robbi Zeck describes Fragonia as "like a candle

carrying the light of dignity". When the life force has wilted and patterns of behaviour leave emotional scarring, Fragonia can be used in a friction massage at the base of the skull and along the spine to release what Pert describes as traumatic memories stored in the autonomic ganglia.[22]

Felicity Warner considers *Agonis fragrans* (Fragonia) one of her sacred oils for end of life care. She describes its ability to "see us through a crisis". For uncertain times and major transitions she considers it a great ally.[23]

Children are often drawn to this oil. I remember the little eight-year-old boy who said to me, "When I feel angry I go to my schoolbag and sniff my Fragonia aromastick and I feel better."

Rosa damascena (Damask rose)

Often called the "queen of flowers", *Rosa damascena* (Damask rose) has been revered for centuries for its exotic, sensual, beautiful aroma. Scent of the angels some say; a conduit to the divine. In Islam the fragrance represents the sacredness of people's souls. With over three hundred chemical constituents it is a very complex oil and a tonic for the whole body, particularly the female reproductive system, purifying and regulating.[24]

Symbol of love, oil of the heart chakra, it is a soul friend. Holmes refers to its totality of treatment for the female body, mind and soul.[25] A gentle but potent antidepressant, it promotes a sense of wellbeing, opens the heart, soothes feelings of anger, fear, anxiety and grief and softens hard attitudes. It helps to heal emotional wounds when rejection or loss has injured our capacity for self love. In the lovely words of Gabriel Mojay, "Bringing warmth to a soul grown cold through abuse or hurt, rose oil can touch the deepest despair, restoring the trust that makes it possible to love again."[26] It is a gift for the sad and the bereaved.

I complete all my treatments with a rose facial. Diluted at 3% in Jojoba oil, I put a few drops on my fingertips and hold the palms of my hands over the client's face for a few seconds. Always there is a deep intake of breath and an almost sighing expiration as if the last vestiges of tension were leaving the body.

It is a beautiful way to finish a treatment connecting to the heart chakra, the centre which reflects our capacity to love. In the big scheme of things, what else really matters?

For the labouring mama, *Rosa damascena* (Damask rose) has been shown to be one of the oils effective for calming anxiety in labour.[27]

What a beautiful scent with which to welcome a new soul to this earth. I have helped countless new mothers with postnatal emotional distress with a spritzer blend of *Rosa damascena* (Damask rose), *Agonis fragrans* (Fragonia) and *Pelargonium graveolens* (Geranium) essential oils.

Cupressus sempervirens (Cypress)

The tall, thin, elegant cypress trees are synonymous with the Mediterranean landscape. In ancient Egypt the wood was used to make sarcophagi. The ancient Greeks dedicated the tree to Hades, god of the underworld, associating it with death and eternity. It was consequently planted around graveyards as a symbol of grief and source of solace. Often called the "oil of transition", *Cupressus sempervirens* (Cypress) is associated with often painful major life changes when we can be beset by fear and discouragement. Its energetics are beautifully described by Robbi Zeck: "When change is imminent, cypress brings structure, strength and a sense of protection... It supports and holds the space for the soul to remain in balance."[28]

I remember the anosmic patient who, although the smell eluded her, was fiercely drawn to the energy of Cypress to help her through traumatic events in her life.

I use it often in our unstable world when people, buffeted by the winds of change, are having to make painful decisions. It always seems to tether and ground them while they work through options.

Vetiveria zizanioides (Vetiver)

Vetiveria zizanioides (Vetiver) is a densely rooted grass whose roots resemble matted dreadlocks. It's a perfect example of the Doctrine of Signatures as it is used to stabilise the ground and prevent erosion, reflecting its use as a powerful sedative helping us to anchor our energies in the physical body during times of mental/emotional instability.[29]

With its smoky, earthy, musky scent, it has been used for thousands of years as a perfume in Indonesia and India. The roots woven into blinds and screens in India provide shade and when doused in water "the cool, sweet scent of their vapour turns scorching winds that dehydrate into moist and balmy breezes".[30] Environmental fragrancing at its best!

Holmes describes it as a classic for burnout and one of the most restorative remedies, "repairing as it does the body's four core systems; the nervous, endocrine, gastrointestinal and immune...this is an

aromatic for chronic deficiencies arising from long term stressors".[31] Known as the oil of "Tranquillity and Abundance", he regards Vetiver as a gift from mother earth representing nurture and self empowerment.

Vetiver also has a reputation for energetic protection. One drop anticlockwise on the solar plexus is said to prevent us from becoming a "psychic sponge".[32]

I am reminded of a lovely young woman who came for a treatment. Normally strong and capable, she was needing to draw on all her resources to cope with the stresses in her life. Vetiver was calling to be used in her blend. Her response was very interesting: "The treatment included the oil vetiver which didn't appeal to me as a scent at the time. However, the next day I felt like I had this force field of protection around me."

Picea mariana (Black spruce)

When I was teaching, the students used to call me "Queen of the Black Spruce" because I adored it so much. To me it is *shinrin yoku* in a bottle. I'm walking in the boreal forests of Canada on my way to witness the aurora borealis. I wish. It's on the bucket list. The oil is divine and arguably has the greatest range of therapeutic effects among the conifers. So much so that Holmes warrants defining it as an adaptagenic having a broad spectrum regulating, normalising effect and influencing the nervous, endocrine and immune systems. It is well known as a booster and regulator of the hypothalamic–pituitary–adrenal (HPA) axis, giving rise to its use for adrenal fatigue. The age old conifers have been with us for eons. When exhaustion defeats us, Black spruce when inhaled can evoke qualities of strength, endurance, willpower and courage. It can connect to ancestral wisdom and enable us to see our journey in a new way.[33]

Pinus sylvestris (Scotch pine)

For me *Pinus sylvestris* (Scotch pine) essential oil is energetically all about self worth, burnout, loss of willpower, guilt and blame. Holmes observes that pine "is for the person whose soul strength has been crushed by severe hardships…and may kindle a spark of courage and motivation to continue on life's journey".[34]

Also regarded as an adaptogen, it is one of the best oils for fatigue and nervous exhaustion. Zeck describes it as validating our unique gifts,

encouraging self worth, generating a "quiet understanding of our unique expression in life" and believing we are worthy of having our dreams come true.[35] I remember distinctly reading this description to a client working through trauma which had left her deeply lacking in a sense of self worth, and the mere act of hearing these words reduced her to tears. Scotch pine played a significant role in her recovery.

A very useful adrenal support massage oil consists of 50ml carrier oil and seven drops each of *Pinus sylvestris* (Scotch pine), *Picea mariana* (Black spruce), *Cupressus sempervirens* (Cypress) and *Citrus sinensis* (Sweet orange) essential oils. Applied to the kidney area twice a day, I have found it very beneficial for chronic fatigue.

Citrus paradisi (Grapefruit)

Like all the citrus oils *Citrus paradisi* (Grapefruit) has a fresh, clean, revitalising sit up and take notice kind of aroma and is useful when we feel drained and a little fed up with life. In TCM the liver is associated with anger. As a liver and lymphatic decongestant, helping to move stagnant qi energy, Grapefruit is therefore excellent for soothing feelings of irritability and frustration when we expect too much of ourselves and others. The resulting guilt and depression can result in comfort eating.[36]

I keep Grapefruit in my aromatic tool kit for one main reason. When my clients circle the emotions they have been feeling in recent months it is surprising how often the word "resentment" rears its ugly head, despite not having appeared throughout the conversation. In situations like this I always add Grapefruit to the blend to mellow out that insidious emotion which can gnaw away at our wellbeing. Holmes regards Grapefruit as "one of the best oils for healing the head-heart connection". It brings a gentle mental clarity as opposed to a sharp spotlight like lemon.[37]

Boswellia carterii (Frankincense)

Offered as a gift to the Christ child and used for millennia in religious ceremonies, *Boswellia carterii* (Frankincense) is deeply spiritual, meditative and calming for the nervous system. It deepens the breath, stills the mind and helps to silence mental chatter. Often called the "decision maker", it helps us to focus the mind and cut ties with the past, to move on. It helps us transcend our earthly worries and takes us to an "otherworldly" place. I often use a drop of Frankincense in a steam inhalation

at the beginning of a treatment because of its ability to do just that, to transport the client beyond the physical.

I use Frankincense for the worriers, the nonstop thinkers, the insomniacs, the anxiety sufferers, the restless, the lost. It intrigues me how often, when clients return for a follow up treatment, they have moved on from indecision to pro action. I have witnessed the power of this oil to calm the lungs of asthmatics and those with bronchiectasis when nothing else alleviates the coughing fits. It's a comfort also in end of life care when it can deepen the breath and connect to the spiritual realm.

Once again the Doctrine of Signatures comes to mind when I see the tears of Frankincense resin solidifying and healing the cuts on the tree, mirroring its ability as a wound healer for mankind, physically and psychologically.[38]

When I think "frankincense" I think "holy".

Eucalyptus radiata (Narrow-leaved peppermint eucalyptus)

There are hundreds of varieties of eucalyptus, a member of the Myrtaceae family commonly associated with pathologies of the respiratory system. High in the molecule 1,8 cineole, often called "the breathing molecule", Eucalyptus has a pungent, stimulating, fresh, camphoraceous aroma immediately refreshing for congested nasal passages. A tonic of the lung qi, "it opens the chest",[39] and is a bronchial decongestant.

On a subtle level this ability to breathe more deeply, to open up the chest area, has the potential to release old grief, old patterns of behaviour, despondency and apathy. When we feel bogged down in details and stagnant energy, restricted in life by predictable routine, eucalyptus can refresh and revitalise the psyche helping us to see things more clearly, to let go of the old and welcome the new.[40]

I use *Eucalyptus radiata* (Narrow-leaved peppermint eucalyptus) for those whose diaries leave no space for down time; for those juggling work and homelife to the detriment of their own wellbeing; for those carrying a heaviness in their chest through unresolved grief; for those who just need to take a deep breath and get off the merry go round.

Angelica archangelica (Angelica)

With its strong structural form up to 2m high reaching to the sky and deep roots sunken into the earth, *Angelica archangelica* (Angelica) emits

a powerful, stabilising energy in its beauty. Long associated with the angelic realms and angelic guidance, it is an oil for the discouraged, those lacking in willpower and self belief, those who have been repeatedly "knocked down". Zeck has one of the best descriptions when she talks about its use to "stand your ground, to assert and express your truth, sending clear messages to others about a particular situation". It is one of Felicity Warner's sacred oils with a very high vibration associated with the warrior Archangel Michael, protecting against negative energies, emotions and situations.[41]

I often use *Angelica archangelica* (Angelica) to anoint the throat chakra, our communication centre, when "speaking up" is important. I remember clearly the family member of a client preparing to go to court to fight for custody of a young child not in the best of circumstances. She was nervous and unsure that she could cope with the judicial surroundings. And so we anointed the throat with *Angelica archangelica* (Angelica) oil and she carried it with her in an aromastick. She spoke up with a fierce protective passion for this young soul; all fear, all doubt left her. Maybe the angels were with her. You decide. She spoke, she won, we cried.

Citrus aurantifolia (Lime)

There's something about *Citrus aurantifolia* (Lime) which leaves the other citruses in its shade. It's intensely aromatic, revitalising, cleansing somehow. Cooling to heated emotions, it has a restorative action on mental fatigue and a spasmolytic effect on the nervous, cardiovascular and musculoskeletal systems. Whether the heat is from a fever or emotionally driven by elation, anger or fear, Lime can bring us to a place of calm.[42]

Proof then that the beautiful young mama to be knew exactly what she needed when she insisted on *Citrus aurantifolia* (Lime) as her oil of choice for inhalation during labour. As a mother of seven I can assure you that if ever we need strength, endurance and an ability to remain in control of our emotions, it's during the profoundly powerful experience of bringing a new life into the world. I can still see this young woman radiant in the bath, the molecules of Lime redolent in the air. What a privilege it was to be there for my daughter.

Zingiber officinalis (Ginger)

We are all familiar with the pungent fiery warming taste of Ginger. If we think of the Doctrine of Signatures we would immediately think

"warming for cold conditions" and we would be right. Traditionally used for nausea, indigestion, cold painful muscles, poor circulation and congestion in the respiratory tract, it is one of the few herbal remedies used for the last two thousand years in the Chinese, Ayurveda and Greek systems of traditional medicine.[43] Regarded as an energy tonic, it warms the metabolism, strengthening the yang energy of the kidneys which of course in TCM are associated with the will.[44]

I use Ginger therefore for those who "have lost the fire in their belly", lacking motivation, self confidence and drive, leading to withdrawal, depression, fatigue and apathy. They have suffered a loss of mental and physical energy over time. They often describe "feeling gutted" about where they are in life or about being hurt by the words and deeds of others. Emotional upset is often felt in the gut and the area of the solar plexus chakra which has to do with our personal power. You can see, therefore, why Ginger works well to activate the metabolism through warmth, settling the digestive system, reinvigorating not just the body but the mind too.

In today's world it's not uncommon for Ginger to come up in the consultation when the relentless treadmill of life brings no respite or fulfilment and there is a loss of energy over time.

Anthemis nobilis (Roman chamomile)

Anthemis nobilis (Roman chamomile) has been around for a long time. According to Holmes it was an "important part of the materia medicas of the medical systems of ancient Egypt, Greece, Islam and Europe".[45] In the Middle Ages it was used as a strewing herb and is indeed wonderful to grow as a chamomile lawn releasing those sedative esters when walked upon. With an enormously high percentage of esters it is of course going to be relaxing to the central nervous system. Associated with treating rigidity both emotionally and physically, its calming effect can help to defuse tense situations and energy stagnation, relaxing smooth and striated muscles, thus providing a physical analgesic, antispasmodic effect as well as a psychological soothing balm. It can "help dissolve those ego defences rooted in anger".[46]

Anthemis nobilis (Roman chamomile) is therefore wonderful for the cranky child, the red-faced temper tantrums, restlessness, anxiety, insomnia. Cooling to the liver qi, associated with anger, it is also called for when we are uptight, inflexible and convinced we are always right. For panic attacks when combined with *Lavandula angustifolia* (Lavender

true) it has no equal in my eyes. I carry with me my soothing roll on with those very oils for those very occasions. I am reminded of its use with *Lavandula angustifolia* (Lavender true) for the babies suffering neonatal abstinence syndrome (NAS) and how their time in the NICU was dramatically reduced, discussed above. Long regarded as the children's herb, it's a must for anyone's herb garden.

Citrus sinensis (Sweet orange)

There's something about *Citrus sinensis* (Sweet orange) that lifts the spirits. Its sweet fresh aroma has a sort of bubbly effect rather like a glass of champagne. There is a plethora of research on the anti-anxiety effects of this oil, such as diffusing into dental waiting rooms, and research too into the anticarcinogenesis effect of essential oils high in limonene such as *Citrus sinensis* (Sweet orange).[47]

So the humble orange packs quite a punch. It is mood enhancing, brings lightness, laughter, helps us connect to our inner child. Zeck describes it as useful when we are "feeling gloomy and unable to see light at the end of the tunnel".[48] Mojay advises it for the perfectionists who can become intolerant and irritable expecting too much of themselves and others.[49] It is a universal favourite with children. I remember the little girl whose behaviour changed at home to one of moodiness and aggression towards her family as though she had picked up some sort of negative energy. She chose *Citrus sinensis* (Sweet orange) for her own therapeutic perfume mist. The result was remarkable. She self treated with her spray whenever she felt angry and within a few days her joyful light hearted nature had returned.

Thymus vulgaris ct linalool (Thyme)

Thyme, as we know, is a hot spicy little herb which should indicate its use according to the Doctrine of Signatures. It is "a powerful tonic of the body's yang energy, reinforcing the functions of the Lungs, Heart, Kidneys and nervous system".[50] It is indicated therefore for apathy, loss of motivation, fatigue, fear, loss of confidence. According to Zeck its dynamic energy "activates a vital force for the positive use of willpower strengthening resolve and assisting in the breaking of negative patterns or habits."[51]

In today's world it is not uncommon to need a drop of *Thymus vulgaris* ct linalool (Thyme) in the blend. Simply surviving is a struggle for

many, resulting in a profound fatigue, lethargy and loss of confidence. A drop of *Thymus vulgaris* ct linalool (Thyme) is like striking the match to rekindle the fire. There are several chemotypes of *Thymus vulgaris* (Thyme). It's important to use the alcohol variants such as ct linalool, ct thujanol and ct geraniol as opposed to ct thymol, which is phenolic and dermocaustic. This little bottle is never far out of reach in these troubled times.

***Santalum album* (Sandalwood)**
***Santalum spicatum* (Australian sandalwood)**

Indian *Santalum album* (Sandalwood) is highly endangered; therefore I use the Australian *Santalum spicatum* (Sandalwood), which is more sustainably produced. This valued oil distilled from the heartwood is cooling to the body and heated emotions. Traditionally used in meditation and prayer, it stills the mind and reduces what Mojay calls "the tyranny of the intellect".[52] I love that description. Sometimes called the "metaphysical rescue remedy", it is called for when we overthink, ruminate and worry obsessively. An excellent skin oil, its cooling, moisturising, anti-inflammatory properties are helpful for dryness and irritation. It is also a very sensual oil, helping us to connect to our emotions in a stabilising harmonious way.[53] For all these reasons it is an essential ingredient in my "Liaison pure joy" massage oil blended for romance, and I can tell you right now it works and has saved many a relationship and enhanced many more!

***Cananga odorata* (Ylang ylang)**

Cananga odorata (Ylang ylang) is credited with harmonising sedative qualities and is widely used to combat stress, anxiety and tachycardia. With its sensuous, seductive euphoric scent it has long been considered an aphrodisiac and was used to perfume the beds of newlyweds in Indonesian culture. Helping to dispel anger, fear and create a sense of loving togetherness, it's not surprising, therefore, that it too is an essential ingredient in my Liaison pure joy oil! I use it to bring out the softer feminine aspect in both men and women, to help them find that sense of self. I use it for the workaholic woman who has lost that. Its heady scent is intense, but blended it can work magic.

Pogostemon cablin (Patchouli)

Scent of the Orient, complex, beautiful, earthy, long lasting, with a history of use in temples and perfumes, you will either love or loathe this musky fragrance of the hippy generation of the 1960s. Deeply hydrating, it supports toned skin and is said to be a tissue regenerator with strong, astringent, cicatrisant properties.[54] Its bracing action on the central nervous system may explain its association with increased libido. *Pogostemon cablin* (Patchouli) teaches us about the sacredness of our senses and sensuality, doorway to the soul.[55] It is a profoundly grounding oil often described as the oil "for dreamers", helping to integrate body and soul.[56] It is of course the third ingredient in my Liaison pure joy oil (the fourth being *Rosa damascena* (Damask rose), oil of the heart chakra, as previously discussed).

Nardostachys jatamansi (Spikenard)

Before I talk about this beautiful oil it is crucial to point out that it is critically endangered and thus we are discouraged from purchasing it now. The little bottle that I have is therefore precious and used highly diluted only as a chakra oil. Diluting does not diminish its effect. In fact when working energetically, the higher the dilution the more potent it is. To counteract the sustainability issue Felicity Warner uses local herbs and has found *Geranium robertianum* (Herb robert) to have similar effects to *Nardostachys jatamansi* (Spikenard), which is very encouraging.

Nardostachys jatamansi (Spikenard) is an ancient and holy oil. Also called Nard oil, it was used by Mary Magdalene to anoint the feet of Jesus. The Cathars used it in a ceremony called Consolamentum to prepare the dying for transition.[57] Its name *jatamansi* means "spirit incarnate" and attests to its association with spiritual issues and contemplation on "the existential mystery of life".[58] I have found it truly holistic, stabilising the heart and mind at times of great personal change. Clients have described it as "like having a big comforting blanket wrapped around them" when I use it to anoint the solar plexus, seat of personal power.

Commiphora myrrha (Myrrh)

Myrrh is distilled from the sticky resin from incisions made in the tree trunk. It was highly prized in ancient cultures, used in the embalming process in Egypt and one of the gifts offered by the Magi to the Christ child. Along with *Boswellia carterii* (Frankincense) and *Nardostachys*

jatamansi (Spikenard) it was one of the three revered sacred essences. It has a deeply calming effect on the mind, reducing obsessive thinking and worry, helping to bring about stillness. It encourages us to let go of fear and painful emotions, to move on with wisdom and forgiveness.[59]

Juniperus communis (Juniper berry)

I love *Juniperus communis* (Juniper berry) not just because it is the main ingredient in gin but because of its ability to cleanse and detoxify. It is a good fluid decongestant and warming to the kidney's yang energy associated with the will. I use it particularly these days for those who are despondent, discouraged, fearful, lacking in willpower and dealing with scattered energy. I use it for those whose energy carries a negative vibe. It helps to purify the atmosphere and dispel unwanted negative thoughts. When there is no joy, it helps to bring stability in times of emotional and spiritual challenge. It's one of my favourite oils with which to begin a treatment, in a steam inhalation. I regard it as trying to wipe the slate clean.

CHAPTER 7

Client Reflections and Case Studies

The names and certain specific details have been changed to maintain confidentiality. The common thread running through these case histories is how much the act of being listened to and cared for in a safe space means to the clients. It is everything.

Sarah (Auckland)

Sarah's story was very much about the plight of the immigrant and the loss of self that can ensue for a time; the feeling of disconnection in a new land, far from family, friends and the piece of earth that had nurtured her. Her energy was "scattered", she had "no direction", "no joy". She felt her life had "contracted". She used words like "idle", "aimless", "no sense of place or belonging". Sarah was a highly intelligent compassionate human being and I could sense that her confidence and self worth had been undermined. I understand perfectly the plight of the immigrant, having been in that situation twice in my life. I understand how we can feel like an appendage to someone else's family tree until we put down our own roots, make our own friends and forge our own path in this new land. It was of the utmost importance, therefore, to make Sarah feel welcome, cared for and validated for the wonderful person she is. She really enjoyed the treatments and interestingly during one session felt a strong connection to ancestral feminine energy and a "sense of empowerment". Here are her words:

"As soon as I stepped into the consultation room I felt cared for by all the small touches: beautifully presented herbal tea, a warm blanket, a warm room. Already it felt like I was entering a safe space where it got to be all about me – something I didn't fully appreciate I needed until it was

happening. I got the sense that I mattered, that this wasn't a transaction but a space of healing. Being engaged in conversation about what was going on for me made me feel seen and cared for.

The consultation felt specially curated for this purpose. I didn't feel rushed or pressured to say anything I didn't want to, which contributed to the safety. I also appreciated the short form I was to fill out because it created a thread of continuity between sessions. Though I am fairly good at this point in my life with naming my emotions, being presented with a list of emotions to choose from made me feel like I was providing information that would help Annie select the right oils. Her clarifying questions about my feelings over the past week were of course crucial in this process. When Annie selected the oils after our conversation, I felt excited and grateful that I would be receiving exactly what I needed during the massage.

The massage itself – the specific process and reliable order of events – was always so relaxing and soothing. The touch, the care, the environment and the oils all combined to make it a beautiful experience. I could tell that Annie treats her process and clients with the greatest respect, which in this day and age of easy distraction and fast paced everything was healing in itself. I was made to feel like I mattered, that this time was for me, and that I deserved to be attentively cared for.

The conversation after the massage was a really nice way to tie up the treatment. Again, I was made to feel like my experience and feelings were central to the process. The care and safety I felt from Annie continued throughout the treatment from start to finish. It gave my nervous system a much needed reprieve and reset."

"The impact of my first experience of working with Annie was spectacular. I arrived stressed, anxious and burnt out. I felt awkward and angular, overloaded with heady intellectualising of my various dilemmas, emotional and professional. The soothing tea in the beautiful consulting room and the infinite unhurried manner whereby Annie sought to find clarity regarding my key issues were balm to my troubled soul. Her questions had integrity and felt authentic and appropriate. The levels of care, time and commitment were extraordinary and my body simply drank it all in. Somehow many of the needed changes in my life were crystallised and made manifest through this session. Thank you Annie." E. (Auckland)

Matthew

Matthew had my card for a year before he appeared on my doorstep. A colleague was a regular client of mine and had encouraged him to make an appointment for stress relief. The word "aromatherapy" does not always attract the male sex, it's often seen as a bit "airy fairy", so it required a bit of courage on his part to take this leap of faith. He looked slightly ill at ease, avoiding eye contact and sat down on the edge of the chair. I encouraged him to sit back and relax and enjoy the herbal tea I had prepared for him fresh from the garden. He was surprised by and interested in this gesture and keen to know what plants were used and why. He visibly relaxed in this comforting environment and so began ten months of monthly conversation during which time Matthew completely fell in love with essential oils and even started to study them himself.

Matthew was a very handsome young man in his thirties working in the area of children's mental health. He was obviously brilliant at his job, completely devoted to those in his care and was loved by everybody. Everybody that is except himself. Growing up gay in a fundamentally Christian family with a homophobic father and emotionally absent mother, Matthew carried deep wounds in the psyche and an ingrained lack of self worth which he carried deep in the solar plexus area, an area so tense that it was almost painful to the touch. He often repeated the words "I feel not good enough, not lovable" despite his stellar career and natural beauty. We would spend three hours every month talking and talking, exploring Matthew's upbringing, the sadness and anger he felt at not being accepted for who he was. We would talk about everything and anything and he loved it. It was the highlight of his month. Matthew became intrigued by the oils, especially their energetic signatures, and would use aromasticks at home on a daily basis or on his way to work. They were based on the oils chosen for his massage treatments to address his deep seated angst.

Slowly we peeled away the emotional layers. It took a long time as the pain was so deeply embedded in his body and mind. At one point I encouraged him to start a three-week protocol of writing two pages a day of positive thoughts focusing on how he would like to feel and to release the untruths deep in his subconscious. I have read that it takes three weeks to change the programming in the subconscious mind, which doesn't distinguish between truth and fiction but will believe what it constantly hears. I have done this myself with great success.

At the same time Matthew told me about a recurring dream that he

had. It was of a baby which was always malformed in some way. True to form Matthew started his writing at home, often while inhaling some of his precious oils, and ten days in he arrived one day and said to me, "I had that dream again. I dreamt I was holding this beautiful, perfect, dark, curly haired, brown-eyed baby, showing it to people saying this is me." I'm not afraid to cry in front of clients when appropriate, and oh yes, we cried. Towards the end of the ten months Matthew rang me and asked if I had an hour free just to talk. He particularly loved the outlook from my consultation room which looked on to a beautiful forest. When he arrived he stood in front of the big picture window and said "I just want you to sit there, say nothing and listen" and for one hour it poured out of him from the depths of his soul: all the injustice, the hurt, the anger, the grief, the despair, the frustration, the wasted years of self hate, it just poured out of him as he spoke to the trees. It was a shedding of a burden he had carried for thirty odd years. It was catharsis of the highest order. It was one of the most profound moments of my life. With tears streaming down our faces I hugged him and simply said, "I am so proud of you."

After ten months Matthew was a changed man. He believed in his self worth. He took off on his overseas experience with a heart that was light and looking for adventure. I haven't seen him in a long while but I believe he is happily in a new relationship. I used *Helichrysum italicum* (Everlasting) a lot to anoint the solar plexus area on Matthew. It is reputed to help undo deep knots in the psyche. It certainly was a factor in soothing away the almost painful tension in that chakra.

"The consultation process was therapeutic in itself; discussing my emotions without judgement, but just acknowledging how I was feeling at that moment. This was also never rushed, so felt genuine. Often all we need is for someone to listen. The oils were then tailored to suit exactly what I needed at that time. I valued the time that was taken to explain each of the oils selected for the treatment, and the benefits that they provided. I have vivid memories of a treatment I had during a time I was dealing with a lot of other people's 'stuff' and struggling to create boundaries for my own emotions. The treatment included the oil vetiver which didn't appeal to me as a scent at the time. However, the next day I felt like I had this force field of protection around me."
B. (Auckland)

"The healing and transformational power of botanical aromatherapy is truly remarkable. I discovered Annie on my journey surviving an acrimonious divorce facing up to countless rounds of litigation. As a trained professional, she always deduced exactly what I needed after a thorough consultation. The result is a very noticeable reaching beyond the physical, causing shifts beyond explanation. I consider Annie one of my 'secret weapons' that has made me the resilient woman that I am today." S. (Auckland)

Beverley

I had known Beverley for a long time. She was 62 years old, a teacher and solo mother. She was normally an extremely optimistic, compassionate person with a happy disposition. She was intelligent, well travelled, resourceful and very independent. She came to me in a state of extreme distress, unable to sleep, rating her self esteem, confidence, happiness and energy levels all as 1 out of 10. The words she used to describe her emotional state were many: "anxious, depressed, tired, angry, helplessness, rage, indignation, self pity, disbelief, sad, overburdened, resentful, critical". She couldn't eat and had no motivation to tend her garden or cook, both passions of hers. She felt "desolate" and that "her core feeling of optimism had been washed away", "like a kick in the solar plexus".

The cause of her extreme distress was a work-related incident which basically attacked her integrity, honesty and ability to do her job. It was a malicious attempt by someone, provoked by jealousy, to discredit her (the accusation was subsequently dismissed).

My therapeutic intent was:

- to dispel the negative energy around her
- to balance her heart/mind turmoil
- to boost her energy and renew her optimism
- to boost her confidence, self esteem and promote forgiveness
- to enable her to be assertive and speak her truth.

The oils were chosen for their energetic signatures as described in the previous chapter and included *Juniperus communis* (Juniper berry) to dispel negativity, *Zingiber officinalis* (Ginger) for energy, *Angelica archangelica* (Angelica) on the throat chakra for assertiveness and *Nardostachys*

jatamansi (Spikenard) on the solar plexus for mental/emotional stability, *Vetiveria zizanioides* (Vetiver) for grounding and *Cymbopogon martinii* (Palmarosa) for self confidence and betrayal.

Beverley shed a few tears during the massage, then relaxed deeply. Afterwards, while having a cup of tea, she gradually began to feel different. "I'd been a stranger and came back to myself," she said.

Her friend talking to her a couple of hours later couldn't believe the change in her. The stress had gone. She felt calm and strong.

The important thing with Beverley was to allow her to vent the intense feelings she had and to take note of the words she used to describe her emotional state, as well as how she rated her self esteem, confidence, happiness and energy levels from 1 to 10. These two protocols gave me a very clear picture of her mental/emotional state and were pointers to choosing appropriate oils.

As always, working with intent on my part was crucial, and heart centred breathing, leading to coherence and a positive electromagnetic energy, would have been picked up by her electromagnetic field, helping her to relax (see the previous discussion on the HeartMath Institute). The importance of the personal conversation was so evident in Beverley's case. Form filling would have been disastrous. She needed the warmth and empathy of a compassionate human being. Above all she needed to voice her distress out loud to help release it from her body. She needed validation.

"I met Annie and aromatherapy over seven years ago when going through a difficult period and the results were amazing. I have since read that smell is the sense that connects us most quickly with our emotions and I am sure that touch must follow second. I find that the essential oils and Annie's intuitive choice (based on a deep theoretical knowledge) are both immediately rejuvenating and subsequently restorative. The combination of touch and smell addresses both the physical and emotional that link deeply with our spiritual wellbeing. I have continued with regular treatments for my health and happiness, especially at those times when life's stressors seem overwhelming. Thank you, Annie, for the care and love you put into every treatment." H. (Auckland)

"The consultation specifically looks at the emotional, physical and mental needs of the client, and with that in depth knowledge allows the therapist to attain a healing mix of oils to bring together inner balance for the client. Most of all I feel listened to and cared for completely; the kindness and empathy is heartfelt." B. (Auckland)

"Sacred anointing with oil – so much more than a massage." H. (Auckland)

Conclusion

This book is essentially a book about connection: connection to one another, to the earth and to all living things, observed through the lens of aromatherapy. Organisational psychologist Richard Davis believes we are losing the cognitive and social skills needed to thrive in our personal and professional lives due to our dependence on technology, reducing our ability to talk to and really connect with one another. He considers it "a major concern".[1] We live in a world obsessed with consumerism, technology and the need to prove everything. Ron Guba talks about "scientific materialism", the fact that evidence is everything, but it is not the full picture.[2] There are things that cannot be dissected and proved in a narrow reductionist manner. They are too complex, too indefinable, too magical. I refer to the profound intelligence of the natural world and the botanical gifts of wellbeing that it gifts us. I refer to what it means to be human: the intricate workings of the body, mind and soul that make us who we are as unique individuals and the spark that can be ignited when we connect with our fellow beings. A spark that can give meaning to our life on earth, a spark that can bring immense joy and happiness, a spark that can heal.

The therapeutic relationship is a unique way in which we can ignite that spark of connectedness, and aromatherapy has the tools to feed that depth of closeness in a myriad of ways. The French verb *sentir* means both "to smell" and "to feel". Our olfactory system is undeniably the gateway to the emotions. We talk about "smelling a rat", "something smells fishy", "something smells divine". We live in a world that is often harsh, driven by the struggle to survive or the ambition to succeed; driven often by greed, intolerance and a lust for power.

> *We have been tribeless and disconnected for so long now.*
> *It's time for us all to come home.*
>
> JOHANN HARI[3]

Appendix: An Insight into the World of Aromatherapy

The following pages explore the fundamentals that you need to know when studying aromatherapy. This is not only for student practitioners to help them to practise well but for those who have no knowledge of this powerful modality and are curious to know more.

1. Aromatherapy explained

In today's world the term aromatherapy has unfortunately been hijacked by marketers of synthetic scent and used to describe everything imaginable from toilet cleaners to shampoos, thus debasing its real meaning and power.

It is in fact a branch of herbal medicine involving the controlled use of essential oils and aromatic plant essences to help promote and maintain physical, psychological and spiritual wellbeing. Their use dates back to ancient civilisations which utilised aromatic plants medicinally and cosmetically.

Avicenna, eleventh-century Persian scholar and physician, is traditionally credited with perfecting the art of distillation, but the discovery of a four thousand-year-old alembic still on the island of Cyprus, by Dr Maria Belgiorno, has shown that people were distilling thousands of years ago and not simply macerating plants in olive oil. "The experiments made with a replica confirmed that the Pyrgos distiller could produce essential oils and scented waters."[1]

The remains of essences such as *Commiphora myrrha* (Myrrh), *Boswellia sacra* (Frankincense) and *Cedrus atlantica* (Cedarwood), used in the mummification process, have been found in Egyptian tombs with their fragrance intact. In essence they were the earliest antiseptics.

The name *aromatherapie* (therapy through the molecules of scent)

was coined early in the twentieth century by René Maurice Gattefossé, a French biochemist, who after burning his hand severely in a laboratory experiment treated it with pure *Lavandula angustifolia* (Lavender true) essential oil and was so impressed by its analgesic, antimicrobial and healing properties that he devoted the rest of his life to studying the chemistry and therapeutic properties of essential oils. In 1937 he wrote the seminal text *Aromatherapy.* His work is carried on today by the Gattefossé Foundation (www.gattefosse.com) which aims to promote the scientific and clinical use of essential oils as part of integrative medicine.

Clinical aromatherapy is a profession and a treatment like any other modality. **The quality of the oils is critical, as is the training of the therapist.** Clinical aromatherapy requires years of ongoing study in the art and science of aromatherapy, including chemistry, anatomy and physiology, the properties of the essential oils and related botanicals, listening and consultation skills. The Diploma of Aromatherapy is simply the beginning/foundation, in my estimation.

Education is key here and fortunately the spread of clinical aromatherapy globally is addressing the misconceptions, thanks in no small measure to the Botanica conferences, the Essence of Clinical Aromatherapy (ECA) seminars and the International Clinical Aromatherapy Network (ICAN) platform, all spearheaded by Rhiannon Lewis of Essential Oil Resource Consultants in Provence. These platforms bring together qualified aromatherapists, doctors, nurses, scientists, researchers and herbalists to share knowledge, research and the successful implementation of essential oils and botanical medicine into their rightful place in integrative healthcare.

> When nausea is relieved through the inhalation of peppermint, insomnia is alleviated through the inhalation of lavender or rose, or candida albicans is killed by tea tree, we are witnessing clinical results – not just the "feel-good" factor. Aromatherapy can work at a clinically significant level.[2]

The story of Abby Jean

I begin every one of my classes with the story of Abby Jean because it illustrates unequivocally the power and real meaning of aromatherapy. It is to be found in *Natural Home Health Care*

Using Essential Oils written by Daniel Pénoël MD and published in 1998 by Osmobiose.

The introduction was written by Abby Jean herself in 1996. Here is a summary of her tale.

Abby Jean, a seven-year-old girl from Auckland, brought up in Australia:

- First seven years of her life plagued by chronic bronchial, pulmonary and ear infections.
- Received **thirty courses of antibiotics** which failed to change this state of permanent infection.
- Her physical and mental health suffered from this constant systemic attack on her body.
- She had allergic reactions to antibiotics, and tetracycline damaged her teeth.
- She suffered severe joint pain.
- Her immune system was weakened by this constant aggression and turned itself on the tissues of her body.
- Her hearing decreased; she lagged behind in school, was thin and had no appetite for life.

In 1986 an x-ray showed yet another serious infection in the maxillary sinuses and deep nasal cavities.

Her ENT specialist prescribed yet another 15-day course of antibiotics.

If there was no improvement in two weeks he suggested surgery to break open the sinuses, release pus and flush the nasal cavities.

Enter Dr Pénoël, French medical doctor and pioneer in medical aromatherapy, who was on a two-year sabbatical in Australia.

He had 15 days to cure an infection that had festered under conventional medical care for seven years.

He developed a plan of inclusive healthcare with the family:

1. **Nutritional correction**: already gluten and dairy free, there was to be no peanut butter or Vegemite, as they are allegedly hard to metabolise, tax the liver and the residues leave the body

through the respiratory mucous membranes, causing congestion. Other foods were eliminated and she drank lots of carrot juice.

2. **Intensive aromatic care**:

- daily two-hour treatments including aromatic aerosols, massage, reflexology, manual drainage; nasal cleansing (Hydrofloss machine).

3. **Home treatments**:

- topical applications using essential oils
- night inhalation of a directional mist of essential oils.

"I was required to eat, drink and breathe essential oils. I was almost bathed in their heady, intense aromas for twenty four hours each day. Before bed I was massaged with them: during the night I breathed them in through an amazing array of twisted and blown glass aerosol equipment. I sprayed my throat with a rosemary oil mixture and swallowed essential oils mixed with honey. At night the beautiful aromas of the essential oils were somewhat diluted by the sauteed onions which encased my feet!" Abby Jean

In two weeks all infection had cleared (before and after photos are in *Natural Home Health Care Using Essential Oils*).

- Essential oils cleared the infection.
- Essential oils and a change in diet brought back vital strength to her body.
- She began to heal properly.
- Over several months, while continuing aromatic treatments along with a strict diet, her body continued to expel the toxins and waste material accumulated from previous medications/infections in a brown mucous discharge found on her pillow each morning.

At the time of her writing (1996) she was symptom free, "a robust teenager" at university.

Her final words were: "Through alternative medicine I have

been able to achieve the healthy lifestyle that was once only a dream. I can only hope that in the future, the alternative medicines which changed my life will be readily available to all, and that the essences of nature will be recognised by all doctors as effective treatments for disease and illness." (*Natural Home Health Care Using Essential Oils,* p.22).

I ask myself often: "Where would Abby Jean be today if aromatic medicine hadn't come into her life?" If still alive, then probably extremely unwell with no quality of life, because allopathic medicine had no answer.

I have told this story so often to bring enlightenment and education to students and sceptics alike, and each time I get a frisson of wonder, joy and satisfaction because it so perfectly illustrates the power of clinical aromatherapy and essential oils, both to clear infection and to strengthen the body's terrain to deal with disease.

2. What are essential oils?

- Essential oils are essences used medicinally and cosmetically in all the ancient civilisations (a 4000-year-old still has been discovered in Cyprus).[3]
- Highly aromatic, volatile substances found in various parts of aromatic plants: leaves, flowers, bark, resins, seeds, roots, fruit, wood.
- Seventy times more potent than the plant itself, a huge amount of plant material is required to produce a tiny amount of essential oil (e.g. approximately 67 rose petals for 1 drop of rose oil). Steam distillation, cold pressing, CO_2 and solvent extraction are methods of extraction.
- They are composed of hundreds of molecules from different chemical groups, giving the plant its characteristic aroma and therapeutic qualities.
- Small molecular size, lipophilic, easily absorbed through the skin.
- They produce physiological reactions in the body.
- These molecules of scent have a direct pathway into the limbic system. There they trigger the release of neurochemicals which affect mood and behaviour.

- Multitalented, they can be sedative, stimulating, antibacterial, antiviral, analgesic, anti-inflammatory, cicatrisant, wound healing, mood enhancing.

The fact that a single essential oil can be used effectively on the physiological level to treat inflammation and infection; on a mood level to help even out mood swings; on a mental level to treat distractability; and on an emotional level to help resolve negativity and emotional conflicts is astonishing in itself. This versatility of treatment applications currently displayed by essential oils clearly engages multiple pathways of therapeutic influence.[4]

- They are Nature's antiseptics, protecting the plant from various pathogens.
- "A plethora of research exists on their antibacterial qualities."[5] Highly relevant in our post antibiotic era.
- Essential oils are used in integrated healthcare to improve mood, reduce stress, relieve anxiety, aid in wound care and pain relief, help fight infection, uplift the spirit and to bring comfort and solace in palliative care.[6]
- Essential oils connect us with our senses and to Nature. They can empower us to deal with everyday ailments before resorting to allopathic medication.

3. Methods of extraction

- **Steam distillation**: steam is forced through plant material, breaks open cells with essential oil which vaporises and is carried across with the steam to a cooling condenser. The mixture condenses back to liquid state (oil and water) and flows into a Florentine vessel where essential oil floats on top and is drawn off. There is an art and science to distillation and small artisanal distillers are highly prized.
- **Cold pressing** of citrus fruit rind. Rind is excoriated or whole fruit crushed. Oil and juice are separated by centrifugal force.
- **Solvent extraction-absolutes**: plant material is macerated in solvent (hexane), then removed, giving a "Concrete". Concrete is washed with alcohol, then distilled to remove it.

- **CO_2 extraction**: under pressure CO_2 transforms into an almost liquid state called supercritical. It is pumped into plant material in a sealed receptacle. With low heat and high pressure, the liquid state encourages the plant material to release the aromatic compounds. When pressure is released, the CO_2 changes back to a gaseous state, leaving the extracted material. The extracts contain more of the plant's original material and have a rich, intense aroma.

4. The chemistry of essential oils and the great functional group theory (FGT) debate

With the understanding that aromatherapy is an art and a science, it is imperative that we learn the basics of essential oil chemistry.

Why?

- To understand how and why essential oils work.
- To choose essential oils for clinical applications.
- To understand purity and safety issues.
- To speak the language of medical and scientific professionals.
- To understand the importance of chemotypes, genetic variations among species producing different chemical constituents (e.g. *Thymus vulgaris* ct linalool, *Thymus vulgaris* ct geraniol, *Thymus vulgaris* ct thuyanol, *Thymus vulgaris* ct thymol, *Thymus vulgaris* ct carvacrol).

Functional group theory is an area of great scientific debate in the aromatherapy world. It alleges that the different chemical families (functional groups) have distinct therapeutic properties unique to them.

Opponents of the theory believe that one cannot generalise and that the individual constituents in each chemical family have their particular therapeutic action. Robert Tisserand and colleagues conclude the following in a paper:

> When studying the action of essential oil constituents in the body, students will find some commonalities within functional groups. Some of these occur because the molecules are similar. Students will also learn about functional groups since they are a basic part of learning essential oil chemistry. But learning functional group theory as a shortcut to

> understanding the complexity of these natural substances is not sensible nor logical, and it cannot be justified.[7]

One of the accepted texts for studying essential oil chemistry is *The Chemistry of Aromatherapeutic Oils* by E. Joy Bowles, a co-author of the above paper.[8] In it she does indeed look at the chemistry of functional groups, and I quote:

> As the functional group(s) of a molecule give it distinct properties, we can group molecules by their different functional groups. Generalisations can be made with caution about the therapeutic properties of molecules based on their functional group structure, but research is needed to discover the specific actions of each different constituent, alone and in synergy with the other constituents in the oil.[9]

While I absolutely agree with the fact that we cannot overgeneralise the properties of functional groups and need to study the effects of individual constituents, it seems to be agreed that there are "some commonalities" and "generalisations can be made with caution" within each chemical family, which in my opinion can be crucial for students to know. For example, we can say with certainty that a phenol is much stronger in antibacterial action than an alcohol and is not to be slathered on the skin without knowledge of the possible dermocaustic effects and how to minimise them.

We can also say, for example, that aldehydes have the potential to be skin sensitising and that essential oils containing oxides, in particular 1,8 cineole, offer great respiratory support through their decongestant, mucolytic, expectorant, spasmolytic activity. In fact 1,8 cineole is often referred to as the "breathing molecule".

Based on Bowle's book and further reading,[10] I have summarised and simplified in the following pages some of the important aspects of essential oil chemistry, bearing in mind that this is simply a starting point for students to at least recognise and have some appreciation of basic chemical components.

The percentage suggested for certain constituents in a specific essential oil is an average, as amounts vary with each distillation depending on climate, terrain and expertise of the distiller.

For further in depth study please note the following courses, two of which are run by authors of the above paper (Bowles and Valussi):

Aromatic Chemistry Certification Course taught by Dr Joy Bowles (www.tisserandinstitute.org/aromatic-chemistry)

Advanced Aromatherapy Science Program with Marco Valussi, BSc (Hons) Herbal Medicine and Benoit Roger, PhD (www.essenceofthyme.com/advanced-aromatherapy-science)

Classes run by Timothy Miller, ND, Mac, Lac, RA on Aroma Chemistry, Aroma Pharmacokinetics, Functional Groups: AromaChemistry's Great Debate (www.naturopathicce.com)

> Chemistry and Scientific Research are complementary to the more subtle aspects of Essential Oils and do not detract from their magic. Indeed it serves to further enhance our deep respect for these remarkable healing tools.[11]

Essential oils are complex mixtures of chemical compounds.

Even trace amounts can affect aroma and therapeutic action.

Plants absorb

- Water H2O (from the ground)
- Carbon dioxide (from the air)

use

- Energy from the sun (photosynthesis)

to make

- Glucose

↓

Primary metabolites
(Carbohydrates, Proteins, Lipids)

↓

To grow

Plants release

- Oxygen and water back to the atmosphere

Many plants make

- Secondary metabolites

↓

Colour pigments and essential oils

Atoms in essential oils	Plus extra atoms	Functional groups
carbon	usually oxygen	alcohols
hydrogen	↓	phenols
	functional groups	ethers
		aldehydes
		lactones
		coumarins
		oxides
		ketones

Organic chemistry

- All living things – people, animals, plants – are composed of carbon compounds.
- Carbon atoms like to a) bond together to form chains and rings and b) bond with hydrogen to form a hydrocarbon.
- An isoprene unit is a branched chain of 5 carbon atoms. This is the basic building block of terpenes.
- Monoterpenes = 2 x isoprene units = 10 carbon atoms.
- Sesquiterpenes = 3 x isoprene units = 15 carbon atoms.
- Diterpenes = 4 x isoprene units = 20 carbon atoms.

The two common pathways that plants use to make essential oils

- The Mevalonate pathway, which produces terpenoids. As we have a terpene pathway in our body, these components are familiar to us; the body knows how to use them. Toxicity risk is very low.
- The Shikimate pathway produces phenylpropanoids which are unfamiliar to us. They have molecules based on the phenyl or benzene ring with 6 x carbon atoms with stable bonds. They have a pronounced aroma and are usually powerful antimicrobials to be used in low dose in the short term. Phenols are part of this group.

Introduction to the functional groups (chemical families) of essential oil chemistry

Monoterpenes, -ene

PROPERTIES/SAFETY

- very common
- antiseptic (a-pinene is antibacterial, antiviral, antifungal, anti-inflammatory)
- tonics/immune stimulants (*Picea mariana* (Black spruce) is fantastic for fatigue)
- rubifacient/skin penetrating/lipophilic, penetrate lipid barriers of stratum corneum. Penetration enhancers for dermally applied drugs
- decongestant; oedema (phellandrenes take fluid out of tissues)
- respiratory (a-pinene is mucolytic, decongestant)
- volatile, great airborne deodorisers
- antitumoral (limonene)
- liver protective (limonene)
- analgesic (myrcene, p-cymene, pinene)
- oxidise easily/possible dermal irritants (citrus/needle oils)
- caution with asthmatics with *Pinus sylvestris* (Scots pine) and pinene rich oils.

Examples	Essential oils
Limonene	All Citrus essences very high 60–70%
	Citrus sinensis (Sweet orange) 94%
	Citrus x paradisi (Grapefruit) 93%
	Myrtus communis (Green myrtle)
	Piper nigrum (Black pepper)
A-pinene	All pines/conifers
	Cupressus sempervirens (Cypress)
	Boswellia sacra (Frankincense)
	Kunzea ambigua (Kunzea)
	Kunzea ericoides (Kanuka)
	Cistus ladaniferus (Rock rose)
P-cymene	*Melaleuca alternifolia* (Tea tree)
	Origanum vulgare (Oregano)
	Thymus vulgaris ct thymol (Thyme)
	Eucalyptus globulus (Blue gum)
Myrcene	*Cymbopogon citratus* (West Indian lemongrass)
	Picea mariana (Black spruce)
	Origanum majorana (Sweet marjoram)
	Juniperus communis (Juniper berry)
Sabinene	*Zingiber cassumunar* (Plai)
	Cinnamomum camphora ct cineole (Ravintsara)
	Origanum majorana (Sweet marjoram)
Y-terpinene	*Melaleuca alternifolia* (Tea tree)
	Origanum majorana (Sweet marjoram)
B-pinene	*Pinus sylvestris* (Scots pine)

Sesquiterpenes, -ene

PROPERTIES/SAFETY

- anti-inflammatory (b-caryophyllene potent, chamazulene formed during distillation)
- calming

- antiviral rhino/influenza viruses (zingiberene)
- antiallergenic
- more stable due to higher molecular size.

Examples	Essential oils
Bisabolene	*Matricaria recutita* (German chamomile)
	Zingiber officinalis (Ginger)
Chamazulene	*Matricaria recutita* (German chamomile)
	Achillea millefolium (Yarrow)
	Tanacetum annuum (Blue tansy)
B-caryophyllene	*Cananga odorata* (Ylang ylang)
	Lavandula angustifolia (Lavender true)
	Syzygium aromaticum (Clove bud)
	Melissa officinalis (Lemon balm)
	Piper nigrum (Black pepper)
	Pogostemon cablin (Patchouli)
Zingiberene	*Zingiber officinalis* (Ginger) 27%
Germacrene	*Cananga odorata* (Ylang ylang)
	Juniperus communis (Juniper berry)
	Melissa officinalis (Lemon balm)
B-phellandrene	*Zingiber officinalis* (Ginger)
	Piper nigrum (Black pepper)
	Laurus nobilis (Bay laurel)
B-sesquiphellandrene	*Zingiber officinalis* (Ginger) 14%
Trans-B-farnesene	*Matricaria recutita* (German chamomile)
Curcumene	*Helichrysum italicum* (Everlasting) 13%
Aromadendrene	*Melaleuca ericifolia* (Rosalina)

Esters, -yl, -ate

Named after their parent molecules, alcohols and acids, e.g. linalool+ acetic acid becomes linalyl acetate.

The alcohol drops the -ol and becomes a -yl. The acid drops the -id and gains an -ate.

PROPERTIES/SAFETY

- usually very calming; regulate, balance the sympathetic nervous system and neuro-endocrine system (linalyl acetate, isobutyl angelate)
- antispasmodic (bornyl acetate is a smooth muscle spasmolytic; isobutyl angelate is "one of the grand antispasmodics of the pharmacopeia")[12]
- terrain supports
- pleasant fruity fragrance
- safe
- exception: methyl salicylate found at 95% in *Betula lenta* (Sweet birch) and *Gaultheria procumbens* (Wintergreen) essential oils. Do not use with blood thinning medication (warfarin, heparin, aspirin), asthmatics or in pregnancy. Readily absorbed through skin; poisoning can occur over time with repeated doses (salicysm). Use at 5% short term on healthy individuals with acute muscular injury for analgesic, anti-inflammatory effects. Don't rub or heat; can cause tissue necrosis. Phenolic ester; transforms into salicylic acid; 1ml = 30 aspirin.[13]

Examples	Essential oils
Linalyl acetate	*Lavandula angustifolia* (Lavender true) 40%
	Lavandula x intermedia (Lavandin)
	Salvia sclarea (Clary sage) 50% to 70%
	Citrus aurantium subsp. *amara* (Petitgrain bigarade) 46% to 70%
	Citrus x limon syn *bergamia* (Bergamot)
	Mentha citrata (Bergamot mint) 60%
Angelates (isobutyl etc.)	*Chamaemelum nobile* (Roman chamomile) 70%
Bornyl acetate	*Salvia rosmarinus* ct verbenone (Rosemary) 2% to 10%
	Picea mariana (Black spruce) 36%
	Inula graveolens (Sweet inula) 50%
Geranyl acetate	*Pelargonium graveolens* (Geranium)
	Cymbopogon martini (Palmarosa) 20%
	Thymus vulgaris ct geraniol (Thyme)
Neryl acetate	*Helichrysum italicum* (Everlasting) 46% to 70%

Terpinyl acetate	*Cupressus sempervirens* (Cypress)
	Laurus nobilis (Bay laurel)
Myrtenyl acetate	*Myrtus communis* (Myrtle) 14%
Menthyl acetate	*Mentha x piperita* (Peppermint) 9%

Monoterpene alcohols (Monoterpenols), -ol

The -OH group[14] can be added to carbon atoms at different places in the molecule, yielding:

Primary alcohols (attached to one carbon atom): pronounced **antifungal** activity. Oxidise to aldehydes, e.g. geraniol, nerol, citronellol.

Secondary alcohols (attached to two carbon atoms): pronounced **antiviral** activity. Oxidise to ketones, e.g. borneol, isoborneol, menthol, thujanol.

Tertiary alcohols (attached to three carbon atoms): **generalised antimicrobials**. Do not oxidise, e.g. linalool, terpinen-4-ol.[15]

PROPERTIES/SAFETY

- strong antimicrobials (see above)
- tonics, terrain supports (terpinen-4-ol increases white cell production)
- antioxidants
- analgesic (menthol is powerful, can be cooling or rubefacient according to dose; linalool, geraniol, a-terpineol)
- antispasmodic (esp. to smooth muscle, geraniol, linalool, menthol, borneol, citronellol)
- sedative (linalool has proven sedating quality)
- generally very safe.

Examples	Essential oils
Linalool	*Lavandula angustifolia* (Lavender true) 35%
	Lavandula x intermedia (Lavandin) 25%
	Salvia sclarea (Clary sage) 15%
	Thymus vulgaris ct linalool (Thyme)
	Agonis fragrans (Fragonia) 12.5%
	Melaleuca ericifolia (Rosalina) 45%
	Cinnamomum camphor ct linalool (Ho leaf) 90%
	Citrus aurantium var *amara flos* (Neroli) 30% to 55%
Geraniol	*Cymbopogon martini* (Palmarosa) 78%
	Pelargonium graveolens (Geranium)
	Thymus vulgaris ct geraniol (Thyme)
	Rosa damascena (Damask rose) 14% to 32%
Menthol	*Mentha x piperita* (Peppermint) 29% to 46%
	Mentha arvensis (Cornmint) 70% to 90%
Nerol	*Helichrysum italicum* (Everlasting)
Terpinen-4-ol	*Melaleuca alternifolia* (Tea tree) 42%
	Origanum majorana (Sweet marjoram) 35%
	Zingiber cassumunar (Plai)
Citronellol	*Pelargonium graveolens* (Geranium) 20%
	Rosa damascena (Damask rose) 18% to 55%
	Eucalyptus citriodora (Lemon scented gum)
Borneol	*Inula graveolens* (Sweet inula) 9%
	Picea mariana (Black spruce) 3%
a-terpineol	*Eucalyptus radiata* (Narrow-leaved peppermint eucalyptus) 35%
	Cinnamomum camphora ct cineole (Ravintsara) 8%
	Agonis fragrans (Fragonia) 7%
trans-thujanol-4	*Thymus vulgaris* ct thuyanol (Thyme)

Sesquiterpene alcohols (Sesquiterpenols), -ol

PROPERTIES/SAFETY

- anti-inflammatory; reduce histamine response or inflammatory mediators (alpha-bisabolol)
- antimicrobial
- immunostimulant
- antispasmodic (farnesol)
- antiviral (santalol, herpes simplex i and ii)
- cellular regeneration
- anti-cancer effects (in vitro, farnesol; nerolidol)[16]
- antimalarial (in vitro, nerolidol)[17]
- skin protective, radiotherapy dermatitis (viridiflorol)
- cellular regeneration (*Commiphora myrrha* (Myrrh), *Pogostemon cablin* (Patchouli), *Cistus ladaniferus* (Rock rose))
- usually viscous, slow flowing
- woody earthy odour; base notes
- GRAS.[18]

Examples	Essential oils
a-bisabolol	*Matricaria recutita* (German chamomile) up to 60%
Nerolidol	*Citrus aurantium* var *amara flos* (Neroli)
Santalols	*Santalum spicatum* (Australian sandalwood) up to 75%
Viridiflorol	*Melaleuca quinquenervia* ct viridiflorol (Niaouli) 30% to 66%
	Kunzea ambigua (Kunzea) 3%
Globulol	*Kunzea ambigua* (Kunzea) up to 20%
Carotol	*Daucus carota* (Carrot seed) 36% to 70%
Patchoulol	*Pogostemon cablin* (Patchouli) 24% to 50%

Diterpene alcohols are normally too big to come across in distillation; the exception is sclareol in *Salvia sclarea* (Clary sage), which is just small enough.

Phenols, -ol

Have a hydroxyl (-OH) group attached to an aromatic or benzene ring. This is the difference between them and alcohols.

PROPERTIES/SAFETY

- powerful antimicrobials; broad spectrum against bacteria/fungi (thymol – lung infections; carvacrol – gut/urinary infections)
- stimulant
- anti-inflammatory (eugenol)
- antioxidant
- antiviral (eugenol, herpes simplex i and ii)
- rubefacient (muscular/joint preparations)
- anesthetic/anti-inflammatory (eugenol)
- anticoagulant (eugenol) contraindicated with anticoagulant medication
- skin and mucous membrane irritants; no more than 3% in blend for topical use
- hepatotoxic in high doses orally
- contraindicated for children and pregnancy
- not for airborne diffusion unless in combination with other oils at less than 15%
- eugenol has such a wide range of actions it has been proposed as an adaptogenic. *Ocimum sanctum* ct eugenol (Holy basil), a confirmed adaptogenic, has eugenol as its main component.

Examples	Essential oils
Carvacrol	*Origanum vulgare* ct carvacrol (Oregano) 30% to 80%
Thymol	*Thymus vulgaris* ct thymol (Thyme) 30% to 48%
Eugenol	*Cinnamomum zeylanicum* (Cinnamon bark) 2% to 13%
	Syzgium aromaticum (Clove bud) 50% to 95%
	Ocimum sanctum (Holy basil) 35% to 67%

Ethers, -ol, -ole, -ether and others

PROPERTIES/SAFETY

- derived from phenols or alcohols
- antispasmodic (smooth muscle of intestines and genitourinary tract; methyl chavicol (also called estragole), methyl eugenol, trans-anethole)
- antibacterial/analgesic (eugenol)
- carminative (organs below the diaphragm)

- sedative (reported psychotropic effects of myristicin and elemicin)
- weak oestrogenic activity (trans-anethole)
- caution regarding use: high dose, long term, can be neuro/hepato toxic and carcinogenic (methyl eugenol, methyl chavicol, safrole, apiole, myristicin)
- do not use eugenol with anticoagulant medication
- do not use *Myristica fragrans* (Nutmeg) with pethidine in childbirth.

Examples	Essential oils
Methyl chavicol (estragole)	*Ocimum basilicum* ct methylchavicol (Tropical basil) 68% to 87%
Anethole	*Foeniculum vulgare* (Sweet fennel) 46% to 89%
	Pimpinella anisum (Aniseed) 70% to 90%
Myristicin	*Myristica fragrans* (Nutmeg) 3% to 11%
Safrole	*Myristica fragrans* (Nutmeg)

Aldehydes, -al, -aldehyde

Powerful fragrance, often lemony. Formed from oxidation of primary alcohols and in turn can oxidise into carboxylic acids under poor storage.

PROPERTIES/SAFETY

- strong antimicrobials
- antifungal (cinnamaldehyde, citral, perillaldehyde)
- sedative (citral, citronellal, valeranal)
- anti-inflammatory/pain relief for joints and muscles (citronellal)
- oxidise readily, so possible dermal irritants; blend with non-irritant oils like *Lavandula angustifolium* (Lavender true)
- mucous membrane irritants (don't use in inhalations)
- anti-melanoma activity (trans-2-hexanal, found in low concentrations in many leaf oils, e.g. *Origanum vulgare* (Oregano), *Origanum majorana* (Sweet marjoram), *Thymus vulgare* (Thyme)).[19]
- very small amounts in diffusion, if at all; can cause itchy eyes.

Examples	Essential oils
Cinnamaldehyde	*Cinnamomum zeylanicum* (Cinnamon bark) 60% to 75%; Cinnamon leaf has much less; don't use dermally; extremely strong
Citral (neral and geranial)	Citrus essences, low amount
	Cymbopogon citratus (West Indian lemongrass)
	Cymbopogon flexuosus (East Indian lemongrass) 70% to 80%
	Melissa officinalis (Lemon balm) 65%
	Backhousia citriodora (Lemon myrtle) 80%
	Litsea cubeba (May chang) 74%
Citronellal	*Eucalyptus citriodora* (Lemon eucalyptus) 80%
	Cymbopogon winterianus (Java citronella) 32%
	Cymbopogon nardus (Ceylon citronella) 5%
Benzaldehyde	*Prunus amygdalus* var *amara* (Bitter almond) large amounts render it toxic

Ketones, -one; exception: camphor (also known as 2-bornanone)
Derived from secondary alcohols by oxidation.

PROPERTIES/SAFETY

- mucolytic (respiratory and genito-urinary) (bornanone, isopinocamphone)
- wound healing/cicatrisant
- antifungal (carvone is powerful, comparable to phenols)
- anti-haematomal (italidiones)
- antiviral, esp. enveloped viruses (thujone, bornanone effective for herpes simplex i; thujone effective for human papilloma virus)
- sedative, stimulate parasympathetic, leading to calming (valeranone, bornanone, thujone)
- safe ketones are: verbenone, fenchone, carvone, jasmone, italidione
- high dose, long term, can be neuro and hepato toxic; can accumulate in body tissues; are very lipohilic; nerves are in a lipid rich environment
- care with thujone, camphor, pinocamphone, isopinocamphone, pulegone
- pulegone, thujone are abortifacient in high doses.

Examples	Essential oils
Bornanone/camphor	*Lavandula latifolia* (Spike lavender) 20%
	Lavandula x intermedia (Lavandin) 12%
	Salvia rosmarinus ct camphor (Rosemary) 12% to 22%
Verbenone	*Salvia rosmarinus* ct verbenone (Rosemary) 1% to 7%
	Cistus ladaniferus (Rock rose) 2%
Italidione	*Helichrysum angustifolium* (Everlasting) 15% to 20%
Carvone	*Mentha spicata* (Spearmint) 65%
Pinocarvone	*Chamaemelum nobile* (Roman chamomile)
Fenchone	*Foeniculum vulgare* (Sweet fennel)
Jasmone	*Jasminum officinale* (Jasmine) 9%
Pulegone	*Mentha pulegium* (Pennyroyal) (do not use)
Thujone	*Salvia officinalis* (Sage) 7% to 50%
Pinocamphone	*Hyssop officinalis* var *decumbens* (Hyssop) a safe hyssop very low in pinocamphone
	Hyssop officinalis (Hyssop) 40%
Menthone	*Mentha x piperita* (Peppermint) 10% to 20%. Do not use Peppermint with children under the age of seven, *Mentha spicata* (Spearmint) is a safer choice
Valeranone	*Nardostachys jatamansi* (Spikenard) 15%. Spikenard is now endangered
Leptospermone	*Leptospermum scoparium* (Manuka) 8% to 19%

Oxides, -ole, -oxide

Oxides are a type of ether. The most common one is 1,8-cineole, also called eucalyptol; a great respiratory supporter.

PROPERTIES/SAFETY

- mucolytic
- expectorant
- decongestant
- spasmolytic
- mental tonic
- skin penetration enhancer
- antimicrobial

- antiviral (peaks of 1,8-cineole found to be antiviral)[20]
- ideal in inhalations for respiratory system
- facilitates gas exchange at alveoli level
- potent analgesic/anti-inflammatory
- care in inhalations with asthmatics
- do not use essential oils containing 1,8-cineole near the mouth or nose of babies
- other oxides mirror their respective alcohols.

Examples	Essential oils
1,8-cineole (eucalyptol)	*Eucalyptus radiata* (Narrow-leaved peppermint eucalyptus) 66%
	Salvia rosmarinus ct cineole (Rosemary) 40% to 57%
	Lavandula latifolia (Spike lavender) 30%
	Myrtus communis (Green myrtle) 29%
	Melaleuca ericifolia (Rosalina) 28%
	Kunzea ambigua (Kunzea) 12%
	Cinnamomum camphora ct cineole (Ravintsara) 55%
	Agonis fragrans (Fragonia) 30%
	Melaleuca quinquenervia ct cineole (Niaouli) 38% to 68%
Bisabolol oxide a and b	*Matricaria recutita* (German chamomile) 16%
Rose oxide	*Rosa damascena* (Damask rose)

Lactones, -lactone, -ine

PROPERTIES/SAFETY

- only found in small amounts
- similar to ketones: antimicrobial, mucolytic, sedative
- can lead to sensitisation.

Examples	Essential oils
Atlantolactone	*Inula graveolens* (Sweet inula)
Nepetalactone	*Nepeta cataria* (Catnip)

Coumarins, -en, -in; type of lactone

PROPERTIES/SAFETY

- infrequently found
- sedative
- anti-arrhythmic (bergamottine)
- furanocoumarins are phototoxic (bergaptene, angelicine)
- blood thinners; do not use with anticoagulant medicines.[21]

Examples	Essential oils
Bergaptene	*Citrus x limon* syn *Citrus bergamia* (Bergamot)
Angelicine	*Angelica archangelica* (Angelica)

5. The absorption and effects of essential oils

- **Glandular** Essential oil constituents use the olfactory mucous membranes and olfactory nerves as a highway into the limbic system of the brain, where they not only impact memory and emotion but stimulate the production of neurochemicals through the hypothalamus and pituitary glands, thus having an effect on the endocrine, nervous and immune systems.
- **Skin** Essential oils are lipophilic and of a small molecular size, enabling them to be absorbed dermally; useful for many skin issues.
- **Respiratory** Essential oils are absorbed via the breath into the lungs; helpful for respiratory illnesses.
- **Circulation** Many essential oils benefit the circulation through dermal and respiratory absorption and reach all parts of the body.[22]

6. Methods of use

- **Diffuser** 5 to 10 drops. Diffuse intermittently, e.g. 15 minutes per hour 2 or 3 times a day, to avoid taxing the nervous system.
- **Steam inhalation** 1 to 2 drops in hot water. Cover head with a towel; inhale for 5 minutes. Using too many drops can impact the mucociliatory pathway, increasing water production, paralysing the villi, making congestion worse.

- **Direct inhalation** 1 drop on a tissue. Aromastick 3 to 20 drops. Direct from bottle.
- **Massage** 2.5% is 12 drops in 25ml of carrier oil. Less for the elderly, compromised, pregnant and young children.
- **Compress** 2 to 10 drops in a bowl of water.
- **Creams/lotions** 0.25% for the face; 1% to 2% for the body.
- **Spritzers** 1% to 2%.
- **Bath** 5 to 10 drops diluted in solubiliser or, for example, 1 tsp of eco bodywash.

7. General guidelines for the safe use of essential oils

- **First and foremost, become educated, from a reliable, respected source**, in the art and science of aromatherapy and the safe use of essential oils. They are not to be feared. They are to be learned about, respected and used following guidelines, as you would for any other medicine. When Dr Jean Valnet, army physician, was interviewed by Christine Scott for the *International Journal of Aromatherapy* in 1993, he said that "it is not necessary to be a doctor to use aromatherapy. But one has to know the power of essential oils in order to avoid accidents and incidents."[23]
- **Join ICAN** (International Clinical Aromatherapy Network), directed by Rhiannon Lewis of Essential Oil Resource Consultants. This is a platform for professional aromatherapists with information you can trust. There is a wealth of information in the library, lectures, spotlight interviews, research, resources and a forum for discussion. It's a no brainer for serious aromatherapists and students.
- **Use only pure unadulterated oils** from a reputable supplier. **Avoid synthetic fragrances.**
- **Do not use essential oils internally unless under the guidance of a qualified clinical aromatherapist.**
- **Should ingestion occur**, do not induce vomiting. Drink full fat milk or a carrier oil such as olive to help dilute the lipophilic essential oil. Seek medical attention if necessary.
- **Do not apply directly to the skin**; dilute with a carrier oil. If sensitisation should occur, discontinue use and wash off thoroughly with warm, unscented soapy water.
- **Keep out of the reach of children.**

- **Avoid contact with eyes and mucous membranes.** (If contact with eyes occurs, wipe with carrier oil and flush liberally with warm water.)
- Do not use the citrus oils of *Citrus limon* (Lemon), *Citrus x limon* syn *Citrus bergamia* (Bergamot) or other **phototoxic** essential oils such as *Angelica archangelica* (Angelica) before exposure to UV light (wait for 12 hours). **Distilled** *Citrus limon* (Lemon), *Citrus paradisii* (Grapefruit), *Citrus medica* (Lime), *Citrus sinensis* (Sweet orange) and *Citrus reticulata blanco* (Mandarin) are deemed safe.
- **Do not use essential oils on infants, children, pregnant women, the elderly or those with serious health problems without sufficient knowledge.**
- **Avoid prolonged exposure** without ventilation.
- **Store essential oils and carrier oils** properly in dark glass bottles away from heat and light, to avoid degradation and rancidity. Decant large quantities into small bottles to reduce oxidisation.

8. Dilution guidelines for essential oils

These are based on 1ml = 20 drops, 5ml = 100 drops (1 tsp). Therefore 1% = 1 drop in 5ml (1 tsp). This is approximate as drops vary according to viscosity and dropper type. For blends this is the total number of drops when all oils are combined.

	5ml	10ml	15ml	20ml	25ml	50ml
0.5%	0.5	1	1.5	2	2.5	5
1%	1	2	3	4	5	10
2%	2	4	6	8	10	20
2.5%	2.5	5	8	10	12	25
3%	3	6	9	12	15	30
4%	4	8	12	16	20	40
5%	5	10	15	20	25	50
Base oil	**5ml**	**10ml**	**15ml**	**20ml**	**25ml**	**50ml**

To calculate the number of drops in a formula: Desired % x vol of product x number of drops per ml (20), e.g. 2.5% of 25ml is 2.5/100 x 25 = 0.625 x 20 = 12 drops

9. Simple, effective, practical treatments for the feet, hands and head

Adapted from my teaching modules 1 and 3 (www.annieprincearomatherapy.co.nz/classes)

Module 1: The principles of aromatic touch: practical applications for the feet and hands

Module 3: Essential oils for the musculoskeletal system addressing pain and inflammation; incorporating an aromatic head massage for release of tension

The benefits of therapeutic touch with or without essential oils have been well documented but not everyone is interested or trained in full body massage. These simple massage techniques for the head, hands and feet, which are easy to learn and can be performed with the client fully clothed, are therefore very useful. I have taught countless students, both health practitioners and lay people, who have found them invaluable for stress reduction, pain relief and relaxation, improving quality of life.

The following are some examples of the benefits from the research available.

- Hand massage was shown to decrease anxiety and increase comfort levels in the elderly in a nursing home providing a "non medical, non pharmacological intervention with no adverse effects".[24]
- A 15-minute hand massage reduced anxiety in a preoperative outpatient unit.[25]
- Hand massage reduced anxiety and positively affected vital signs in patients before a venipuncture procedure.[26]
- A 5-minute aroma hand massage for 7 days (a blend of *Citrus x limon* syn *bergamia* (Bergamot), *Lavandula angustifolia* (Lavender true), *Boswellia sacra* (Frankincense) 1:1:1 at 1.5% dilution in *Prunus amygdalus dulcis* (Sweet almond oil)) "showed more significant differences in the changes in pain score and depression than the control group" for hospice patients with terminal cancer.[27]
- A 20-minute foot and hand massage was shown to be "an effective, inexpensive, low risk, flexible and easily applied strategy for

postoperative pain management… Massaging the feet and hands stimulates the mechanoreceptors that activate the 'non painful' nerve fibers."[28]

- Harvard Health Education describe foot massage as "the pause that refreshes and is good for you", improving circulation, stimulating muscles, reducing tension and easing pain.[29]
- A meta-analysis study on the efficacy of foot massage for pain relief of laparoscopic cholecystectomy showed significantly lower pain scores and reduced need for additional analgesia after 60 minutes.[30]
- Foot massage along with patient education in patients undergoing coronary artery bypass graft surgery was shown to decrease anxiety, fatigue, pain and improve quality of life.[31]

Feet

Aromatic footbath

Don't underestimate the benefits of this old fashioned, deeply relaxing, under-utilised, simple aromatic treatment. Foot soaks have been shown to improve circulation by dilating the blood vessels, thus reducing pain, improving sleep and activating the parasympathetic nervous system to induce stress reduction.[32] A reduction in physical and psychological stress was reported in terminal cancer and stroke patients after aromatic massage and footbaths.[33]

1. Choose a bowl or basin deep enough to hold sufficient water to cover both feet and ankles.
2. Fill with warm to hot water. Check appropriate temperature. Fresh herbs, flowers, hydrosols, crystals may be added. 1 tbsp Epsom Salt is detoxifying and a good source of magnesium.
3. **Add 3 x drops of chosen essential oils.** To disperse fully add to 1 tsp solubiliser or 1 tsp of eco bodywash. *Lavandula angustifolia* (Lavender true) is usually a safe, multipurpose oil, as is *Melaleuca alternifolia* (Tea tree). The latter is helpful for treating athlete's foot.
4. **Soak for 10 minutes.**
5. Keep client warm. Dry feet thoroughly. Wrap in warm towel or put on socks. Follow with aromatic foot massage.

Aromatic foot scrub

Leaves the skin exfoliated and feeling beautifully smooth. Aids the absorption of essential oils in the footbath and foot massage. Avoid on damaged skin or the fragile skin of the elderly and young children.

1. **2 tsp x *Prunus dulcis* (Sweet almond oil) / 2 tsp x salt / 1 drop x appropriate essential oil.** Mix together in a small dish. Suggestion: 1 drop x *Citrus limon* (Lemon) essential oil; good for the circulation, uplifting, cleansing refreshing aroma.
2. After soaking feet in foot bath for 10 mins, pat dry, rub scrub very gently over each foot and lower leg, with effleurage strokes, for **1 to 2 mins**, rinse off in footbath. Dry thoroughly. Proceed with aromatic foot massage.

Aromatic foot massage

Based on my reflexology and relaxation massage training, this simplified sequence of movements using a gentle pressure is divided into the different anatomical parts of the foot for ease of learning. **Quick to learn, deeply relaxing, suitable for young and old.**

A PREPARATION

- **Wash hands** before and after treatment.
- **Choose appropriate oils.** Suggestion: 10ml x *Prunus dulcis* (Sweet almond oil), 2 drops x *Lavandula angustifolia* (Lavender true) essential oil.
- **Connect with client**: greeting, gentle hand on shoulder; ask permission, ensure warmth; make eye contact while gently holding foot in both hands.
- **Technique**: treat one foot at a time. **Duration is approximately 15 minutes for both feet**:
  - movements are SLOW, **maintain contact by holding foot in between strokes**
  - pressure 4/5 out of 10 = light/medium lotioning
  - number of strokes = 5; this allows the body to acknowledge the touch, feel comfortable and relax into it.
- **If using massage table** place bolster or pillow under the knees to support the lower back.

B OIL APPLICATION

- **Right foot**: coat palms with a little oil, hold foot in palm of one hand and **apply oil gently** with effleurage strokes to lower leg and foot, alternating hands (5 times).
- **Slide both hands upwards** from ankle to knee, separate, slide down the sides of the leg to foot and squeeze gently (5 times).

C ANKLE

- **Achilles tendon stretch**: heel in left hand, right hand holding top of foot, **gently** pull heel towards you and push foot forward. Release and repeat. Do not tilt foot (5 times).
- **Ankle loosening**: edge of hands under ankle, slicing movements back and forth (count of 5).
- **Ankle rotation**: holding foot in one hand, **gently rotate** with other (5 times in both directions). A subtle movement felt along the line on top of foot from ankle to ankle.

D FOOT

- **Gentle friction with palms** on sides of foot (count of 5).
- **Stretch foot out** by placing both hands on top of foot, thumbs underneath, and slide horizontally across the top, keeping fingers flat (5 times).
- **Sole**: with both hands on top of foot, use thumbs to slide horizontally across sole of foot, working down from toes to heel (5 times in each area: ball of foot, arch, heel). You can use a little more pressure here.
- **Solar plexus point K1**: make thumb circles in a clockwise direction on solar plexus point situated at top angle of v shape on sole of foot (5 times). With thumb on solar plexus point and first finger on top of foot in dip between big toe and second toe **L3**, press gently and hold (count of 5). These are renowned relaxation points.
- **Circle inner and outer ankle** bones with flat fingers (5 times).

E TOES

- **Toe stroke**: hold big toe between thumb and first finger; using thumb and forefinger of other hand, stroke each toe upwards, finishing with gentle pressure on tip of toe (5 times). Release big toe and do the same. (The psy point at base of big toe, facing second toe, is related to psychological wellbeing; "psychological trauma accumulates causing a buildup of microcrystals that need to be worked on to set the spirit free".)[34]
- **Toe rotation/toe pull**: with two fingers at base of toe joint and thumb behind, **gently rotate** (5 times in both directions), finishing with a **very gentle pull**.

F TO FINISH

- Coat palms with **a little oil, hold foot in palm of one hand and apply oil gently** using effleurage strokes to lower leg and foot, alternating hands (5 times).
- **Slide hands upwards** from ankle to knee, separate, slide down the sides of the leg to foot and squeeze gently (5 times).
- **Hold foot** gently (count of 5).
- **Wrap foot** in warm towel or sock.
- **Repeat** sequence to **left foot**.
- **Glass of water** to drink on completion of treatment.

Hands

Aromatic hand massage

Based on my reflexology and relaxation massage training, this simplified sequence of movements using a gentle pressure is easy to learn, deeply relaxing, suitable for young and old.

A PREPARATION

- **Wash hands** before and after treatments.
- **Choose appropriate oils.** Suggestion: 5ml x *Prunus dulcis* (Sweet almond oil), 1 drop x *Lavandula angustifolia* (Lavender true) essential oil.
- **Connect with client**: greeting, gentle hand on shoulder; make sure they are warm, ask permission, gently hold hand in both hands, make eye contact.

- **Technique**: treat one hand at a time. **Duration is approximately 10 minutes for both hands**:
  - movements are SLOW; maintain contact by holding hand in between strokes
  - pressure 4/5 out of 10 = light/medium lotioning
  - number of strokes = 5; this allows the body to acknowledge the touch, feel comfortable and relax into it.

B OIL APPLICATION

- **Right hand**: Coat palms with a little oil and, using handshake hold, **apply oil gently** with flat palm and effleurage strokes to lower arm and hand squeezing hand gently between palms (5 times).

C HAND

- Holding the hand in your hands, **use thumbs to slide horizontally across the top of the hand**, working downwards from wrist to knuckles (5 times).
- Using handshake hold, **stroke little finger** upwards, pulling **very gently** (5 times); **circle joints slowly** 5 times, working up the finger joints.
- (3 knuckles) Finish with gentle pressure on tip of finger.
- **Repeat for all fingers.**
- Release thumb and hold hand. Repeat **stroking and joint circles on thumb** (5 times) (2 knuckles).
- Turn hand over, **palm upwards**. Link your little fingers between client's little finger and thumb. **Using your thumbs, stretch out the palm** using horizontal strokes downward from wrist to fingers (5 times). **Make circles** in centre of palm with your thumbs (count of 15). Very relaxing solar plexus point, hence longer time.

D TO FINISH

- Coat palms with a little oil and, using handshake hold, **apply oil gently** with flat palm and effleurage strokes to lower arm and hand, squeezing hand gently between palms (5 times).
- **Hold hand** between your hands (count of 5).
- **Wrap hand** in warm towel.

- **Repeat** sequence for **left hand.**
- **Glass of water** to drink on completion of treatment.

Aromatic hand soak

Bowl of warm water and **2 drops x appropriate essential oils**. Suggestions: *Lavandula angustifolia* (Lavender true) or *Kunzea ambigua* (Kunzea) essential oil; the latter is useful for arthritic fingers and is TGA approved for muscular pain and inflammation.[35] (1 tsp x solubiliser optional to disperse fully.)

- Soak hand for 5 minutes.
- Dry and follow with aromatic hand massage.

Aromatic compress

Bowl of warm water and 2 to 5 drops of appropriate essential oils.

- Soak flannel, squeeze excess water out.
- Place on hand for 5 minutes, and follow with aromatic hand massage.

Head

Aromatic head massage

A delicious treatment, utilising essential oils and potent acupressure points, for the release of stress and tension in the head, neck, shoulders and face.

A PREPARATION

- Chair; quiet, welcoming space.
- Essential oils:
    - **smelling salts**, 5 drops of essential oil in a 5ml bottle of Epsom salts
    - **for the head, neck and shoulders, a warmed essential oil blend** 1% (2 drops in 10ml of carrier oil). Suggestions:
      Lavandula angustifolia (Lavender true)
      Salvia rosmarinus ct cineole (Rosemary)
      Citrus limon (Lemon)
      Mentha x piperita (Peppermint)
      These are useful for headaches. Choose one or two for the blend. Maximum 2 drops total.

  - **for the face** a 1% blend of *Rosa damascena* (Damask rose): 1 drop in 5ml of *Simmondsia chinensis* (Jojoba) carrier oil.
- **Spritzer or hydrosol** to spray aura around client to complete the treatment.
- **Towel** for client to wrap around chest area, if exposing skin (treatment can be given with clothes on without oil).
- **Remove jewellery. Wash hands.**
- **Maintain contact with client throughout treatment.**
- **Smooth hands down hair and over shoulders between movements.**
- **Pressure is gentle but firm. Work SLOWLY.**

B CONNECT WITH CLIENT

- Smelling salts, client to take three deep breaths.
- Rest hands on forehead and base of skull (count of 10).
- Rest hands on shoulders (count of 10).

C NECK, SHOULDERS, BACK

- **Apply essential oil blend** over neck, shoulders and upper back, using effleurage strokes (1 to 2 minutes).
- **Neck stretch**: with left hand cradle and pull head to left side, pressing right shoulder down for a gentle stretch (count of 10). Repeat to other side.
- **Lean on shoulders with forearms**, gentle pressure (count of 10).
- **Smoothing out**: forearms move from base of neck to shoulders (x 6).
- **Massage trapezius**, squeezing between thumbs and fingers, moving from neck to shoulders (x 6).
- **Smooth hands down hair and over shoulders.**
- **Slow, deep thumb circles down thoracic vertebrae** from collar line to base of scapula (x 6).
- **Smooth hands down hair and over shoulders.**
- **Neck grasp and slide**: with one hand on forehead, slide other up from base of neck to hairline, thumb and forefinger either side of neck, grasping, pulling back at centre (x 6).
- **Smooth hands down hair and over shoulders.**
- **Shiatsu neck points**: support head with one hand:
  - Using thumb and forefinger massage points slowly, deeply,

either side of cervical vertebrae from hairline to collar line (x 6).
    - Press thumb into GV16 (hollow at base of skull) (count of 10).
    - Press thumb and forefinger into GB20 (hollows at base of skull either side of GV16 between the two large vertical muscles) (count of 10).
- Smooth hands down hair and over shoulders.
- Repeat grasp and slide for neck (x 6).

D SCALP

- **Shampooing hair** with warm oil into the roots (oil optional); deep, slow, circular movements, tugging hair slightly (x 6). **Smooth hands**
- **Friction up and down over temporalis muscle** above ear to release tension. Fingers extended and together. Head supported. Firm movement (count of 10). Trigger points in the temporalis muscle can be a common cause of headaches with referred pain in the temple area, along the eyebrow and into the upper teeth.
- Repeat on other side (count of 10). **Smooth hands**
- **Shampooing hair**; deep, slow, circular movements, tugging hair slightly (x 6). **Smooth hands**
- **Rub scalp briskly all over with fingertips** (count of 10). **Smooth hands**
- **Ruffling**: separate fingers and ruffle in wave-like motion through hair from front to back with fingertips and nails (x 6). **Smooth hands**
- **Pressure points over entire scalp.** Relieves pressure, clears nerve pathways. Using both hands, press pads of fingers and thumb into scalp, then release. Work from hairline to base of skull. Reposition fingers at base of skull to press into occiput (x 6). **Smooth hands**
- **Compress, lift, hold, release**; using ball of hands over ears, squeeze, lift and release scalp (x 6). **Smooth hands**
- **Compress, lift, hold, release**; hands on forehead and back of head. Same technique (x 6). **Smooth hands**
- **Shampooing hair**, deep, slow, circular movements, tugging hair slightly (x 6). **Smooth hands**
- **Rub scalp briskly all over with fingertips** (count of 10). **Smooth hands**

E FACE

- **Face oil.** Put a few drops of Rose oil blend in palms of hand. Hold over client's nose (count of 10).
- **Support client's head against your chest.** Put rolled towel against neck.
- **Sweep hands alternately across forehead** (x 6).
- **Massage temples** (count of 10).
- **Sweep hands under chin, up sides of face/cheeks to temple in an "s" movement** (x 6).
- **Massage Yin Tang**, third eye point between eyebrows, with middle fingers and **slide thumbs across forehead to temples** (x 6).
- **Press forefinger pad gently into B2 (edge of inner eye socket), squeeze along eyebrow with forefinger and thumb** (x 6).
- **Massage cheeks** with circular movements outwards from nose (count of 10).
- **Gently pull earlobes** downwards and massage inside and out, up to top of ear, pulling gently (x 6).
- **Massage mastoid bones behind ears** and press upwards (count of 10).
- **Finish with sweep of hands in an "s" movement over chin, cheeks, and back up to rest on temples** (x 6). **Smooth hands**

F TO FINISH

- Place left hand on forehead, right hand at base of skull. Hold (count of 10).
- Smooth hands down hair and over shoulders (x 6).
- Rest hands on shoulders (count of 10).
- Aura spray around client with essential oil spritzer or hydrosol.
- Recipient to take home smelling salts.

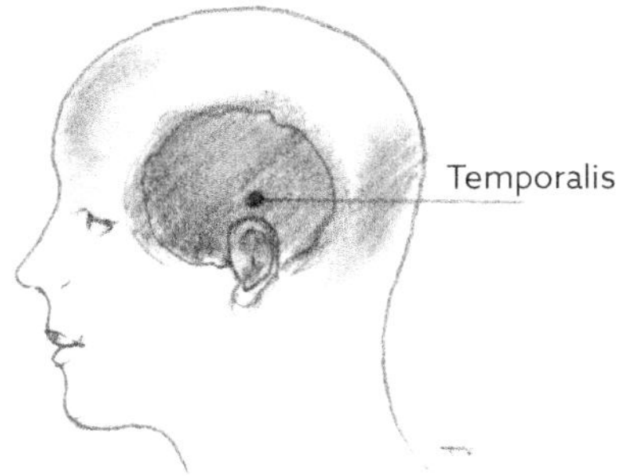

Diagram of head showing temporalis muscle by T.M. Prince

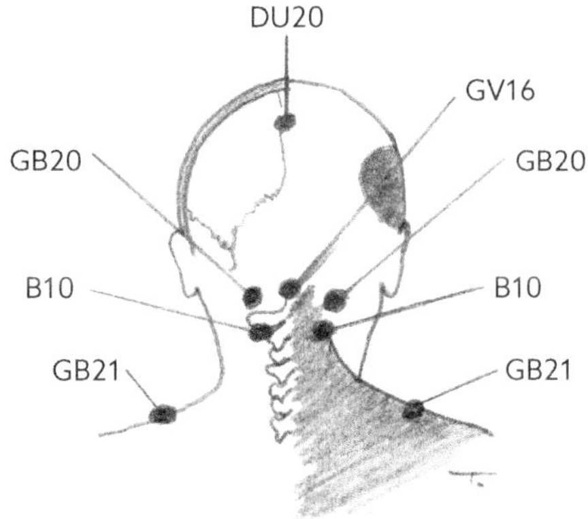

Diagram of acupressure points GB20 and GV16 for relieving headaches by T.M. Prince

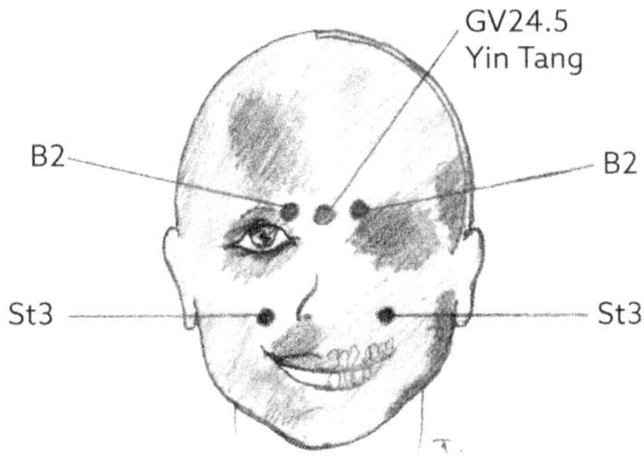

Diagram of acupressure points Yin Tang and B2 for relieving headaches by T.M. Prince

10. Hydrosols and the alchemy of distillation

Alchemy has been defined as "a seemingly magical process of transformation, creation or combination".[36] It was associated in the middle ages with attempts to turn base metals into gold using the elements of earth, metal, fire, water and air.

In the alchemy of distillation:

- Earth represents the plants.
- Metal is the copper alembic.
- Fire heats the still.
- Water makes the steam, cools it and is in the cellular water of the plants.
- Air is represented by the vapour that turns into the essential oil.

It is indeed a wondrous process and Ann Harman describes beautifully the magic of the hydrosol in these words:

A hydrosol starts as a seed
It absorbs the sun and drinks the rain
It frolics with the wind, sings with the birds, sleeps with the moon.
When harvest arrives it dances with the alembic
To become one with fire and water.
It rises as vapour and returns as liquid[37]

What is a hydrosol (hydrolat)?

- The term comes from the Latin *hydro* meaning water, *sol* meaning solution.
- It is the condensate water produced during the steam or hydro distillation of plant material.
- It contains between 0.05 and 0.2 ml of EO per litre, and water soluble acids.
- It is often referred to as the homeopathy of aromatherapy.
- The essential oils are frequently found in solution, i.e. not visible on the surface and not separated out from the water.
- According to Catty the hydrosol contains all of the plant in every drop just like a hologram. She has described them as "herbal espressos, the supercharged version of herbal tea".[38]
- Hydrosols have a wide range of pH but are always on the acid end of the scale, ranging from 2.9 to 6.5, and are in harmony with the acid mantle of the skin, which is 4.5 to 6.2.

- Water to which essential oils have been added with or without a dispersant is **not** a hydrosol.
- These cellular waters are extremely safe to use for everyone from babies to the elderly and infirm.

Ancient stills

In 2005, on the island of Cyprus, Dr Maria Belgiorno discovered a 4000-year-old alembic still during the excavation of "the world's oldest perfume factory" at Pyrgos. Using a replica of the alembic, she proved that they were indeed distilling plants for essential oils and hydrosols, not just infusing them in olive oil.[39]

Ways to use hydrosols

- Can be used in the same way as tinctures in homeopathy. A single drop can be diluted in quantities of distilled water and succussed to distribute the energy of the hydrosol throughout the water.
- Gentle and safe in their pure state, and highly effective in extremely low dilutions. Perfect for infants, children and invalids.
- Can be used for health and pleasure in the following ways:
  - consumed as tonics (2 tbsp in 1 litre of water per day for 21 days)
  - put into baths, shampoos, hair rinses, creams, lotions, skin toner sprays
  - added to food, herbal teas, champagne, cocktails!
  - used as a mist for table bed linen, or when ironing clothes.

Hydrosols suitable as eye washes

- *Anthemis nobilis* (Roman chamomile)
- *Matricaria recutita* (German chamomile)
- *Myrtus communis* (Green myrtle)
- *Centaurea cyanus* (Cornflower)

According to Catty these are the only four hydrosols suitable for eye washes to treat red, sore eyes, inflammation, conjunctivitis. I personally have found *Myrtus communis* (Myrtle) like a miracle worker for tired, sore eyes and hayfever.

Hydrosols have in recent years become a valued part of the aromatherapist's medicine cabinet. **If producing them for sale, the guidelines**

are very strict with regard to hygiene, bottling, transportation and testing for microbes. As they have no preservative added, keeping everything sterile is essential. The shelf life is approximately one year.

If you have a small garden or even a few pots of aromatic plants I would encourage you to get a small 2.5 litre still and make your own for your own use. You will find that by growing and distilling your own plants you will make divine hydrosols which you can then drink as tonics or use in a myriad of ways as suggested above. I have been doing this for years.

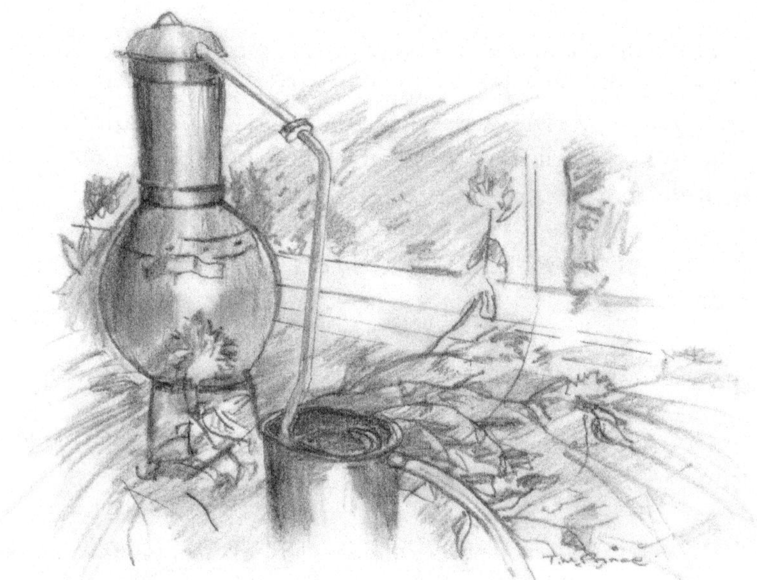

Distilling Monarda fistulosa (Bee balm) on my baby 2.5 litre still called "Paddy" by T.M. Prince

Distillation is an art as well as a science and, as with everything, the energy we put into it has an effect on the end result.

Preparation

- Prepare a clean, sterile, safe, uncluttered environment.
- Prepare yourself mentally with good intention and focus.
- Preferably grow your own plants.
- From harvest to distillation our mindfulness adds "vital healing energy to the medicinal waters".[40]

- We work with our five senses:
  - Watching the plants, the oil, the water.
  - Listening to the song of the still as the steam hums and wends its way to the condenser.
  - Smelling the oil and the waters.
  - Tasting the hydrosols.
  - Touching the plants and patting the still to determine the temperature.
- Copper alembics give a sweeter hydrosol and have antimicrobial properties.

To learn more about the process of distillation and hydrosols I would refer you to the following texts and to www.alembics.co.nz, who have online and in person courses. I consider Catty's and Harman's books essential texts for the home distiller for "how to produce" and "how to use" hydrosols.

Catty, S. 2001 *Hydrosols: The Next Aromatherapy.* Vermont: Healing Arts Press.

Harman, A. 2015 *Harvest to Hydrosol.* Fruitland, WA: IAG Botanics.

Harman, A. 2023 *Harvest to Hydrosol*, 2nd edition. Fruitland, WA: IAG Botanics.

Price, L. and Price, S. 2004 *Understanding Hydrolats.* Edinburgh: Elsevier.

Rose, J. 1999 *375 Essential Oils and Hydrosols.* Berkeley, CA: Frog.

Rose, J. 2001 *Hydrosols & Aromatic Waters.* San Francisco: Jeanne Rose Aromatherapy.

Hydrosol snapshots

The following snapshots are a summary of some of the benefits, properties and uses of various common hydrosols taken from Suzanne Catty's wonderful book *Hydrosols: The Next Aromatherapy.* It may inspire you to have a go at distilling your own. Suzanne spent years immersing herself in the world of hydrosols, consuming gallons, researching and documenting their effects on herself, friends, family, clients and animals. In my opinion she was a groundbreaker in putting hydrosols on the

map. I personally love her book. She discusses 68 in total. Here are a few reprinted with her kind permission.

Achillea millefolium (Yarrow)

- strongly aromatic; stable (2 years)
- potent hydrosol
- digestive aid, eliminates gas, spasms
- aids digestion of fatty foods, heartburn, hepato stimulant, cholagogue
- cooling for fevers
- anti-inflammatory, compress/sitz bath for haemorrhoids, endometriosis with *Cistus ladaniferus* (Rock rose)
- stabilises body fluids
- diuretic
- great balancer physical/mental
- anti-inflammatory, skin damage from wind, sun, thread veins
- styptic, cleans wounds
- animals like it (skin, digestive problems)
- provides mental calm, helps one find peace
- highly energetic
- spiritual work
- cleansing
- anti-allergic, internally for hay fever

Angelica archangelica (Angelica)

- distinctly sedative, grounding
- for anxiety, high stress
- energetically said to bridge heaven and earth, connecting seventh chakra to the base
- exhibits a phenomenal energy field
- intention of use very important for vibrational healing

Anthemis nobilis (Roman chamomile)

- stable (2 years)
- one of the best all purpose waters with *Lavandula angustifolia* (Lavender true) and *Melissa officinalis* (Melissa)
- number one for baby care from birth, in bath water/mist bedding

- wash for breast area, prevents cracked nipples, relaxing for feeding
- diaper rash, diluted 50/50 with Lavender water
- homemade wet wipes
- teething, 2 to 3 drops in bottle of water calms diarrhoea
- rub gums with 2 to 3 drops
- sleep, spritz blankets
- stress reduction, insomnia, calming to nervous system/pets
- skin care, rashes, acne, sensitivity
- best all in one make up remover
- fairly astringent, not long term on dry skin
- combine with *Citrus aurantium* var *amara (flos)* (Neroli) for acneic conditions
- combine with *Lavandula angustifolia* (Lavender true) or *Pelargonium graveolens* (Rose geranium) for dry skin
- one of four hydrosols safe for eyes; the others being *Matricaria recutita* (German chamomile), *Myrtus communis* (Myrtle), *Centaurea cyanus* (Cornflower)
- conjunctivitis, wash, compress

Boswellia carterii (Frankincense)

- taking a drop results in a feeling of energy expansion
- deepens the breath, opens the airways
- can dry up excess mucus in the lungs
- fantastic for the skin, especially in high humidity
- use with *Cistus ladaniferus* (Rock rose) for wrinkle treatments
- internally is drying and diuretic
- gargle for mouth infections

Centaurea cyanus (Cornflower)

- moderately stable (12 months)
- eyewash; *Anthemis nobilis* (Roman chamomile), *Matricaria recutita* (German chamomile), *Myrtus communis* (Myrtle) are also safe for the eyes
- compress, tired itchy eyes, with *Cistus ladaniferus* (Rock rose) compress for fine lines
- tones crepey, devitalised skin

- dry climates on aircraft, with *Pelargonium graveolens* (Rose geranium), moisturising
- scalp/hair, massage in/add to shampoos, gives shine
- general tonic
- douche for uterine tract infections (UTIs) with *Melaleuca alternifolia* (Tea tree)
- reduces fever, internal/topical, safe for infants
- hot flushes, may contain phytohormones
- avoid first trimester pregnancy

Cistus ladaniferus (Rock rose)

- very stable (2+ years)
- highly astringent, cicatrisant, styptic
- stops bleeding almost on contact
- cleans wounds
- powerful antiwrinkle treatment, mist face 2 x a day, plumps cells, reduces fine lines
- good aftershave with *Matricaria recutita* (German chamomile), *Myrtus communis* (Myrtle)
- amelioration of endometriosis with *Helichrysum italicum* (Everlasting) and *Achillea millefolium* (Yarrow)
- powerfully energetic, healing to mind, body, spirit, emotional distress, shock; one of Bach Flowers in Rescue Remedy
- oral use only for specific conditions because of low pH (wound, scar healing properties)
- post-operative, internal healing and bleeding, endometriosis, Crohn's, bleeding

Citrus aurantium var amara (Neroli, Orange blossom)

- sublime aroma, floral, fruity, luscious; one of the most complex smelling hydrosols
- major antistress, calming agent
- mildly sedative to the central nervous system (CNS)
- stops caffeine jitters
- use for hysterics in children and those with attention deficit hyperactivity disorder (ADHD)
- supports the physical and emotional bodies when detoxifying or quitting an addictive habit

- digestive aid, relieves heartburn
- astringent; wonderful for delicate, sensitive oily skin
- avoid on very dry skin or blend in low dilution (20%) with *Lavandula angustifolia* (Lavender true), *Pelargonium graveolens* (Rose geranium) or *Rosa damascena* (Damask rose)
- combine with *Cistus ladaniferus* (Rock rose) as a toner for acne or irritations
- use in a face mask with clay and honey
- a natural perfume for the scent sensitive

Cupressus sempervirens (Cypress)

- very diuretic internally and topically
- use for water retention in tissues and joints
- moderately astringent and styptic
- useful for acne, thread veins, varicose veins, haemorrhoids
- spray on tired heavy legs or use in footbath
- cleanses, detoxifies the system
- avoid in first trimester of pregnancy or in cases of renal or kidney disease because of diuretic detoxifying properties
- antitussive, expectorant qualities for the respiratory system

Daucus carota (Wild carrot seed)

- a comforting, earthy, musky aroma; appeals to men and women
- supports the liver, gallbladder and kidneys
- use with clay to clean the bowels or as part of illness recovery after viral infections
- soothes skin rashes, inflammation, damaged skin
- calming for eczema, psoriasis
- promotes the growth of healthy new cells
- overall restorative tonic
- delicious in soups, juices, sauces, salad dressings

Elettaria cardamomum (Cardamon pod)

- calms spasm and bloat in the digestive tract
- very relaxing; with honey a great bedtime drink
- wonderful in savoury or sweet dishes; not overpowering
- apparently has distinct aphrodisiac properties!

***Eucalyptus globulus* (Eucalyptus)**

- first line of defence against respiratory problems: coughs, colds, chest infections, hayfever
- makes a good gargle, mouthwash or cough syrup with or without essential oils
- can be used in inhalations
- avoid with children under four years of age

***Helichrysum italicum* (Everlasting)**

- stable (2 years)
- bruising, scar tissue with EO and rosehip oil
- anti-inflammatory, cicatrisant, mature sensitive skin
- with *Cistus ladaniferus* (Rock rose) for endometriosis/wound healing
- detoxifies liver (30ml in 1 litre water per day) with *Silybum marianum* (Milk thistle)
- mouthwash, gingivitis, 1 tbsp hydrosol in 1 tbsp water 2 x a day

***Inula graveolens* (Elecampane)**

- number one choice for conditions affecting the respiratory system
- stops coughing fast
- mucolytic, remarkable respiratory system tonic
- make into a cough syrup with essential oils and honey
- valuable cardiovascular tonic; calming, regulating
- douche for thrush, leukorrhea, vaginitis
- infected wounds; oily congested skin

***Juniperus communis* (Juniper berry)**

- a powerful diuretic, pushes fluid out of tissues
- promotes kidney function; not to be used when there are serious kidney problems, an overactive bladder or in first trimester of pregnancy
- use for gout, oedema, rheumatic and arthritic conditions
- cleanses both the physical and etheric body
- highly energetic, one of the best for vibrational work

- spray in the treatment room to clear "vibes"
- apply one drop to palm of your hand, rub together and wipe through auric field to cleanse yourself
- use with intention, very protective against inappropriate energies

Laurus nobilis (Bay laurel)

- can be unstable (8 months' shelf life)
- one of the most delicious hydrosols
- first choice as lymphatic cleanser, three-week protocol 2 tbsp in 1 litre water daily
- not in cases of cancer; use *Comptonia peregrina* (Sweet fern) or *Ledum groenlandicum* (Greenland moss) or apply 1 drop to tumours
- broad acting antiseptic, immune booster, tonic
- take internally with *Melaleuca alternifolia* (Tea tree) or *Myrtus communis* (Green myrtle) and use EO topically to prevent infection
- digestive, aids peristalsis, gas
- mouthwash with *Helichrysum italicum* (Everlasting) for gingivitis
- emotionally comforting
- avoid internally in case of cancer diagnosis

Lavandula angustifolia (Lavender true)

- famed for its regenerative effects on fragile or damaged skin
- mist the face and neck to combat dry atmospheres
- indispensable for skincare when travelling
- use for sunburn, rashes, bites
- cooling, calming to body, mind and spirit
- safe for use with babies and children
- use for cranky children, to clean baby's bottom, cuts and scratches
- a refreshing room spray
- combine with *Mentha x piperita* (Peppermint) and *Salvia officinalis* (Sage) as a spray for hot flushes
- use in a compress for neck, shoulders, forehead for headaches, tension and stress

Lippia citriodora (Lemon verbena)

- stable (18 months)
- powerful mental relaxant, stress buster
- distinctly sedative
- use as tea or in foot bath
- pre-exam jitters, stage fright, knot in stomach
- boosts confidence, self esteem
- general tonic
- stimulates endocrine system, esp. thyroid, pancreas
- reduces cramps
- antiviral, prophylactic during flu season
- cleans digestive system with *Achillea millefolium* (Yarrow)
- strong anti-inflammatory
- affinity for mucous membrane (mouth and nose, sniff drops up nostril)
- mouthwash
- combine with *Cistus ladaniferus* (Rock rose), *Boswellia carterii* (Frankincense) or *Centaurea cyanus* (Cornflower) to refine skin texture, reduce pore size
- good aftershave with *Lavandula angustifolia* (Lavender true), *Mentha x piperita* (Peppermint), *Santalum album* (Sandalwood)
- a rare, costly EO, low yielding, therefore waters are highly energetic; much of the plant's life force remains in water soluble compounds like a hologram
- combined with vibrational healing techniques, it can be extraordinary
- pH close to acid mantle of skin

Matricaria recutita (German chamomile)

- stable (14 months)
- major anti-inflammatory, internally/externally
- burns, blisters with *Lavandula angustifolia* (Lavender true) rashes, itchiness, eczema
- compress for inflamed swollen veins
- cleanser for sensitive, problem skin, reasonably antibacterial
- douche, candida, UTI
- instantly anxiolytic, balances ANS
- good aftershave

- extremely energetic
- powerfully calming, emotionally comforting, soothes the beast within

Melissa officinalis (Lemon balm)

- very stable (2 years)
- calming to body more than mind
- stress, anxiety, childhood hysterics
- ADHD, 30ml in 1 litre water per day
- morning sickness: can add *Mentha x piperita* (Peppermint), *Cinnamomum zeylanicum* (Cinnamon hydrosols)
- suitable for babies, 1 tsp in bath
- cradle cap with *Matricaria recutita* (German chamomile) or *Achillea millefolium* (Yarrow)
- prophylactic in flu season, three-week protocol, 30ml in 1 litre water per day
- immune stimulating
- hypotensive
- aids digestion
- antioxidant, anti-inflammatory, skin clarifier, rashes, eczema
- antiageing, after sun, body care
- pronounced antiviral properties due to aldehydes
- herpes, undiluted 6 to 10 x a day and ½ tbsp internally at each application, works fast

Mentha x piperita (Peppermint)

- unstable after 12 months
- digestive, anti-inflammatory par excellence
- mind stimulant
- Crohn's, irritable bowel syndrome (IBS), combine with *Ocimum basilicum* (Basil) for spasm
- cleanser for digestive tract, mild antibacterial
- combine with *Anthemis nobilis* (Roman chamomile) for parasite cleanse
- motion sickness, small sips 50/50 dilution
- acne treatment, detoxify liver and colon, internal protocol 3 weeks and compress 2 x day if skin red, inflamed
- itches, bites, stings, allergic reactions

- anti-inflammatory, stiff muscles, aches, pains; cooling in hot water, warming in cold, alternate the two
- spritz decollete as toner for bustline
- mental stimulant, spritz on face during hot weather
- hot flushes
- aids concentration
- not to be used with drugs/alcohol, seems to heighten effect
- avoid with children under three years old

Monarda fistulosa (Purple bee balm)

- taste is sharp, spicy, mildly analgesic
- monardas are traditional healing plants of the Native Americans
- *Monarda fistulosa* (Purple bee balm) resembles *Thymus vulgaris* ct geraniol (Thyme) in its chemistry
- use as you would the corresponding thyme
- diuretic, good for fungal infections

Myrtus communis (Green myrtle)

- one of only four hydrosols recommended for the eyes (the others being *Anthemis nobilis* (Roman chamomile), *Matricaria recutia* (German chamomile) and *Centaurea cyanus* (Cornflower))
- mucolytic, expectorant, congested sinuses
- can be used as a prophylactic for recurring chest infections
- useful for asthmatics when triggered by allergens
- useful for colon health in colonics
- a good general health tonic

Ocimum basilicum ct methyl chavicol (Basil)

- extremely effective digestive aid; stimulates peristalsis, reduces spasms in gastrointestinal tract
- considered balancing to the autonomic nervous system
- brings a sense of calm; reduces physical tension in the body
- intense flavour, the scent is strongly liquorice; in dilution the real basil flavour comes out with only a hint of liquorice

Pelargonium graveolens (Rose geranium)

- moderately stable
- favourite all round skincare for young and old
- balancing, adaptogenic for oily, dry acneic and sensitive skin
- make up remover
- humectant, microclusters similar to *Cistus ladaniferus* (Rock rose)
- combine with raw honey for wind damaged, overly dry skin
- anti-inflammatory, very cooling, sunburn, rashes, bites, where heat, redness, broken capillaries, rosacea, with *Matricaria recutita* (German chamomile), *Cistus ladaniferus* (Rock rose) or *Centaurea cyanus* (Cornflower) for dramatic results
- cleans wounds, stops bleeding
- children love it
- hot flushes, spritz
- balances emotions and endocrine system, eases premenstrual syndrome (PMS), menopausal symptoms, esp. when combined with Omega-3 and Omega-6 EFAS or with internal use of EO *Vitex agnus-castus*
- "feel good" hydrosol, balances male/female energy
- lovely perfume on its own, avoid with children under three years old

Picea mariana (Black spruce)

- number one choice for the adrenal glands
- can be used with the essential oil in a three-week protocol at the change of seasons
- use in a cold double compress for relief of pain and inflammation (cold hydrosol compress followed by dry, warm wool wrap)
- a stimulating and restorative body spray, good aftershave
- connects us with nature and the ancient wisdom of the trees

Rosa damascena (Damask rose)

- divine aroma
- good for almost anything
- great for the skin, especially dry, mature, sensitive
- cooling, mildly astringent
- hormone balancer

- affinity with the heart/grief
- promotes balance and emotional processing

***Salvia rosmarinus* ct cineole (Rosemary)**

- shelf life 18 to 20 months (depends on chemotype)
- great antioxidant
- mental/physical stimulant/memory
- mild circulatory stimulant, flushes uric and lactic acid from muscle tissue
- combine with *Mentha x piperita* (Peppermint) as a rub over sore muscles/joints
- good for hair growth and shine, rub into scalp with *Cedrus atlantica* (Atlas cedarwood)
- headaches
- heart tonic

***Salvia sclarea* (Clary sage)**

- flavour and smell is "Earl Grey" tea like
- the "woman's choice" water, a life affirming beverage
- use for hormone related cramps, bloating, moodiness
- use in a three-week protocol to help regulate the menstrual cycle
- menopausal symptoms respond well, esp. hot flushes, in synergy with *Salvia officinalis* (Sage) hydrosol; do not use *Salvia officinalis* (Sage) if hypertensive
- astringent and toning for oily skin
- can be used with *Anthemis nobilis* (Roman chamomile) as a make up remover
- is a euphoriant, antidepressant and some say aphrodisiac
- profoundly energetic, use for emotional trauma and heartache

***Thymus vulgaris* ct thymol (Thyme)**

- the big gun of the thyme family
- antibacterial, antifungal, antiseptic
- very hot to taste, can cause burning sensation on tongue if undiluted, though not dermocaustic like the oil
- makes a great gargle or mouthwash for throat infections

- take 1 tbsp of the diluted hydrosol (60:40 hydrosol to water) in 1 tsp honey every hour in the acute stage of colds or flu
- makes a delicious drink; great in soups, stews and vegetarian dishes

Tilea europaea (Linden flower)

- shelf life 12 to 14 months
- considered a magic tree by many cultures
- distinctly sedative, true stress buster, energetically very alive
- insomnia, anxiety, nervous exhaustion; mist sheets
- useful when body wants to stop and mind keeps whirring
- the "mother" of hydrosols, provides emotional comfort
- good choice for babies and animals
- synergy with *Anthemis nobilis* (Roman chamomile) is extraordinary
- calming to nerves internally and externally (shingles)
- skin, dry eczema, itchy eruptions
- headaches, migraine, compress
- sunstroke with *Lavandula angustifolia* (Lavender true) or *Matricaria recutita* (German chamomile)
- cools body and soul; 15ml for deep meditative state/dream work

Endnotes

Chapter 1

1 Steinbeck, J. 1997 *Travels with Charley: In Search of America.* New York: Penguin, p.38.

2 Ajansı, A. 2022 "ANALYSIS – 2023: challenging year ahead for world." www.aa.com.tr/en/world/analysis-2023-challenging-year-ahead-for-world/2772301; CIDOB 2022 "The world in 2023: ten issues that will shape the international agenda." www.cidob.org/en/publications/publication_series/notes_internacionals/283/the_world_in_2023_ten_issues_that_will_shape_the_international_agenda/(language)/eng-US; United Nations 2023 *World Economic Situation and Prospects 2023.* https://desapublications.un.org/publications/world-economic-situation-and-prospects-2023; American Psychological Association n.d. "COVID-19: information and resources for psychologists, health care workers, and the public." www.apa.org/topics/covid-19.

3 American Psychological Association n.d. "Stress in America." www.apa.org/news/press/releases/stress; Psychology Today n.d. "Loneliness." www.psychologytoday.com/us/basics/loneliness; Cigna Group n.d. "Loneliness in America." https://newsroom.thecignagroup.com/loneliness-in-america; Wooll, M. 2021 "You know you need human connection. Here's how to achieve it." www.betterup.com/blog/human-connection; DCMS 2021 "Loneliness minister: it's more important than ever to take action." www.gov.uk/government/news/loneliness-minister-its-more-important-than-ever-to-take-action.

4 Putnam, R. 2001 *Bowling Alone: The Collapse and Revival of American Community.* New York: Simon and Schuster, pp.111–12.

5 Cacioppo, J.T. and Patrick, W. 2009 *Loneliness.* New York: W.W. Norton, p.247.

6 Hari, J. 2018 *Lost Connections.* London: Bloomsbury, p.109.

7 O'Donohue, J. 1998 *Eternal Echoes: Exploring Our Hunger to Belong.* London: Bantam Press, p.xvi.

8 O'Donohue, J. 2008 *To Bless the Space between Us.* New York: Doubleday, p.194.

9 Murthy, V. 2020 *Together: The Healing Power of Human Connection in a Sometimes Lonely World.* New York: HarperCollins; pp.xv, 151, 10.

10 Murthy, V. 2023 "To Be a Healer." The On Being Project. www.youtube.com/watch?v=DGgESbMigLE.

11 Rankin, L. 2020 *Mind over Medicine*, revised edition. Sydney: Hay House Australia, p.91.

12 WHO 2023 "Depressive disorder (depression)." www.who.int/news-room/fact-sheets/detail/depression.

13 Community and Public Health New Zealand n.d. "Improving community mental health and wellbeing." www.cph.co.nz/your-health/mental-illness.

14 Ministry of Social Development 2016 *The Social Report 2016: Te pūrongo oranga tangata.* https://socialreport.msd.govt.nz/documents/2016/msd-the-social-report-2016.pdf.
15 American Psychological Association n.d. "Resilience." www.apa.org/topics/resilience.
16 Van der Kolk, B. "Resilient Pathways Summit." https://spiritualgrowthevents.com/events/global-resilience-summit.
17 World of Health 2019 "Holistic wellness – 5 pillars of holistic wellbeing." http://theworldofhealth.co.uk/blog/holistic-wellness-5-pillars-of-holistic-wellbeing.
18 Schnaubelt, K. 1999 *Medical Aromatherapy: Healing with Essential Oils.* Berkeley, CA: North Atlantic Books, p.vii.
19 Lown, B. 1996 *The Lost Art of Healing.* New York: Ballantine Books, p.xvi.
20 Rankin, L. 2020 *Mind over Medicine*, revised edition. Sydney: Hay House Australia, p.67.
21 Pert, C.B. 1997 *Molecules of Emotion.* New York: Scribner, p.274.
22 Eggleton, S. 2022 "Essential Oils, Aromatherapy, and Self-Care during the COVID-19 Pandemic." Aeroscena. www.aeroscena.com/blogs/scent-science/essential-oils-aromatherapy-covid-19.
1 Turkle, S. 2015 *Reclaiming Conversation: The Power of Talk in a Digital Age.* New York: Penguin, p.3.

Chapter 2

2 Mcleod, S. 2024 "Maslow's Hierarchy of Needs." https://simplypsychology.org/maslow.html.
3 Brown, B. 2021 *Atlas of the Heart.* New York: Random House, p.169.
4 Waldinger, R. and Schulz, M. 2023 *The Good Life and How to Live It: Lessons from the World's Longest Study on Happiness.* London: Rider.
5 Lieberman, M. 2013 "Why we are wired to connect." *Scientific American.* www.scientificamerican.com/article/why-we-are-wired-to-connect.
6 Hari, J. 2018 *Lost Connections.* London: Bloomsbury, p.88.
7 Cleveland Clinic 2018 "What happens in your body when you're lonely?" https://health.clevelandclinic.org/what-happens-in-your-body-when-youre-lonely.
8 Holt-Lunstad, J. Smith, T.B., Baker, M., Harris, T. and Stephenson, D. 2015 "Loneliness and social isolation as risk factors for mortality: a meta-analytic review." *Perspectives on Psychological Science*, 10(2), 227–37.
9 Turkle, S. 2015 *Reclaiming Conversation.* New York: Penguin.
10 Turkle, S. 2015 *Reclaiming Conversation.* New York: Penguin, p.13.
11 Turkle, S. 2015 *Reclaiming Conversation.* New York: Penguin, p.21; Przybyliski, A. and Weinstein, N. 2012 "Can you connect with me now? How the presence of mobile communication technology influences face to face conversation quality." *Journal of Social and Personal Relationships*, 30(3), 237–46.
12 Neuroscience News 2023 "Zoom conversations vs in-person: brain activity tells a different tale." https://neurosciencenews.com/zoom-conversations-social-neuroscience-24996.
13 Cited in Turkle, S. 2015 *Reclaiming Conversation.* New York: Penguin, Introduction.
14 Turkle, S. 2015 *Reclaiming Conversation.* New York: Penguin, p.14.
15 Sacks, J. 2002 "Listening is the greatest gift we can give to a troubled soul." *The Times*, 14 December. www.rabbisacks.org/archive/listening-is-the-greatest-gift-we-can-give-to-a-troubled-soul.

16 Pennington, A. 2023 *The Top Ten Traits of Highly Resilient People*, 2nd edition, Kindle; "Resilient Pathways Summit. Day Two. Theme: Relational Resilience and Trauma." https://spiritualgrowthevents.com/events/global-resilience-summit.
17 Firestone, L. 2016 "The importance of the relationship in therapy." *Psychology Today*. www.psychologytoday.com/nz/blog/compassion-matters/201612/the-importance-the-relationship-in-therapy; Lambert, M.J. and Barley, D.E. 2001 "Research summary on the therapeutic relationship and psychotherapy outcome." *Psychotherapy: Theory, Research, Practice, Training*, 38(4), 357–61; Horvath, A.O. 2001 "The alliance." *Psychotherapy: Theory, Research, Practice, Training*, 38(4), 365–72.
18 Rankin, L. 2020 *Mind over Medicine*, revised edition. Sydney: Hay House Australia, p.xxviii.
19 Rankin, L. 2020 *Mind over Medicine*, revised edition. Sydney: Hay House Australia, p.xxxiii.
20 Rankin, L. 2020 *Mind over Medicine*, revised edition. Sydney: Hay House Australia, p.xxxvi.
21 Rankin, L. 2020 *Mind over Medicine*, revised edition. Sydney: Hay House Australia, p.xxvii.
22 Rankin, L. 2020 *Mind over Medicine*, revised edition. Sydney: Hay House Australia, p.67.
23 Rankin, L. 2020 *Mind over Medicine*, revised edition. Sydney: Hay House Australia, p.xxxix.
24 Van der Kolk, B. 2014 *The Body Keeps the Score*. New York: Viking Penguin, p.234.

Chapter 3

1 Lown, B. 2008 *Conversations with Maine*. www.youtube.com/watch?v=QHD4NB-8LHc.
2 Lown, B. 1996 *The Lost Art of Healing*. New York: Ballantine Books, p.xiv.
3 Lown, B. 1996 *The Lost Art of Healing*. New York: Ballantine Books, p.78.
4 Bilchik, B.Z. 2021 "A Personal Tribute to Dr. Bernard Lown." Lown Cardiology Group. www.lowngroup.org/a-personal-tribute-to-dr-bernard-lown.
5 Lown, B. 1996 *The Lost Art of Healing*. New York: Ballantine Books, p.90.
6 O'Donohue, J. 2008 *The Inner Landscape of Beauty*. https://onbeing.org/programs/john-odonohue-the-inner-landscape-of-beauty.
7 O'Donohue, J. 1997 *Anam Cara: Spiritual Wisdom from the Celtic World*. London: Bantam Press, p.173.
8 Verghese, A. 2013 The Doctor-Patient Relationship with Abraham Verghese. www.youtube.com/watch?v=VNrWb9w6JWE.
9 Hannon, P. 2020 "Five practices that foster doctor-patient bonds." https://scopeblog.stanford.edu/2020/01/13/five-practices-that-foster-doctor-patient-bonds.
10 Youngson, R. 2015 *Hearts in Healthcare Global Compassion*. www.youtube.com/watch?v=WX74al4UaZM&t=7s.
11 Lown, B. 1996 *The Lost Art of Healing*. New York: Ballantine Books, p.xv.
12 Johns, S. 2019 "Interview: Abraham Verghese on transforming medical education." www.imperial.ac.uk/news/193571/interview-abraham-verghese-transforming-medical-education.
13 Lown, B. 1996 *The Lost Art of Healing*. New York: Ballantine Books, p.78.
14 Mercer, S.W., Maxwell, M., Heaney, D. and Watt, C.G. 2004 "The consultation and relational empathy [CARE] measure: development and preliminary validation and reliability of an empathy-based consultation process measure." *Family Practice*, 21(6), 699–705.

Chapter 4

1 Nayar, V. 2013 "The power of intent." https://hbr.org/2013/02/the-power-of-intent; McTaggart, L. 2007 *The Intention Experiment: Using Your Thoughts to Change Your Life and the World.* New York: Free Press.

2 Backster, C. 1968 "Evidence of a primary perception in plant life." *International Journal of Parapsychology*, 10(4), 329–48.

3 Radin, D.I. and Schlitz, M.J. 2005 "Gut feelings, intuition and emotions: an exploratory study." *Journal of Alternative and Complementary Medicine*, 11(5), 85–91; Stone, J. 2003 *Course Handbook: Training in Compassionate-Loving Intention*; Stone, J. *et al.* in press "Effects of a compassionate/loving intention as a therapeutic intervention by partners of cancer patients: a randomised controlled feasibility study"; McTaggart, L. 2007 *The Intention Experiment: Using Your Thoughts to Change Your Life and the World.* New York: Free Press, p.61.

4 Cade, M. and Coxhead, N. 1986 *The Awakened Mind*, 2nd edition. Shaftesbury: Element; Fahrion, S. *et al.* 1992 "EEG amplitude, brain mapping and synchrony in and between a bioenergy practitioner and client during healing." *Subtle Energies and Energy Medicine*, 3(1), 19–52; McCraty, R. *et al.* 1998 "The electricity of touch: detection and measurement of cardiac energy exchange between people", in K.H. Pribham (ed.) *Brain and Values: Is a Biological Science of Values Possible?* Mahwah, NJ: Lawrence Earlbaum, pp.359–79.

5 Pénoël, D. and Pénoël, R.M. 1998 *Natural Home Health Care Using Essential Oils.* La Drome, France: Editions Osmobiose, p.229.

6 Youngson, R.A. 2012 *Time to Care.* Raglan, NZ: Rebelheart Publishers, p.133.

7 O'Donohue, J. 2008 *The Inner Landscape of Beauty.* https://onbeing.org/programs/john-odonohue-the-inner-landscape-of-beauty.

8 Van der Kolk, B. 2014 *The Body Keeps the Score.* New York: Viking Penguin, pp.80–1; "Resilient Pathways Summit. Day Two. Theme: Relational Resilience and Trauma." https://spiritualgrowthevents.com/events/global-resilience-summit.

9 Youngson, R.A. 2012 *Time to Care.* Raglan, NZ: Rebelheart Publishers, p.133.

10 Nightingale, F. 1859 *Notes on Nursing: What It Is and What It Is Not.* London: Harrison and Sons; Riegel, F., da Graça Oliveira Crossetti, M., Martini, J.G. and Gonçalves Nes, A.A. 2021 Florence Nightingale's theory and her contributions to holistic critical thinking in nursing." *Revista Brasileira de Enfermagem*, 74(2).

11 O'Donohue, J. 2008 *To Bless the Space between Us.* New York: Doubleday, pp.216, 217, 203.

12 In Centeno, C. 2021 "Listening as a diagnostic tool in medicine." Regenex. https://regenexx.com/blog/listening-as-a-diagnostic-tool-in-medicine.

13 O'Donohue, J. 2008 *To Bless the Space between Us.* New York: Doubleday, p.185.

14 O'Donohue, J. 2008 *To Bless the Space between Us.* New York: Doubleday, pp.186, 209.

15 Lown, B. 1996 *The Lost Art of Healing.* New York: Ballantine Books, p.31.

16 Youngson, R.A. 2012 *Time to Care.* Raglan, NZ: Rebelheart Publishers, p.114.

17 Murtagh, J. 1998 *General Practice.* Sydney: McGraw-Hill, as cited in S. Battaglia 2005, *The Complete Guide to Aromatherapy*, 2nd edition. Brisbane: The International Center of Holistic Aromatherapy, p.347.

18 Oprah 2010 "Oprah talks to Thich Nhat Hanh." www.oprah.com/spirit/oprah-talks-to-thich-nhat-hanh.

19 Turkle, S. 2015 *Reclaiming Conversation.* New York: Penguin, p.39.

20 Turkle, S. 2015 *Reclaiming Conversation.* New York: Penguin, p.227.

21 Pert, C. B. 1997 *Molecules of Emotion.* New York: Scribner, p.274.

22 Van der Kolk, B.A. 2015 *The Body Keeps the Score.* New York: Penguin, p.217.

23 O'Donohue, J. 2008 *To Bless the Space Between Us.* New York: Doubleday, p.209.

24 Tanzi, R. and Chopra, D. 2017 *The Healing Self: Supercharge Immune System and Stay Well for Life.* London: Penguin Random House; Van der Kolk, B.A. 2015 *The Body Keeps the Score.* New York: Penguin, p.65.
25 Broom, B. 2018 *Meaning-Full Disease: How Personal Experience and Meanings Cause and Maintain Physical Illness.* Oxford: Routledge.
26 Van der Kolk, B.A. 2015 *The Body Keeps the Score.* New York: Penguin, p.207.
27 Pert, C.B. 1997 *Molecules of Emotion.* New York: Scribner, p.274.
28 Pert, C.B. 1997 *Molecules of Emotion.* New York: Scribner, p.261.
29 Pert, C.B. 1997 *Molecules of Emotion.* New York: Scribner, p.306.
30 Pert, C.B. 1997 *Molecules of Emotion.* New York: Scribner, p.293.
31 Walton, T. as cited in MacDonald, G. 2014 *Medicine Hands: Massage Therapy for People with Cancer*, 3rd edition. Findhorn: Findhorn Press, p.122.
32 Bauermeister, E. 2020 *The Scent Keeper: A Novel.* New York: Saint Martin's Griffin, p.65.
33 Holmes, P. 2016 *Aromatica: A Clinical Guide to Essential Oil Therapeutics*, vol. 1. London: Singing Dragon, p.26.
34 Lizarraga-Valderrama, L.R. 2021 "Effects of essential oils on central nervous system: focus on mental health." *Phytotherapy Research*, 35(2), 657–79.
35 Cook, N. 2008 "Aromatherapy: reviewing evidence for its mechanisms of action and CNS effects." *British Journal of Neuroscience Nursing*, 4(12), 595–601; Ouldred, E. and Bryant, C. 2008 "Dementia care pt 2: understanding and managing behavioural challenges." *British Journal of Nursing*, 17(4), 242–7.
36 Proust, M. 2016 (1913–27) *À la Recherche du temps perdu*, trans. C.K. Scott-Moncrieff and S. Schiff. New York: Centaur.
37 Pert, C.B. 1997 *Molecules of Emotion.* New York: Scribner, p.27.

Chapter 5

1 McLendon, R. "How biophilia can improve your life." Treehugger. www.treehugger.com/how-biophilia-can-improve-your-life-4868182.
2 McLendon, R. "How biophilia can improve your life." Treehugger. www.treehugger.com/how-biophilia-can-improve-your-life-4868182.
3 Sudimac, S. *et al.* 2022 "How nature nurtures: amygdala activity decreases as the result of a one-hour walk in nature." *Molecular Psychiatry*, 27, 4446–52; Tost, H. *et al.* 2015 "Environmental influence in the brain, human welfare and mental health." *Nature Neuroscience*, 18(10), 1421–31; Peen, J. *et al.* 2007 "Is the prevalence of psychiatric disorders associated with urbanization?" *Social Psychiatry and Psychiatric Epidemiology*, 42(12), 984–9.
4 Wilson, E.O. 1984 *Biophilia*, revised edition. Cambridge, MA: Harvard University Press.
5 McLendon, R. "How biophilia can improve your life." Treehugger. www.treehugger.com/how-biophilia-can-improve-your-life-4868182; Sudimac, S. *et al.* 2022 "How nature nurtures: amygdala activity decreases as the result of a one-hour walk in nature." *Molecular Psychiatry*, 27, 4446–52; Takayama, N., Morikawa, T. and Bielinis, E. 2019 "Relation between psychological restorativeness and lifestyle, quality of life, resilience, and stress-coping in forest settings." *International Journal for Environmental Research in Public Health*, 16, 1456; Park, B.J. *et al.* 2010 "The physiological effects of Shinrin-yoku (taking in the forest atmosphere or forest bathing): evidence from field experiments in 24 forests across Japan." *Environmental Health Preventative Medicine*, 15, 18–26; Lee, J. *et al.* 2009 "The restorative effects of viewing real forest landscapes: based on a comparison with urban landscapes." *Scandinavian Journal of Forest Research*, 24, 227–34.

6 McLendon, R. "How biophilia can improve your life." Treehugger. www.treehugger.com/how-biophilia-can-improve-your-life-4868182; Kaplan, R. and Kaplan, S. 1995 *The Experience of Nature: A Psychological Perspective.* Ann Arbor, MI: Ulrich's Bookstore, pp.177–200.

7 Arvay, C. 2018 *The Biophilia Effect: Exploring the Healing Power of Nature.* Sounds True.

8 Berto, R. 2014 "The role of nature in coping with psycho-physiological stress: a literature review on restorativeness." *Behavioral Science (Basel)*, 4(4), 394–409; Takayama, N., Morikawa, T. and Bielinis, E. 2019 "Relation between psychological restorativeness and lifestyle, quality of life, resilience, and stress-coping in forest settings." *International Journal of Environmental Research Public Health*, 16, 1456.

9 Suskind, P. 1986 *Perfume: The Story of a Murderer.* New York: Knopf, pp.86–7.

10 Karan, D., quoted in "How to use perfume – a complete guide." COSIQ. https://mycosiq.com/blogs/news/how-to-use-perfume-a-complete-guide.

Chapter 6

1 Tompkins, P. and Bird, C. 1975 *The Secret Life of Plants.* Harmondsworth: Penguin, back cover blurb.

2 Tompkins, P. and Bird, C. 1975 *The Secret Life of Plants.* Harmondsworth: Penguin, p.43.

3 Montgomery, P. 2008 *Plant Spirit Healing.* Rochester, VT: Bear & Company, pp.xii, xiii.

4 Cited in Graves, J. 2012 *The Language of Plants. A Guide to the Doctrine of Signatures.* Great Barrington, MA: Lindisfarne Books, p.xiii.

5 Davis, P. 1991 *Subtle Aromatherapy.* Saffron Walden, UK: C.W. Daniel, p.3.

6 Birkmeyer, F. 2022 "Aromatic molecules, medicine of the soul and the alchemical journey." Blog, 13 September. aromagnosis.com

7 Warner, F. 2018 *Sacred Oils.* London: Hay House.

8 Maury, M. 1989 *The Secret of Life and Youth.* Saffron Walden, UK: C.W. Daniel, p.94.

9 Holmes, P. 2016 *Aromatica Vol. 1: Principles and Profiles.* London: Singing Dragon; Holmes, P. 2019 *Aromatica Vol. 2: Principles and Profiles.* London: Singing Dragon; Mojay, G. 1997 *Aromatherapy for Healing the Spirit.* Rochester, VT: Healing Arts Press; Zeck, R. 2014 *The Blossoming Heart*, 3rd edition. Invermay, Australia: Aroma Tours; Warner, F. 2018 *Sacred Oils.* London: Hay House.

10 Graves, J. 2012 *The Language of Plants, A Guide to the Doctrine of Signatures.* Great Barrington, MA: Lindisfarne Books; Lavabre, M. 1997 *Aromatherapy Workbook*, revised edition. Rochester, VT: Healing Arts Press.

11 Cited in Graves, J. 2012 *The Language of Plants, A Guide to the Doctrine of Signatures.* Great Barrington, MA: Lindisfarne Books, p.38.

12 Graves, J. 2012 *The Language of Plants, A Guide to the Doctrine of Signatures.* Great Barrington, MA: Lindisfarne Books, p.35.

13 Mojay, G. 1997 *Aromatherapy for Healing the Spirit.* Rochester, VT: Healing Arts Press; Holmes, P. 2016 *Aromatica Vol. 1: Principles and Profiles.* London: Singing Dragon; Holmes, P. 2019 *Aromatica Vol. 2: Principles and Profiles.* London: Singing Dragon.

14 Pénoël, D. and Pénoël, R.M. 1998 *Natural Home Health Care Using Essential Oils.* La Drome, France: Osmobiose, p.138.

15 Adams, E. 2017 "Pediatric experts find aromatherapy effective for promoting infant healing, NAS recovery." University of Kentucky News. https://uknow.uky.edu/uk-healthcare/pediatric-experts-find-aromatherapy-effective-promoting-infant-healing-nas-recovery.

16 Zeck, R. 2014 *The Blossoming Heart*, 3rd edition. Invermay, Australia: Aroma Tours, p.95.
17 Moss, M. 2014 "Halfway to Scarborough Fair? The cognitive and mood effects of rosemary and sage aromas." *International Journal of Clinical Aromatherapy*, 9(1&2), 1–7.
18 Mojay, G. 1997 *Aromatherapy for Healing the Spirit.* Rochester, VT: Healing Arts Press, p.115.
19 Price, S. and Price, L. 2012 *Aromatherapy for Health Professionals*, 4th edition. Amsterdam: Elsevier, p.212.
20 Davis, P. 1988 *Aromatherapy, an A to Z.* Saffron Walden: C.W. Daniel, p.141; Mojay, G. 1997 *Aromatherapy for Healing the Spirit.* Rochester, VT: Healing Arts Press, p.71.
21 Mojay, G. 1997 *Aromatherapy for Healing the Spirit.* Rochester, VT: Healing Arts Press, p.70.
22 Zeck, R. 2014 *The Blossoming Heart*, 3rd edition. Invermay, Australia: Aroma Tours, p.86; Pert, C.B. 1997 *Molecules of Emotion.* New York: Scribner, p.143.
23 Warner, F. 2018 *Sacred Oils.* London: Hay House, p.98.
24 Maury, M. 1989 *The Secret of Life and Youth.* Saffron Walden: C.W. Daniel, p.86; Holmes, P. 2019 *Aromatica Vol. 2: Principles and Profiles.* London: Singing Dragon, p.378.
25 Holmes, P. 2019 *Aromatica Vol. 2: Principles and Profiles.* London: Singing Dragon, p.378.
26 Mojay, G. 1997 *Aromatherapy for Healing the Spirit.* Rochester, VT: Healing Arts Press, p.113.
27 Burns, E. *et al.* 2000 "The use of aromatherapy in intrapartum midwifery practice: an observational study." *Complementary Therapy Nursing Midwifery*, 6(1), 33–4.
28 Zeck, R. 2014 *The Blossoming Heart*, 3rd edition. Invermay, Australia: Aroma Tours, p.80.
29 Holmes, P. 2016 *Aromatica Vol. 1: Principles and Profiles.* London: Singing Dragon, p.355.
30 Mojay, G. 1997 *Aromatherapy for Healing the Spirit.* Rochester, VT: Healing Arts Press, p.124.
31 Holmes, P. 2016 *Aromatica Vol. 1: Principles and Profiles.* London: Singing Dragon, p.359.
32 Davis, P. 1991 *Subtle Aromatherapy.* Saffron Walden: C.W. Daniel, p.224.
33 Holmes, P. 2016 *Aromatica Vol. 1: Principles and Profiles.* London: Singing Dragon, pp.141–8; Zeck, R. 2014 *The Blossoming Heart*, 3rd edition. Invermay, Australia: Aroma Tours, p.128.
34 Holmes, P. 2019 *Aromatica Vol. 2: Principles and Profiles.* London: Singing Dragon, p.436.
35 Zeck, R. 2014 *The Blossoming Heart*, 3rd edition. Invermay, Australia: Aroma Tours, p.118.
36 Zeck, R. 2014 *The Blossoming Heart*, 3rd edition. Invermay, Australia: Aroma Tours, p.91; Mojay, G. 1997 *Aromatherapy for Healing the Spirit.* Rochester, VT: Healing Arts Press, pp.80–1.
37 Holmes, P. 2019 *Aromatica Vol. 2: Principles and Profiles.* London: Singing Dragon, p.231.
38 Mojay, G. 1997 *Aromatherapy for Healing the Spirit.* Rochester, VT: Healing Arts Press, p.74; Davis, P. 1991 *Subtle Aromatherapy.* Saffron Walden: C.W. Daniel, p.205; Holmes, P. 2019 *Aromatica Vol. 2: Principles and Profiles.* London: Singing Dragon, pp.212–16.
39 Mojay, G. 1997 *Aromatherapy for Healing the Spirit.* Rochester, VT: Healing Arts Press, p.69.

40 Holmes, P. 2016 *Aromatica Vol. 1: Principles and Profiles.* London: Singing Dragon, p.183; Zeck, R. 2014 *The Blossoming Heart*, 3rd edition. Invermay, Australia: Aroma Tours, p.82.

41 Zeck, R. 2014 *The Blossoming Heart*, 3rd edition. Invermay, Australia: Aroma Tours, p.64; Warner, F. 2018 *Sacred Oils.* London: Hay House, p.69.

42 Mojay, G. 1997 *Aromatherapy for Healing the Spirit.* Rochester, VT: Healing Arts Press; Zeck, R. 2014 *The Blossoming Heart*, 3rd edition. Invermay, Australia: Aroma Tours.

43 Holmes, P. 2016 *Aromatica Vol. 1: Principles and Profiles.* London: Singing Dragon, pp.200–6.

44 Zeck, R. 2014 *The Blossoming Heart*, 3rd edition. Invermay, Australia: Aroma Tours, p.90; Mojay, G. 1997 *Aromatherapy for Healing the Spirit.* Rochester, VT: Healing Arts Press, pp.78–9.

45 Holmes, P. 2016 *Aromatica Vol. 1: Principles and Profiles.* London: Singing Dragon, p.309.

46 Holmes, P. 2016 *Aromatica Vol. 1: Principles and Profiles.* London: Singing Dragon, p.310.

47 Lehrner, J. *et al.* 2000 "Ambient odour of orange in a dental office reduces anxiety and improves mood in female patients." *Physiology and Behaviour*, 71(1/2), 83–6; Chidambara Murthy, K. *et al.* 2012 "D-limonene rich volatile oil from blood oranges inhibits angiogenesis, metastasis and cell death in human colon cancer cells." *Life Sciences*, 91(11/12), 429–39.

48 Zeck, R. 2014 *The Blossoming Heart*, 3rd edition. Invermay, Australia: Aroma Tours, p.110.

49 Mojay, G. 1997 *Aromatherapy for Healing the Spirit.* Rochester, VT: Healing Arts Press, p.102.

50 Mojay, G. 1997 *Aromatherapy for Healing the Spirit.* Rochester, VT: Healing Arts Press, p.122.

51 Zeck, R. 2014 *The Blossoming Heart*, 3rd edition. Invermay, Australia: Aroma Tours, p.130.

52 Mojay, G. 1997 *Aromatherapy for Healing the Spirit.* Rochester, VT: Healing Arts Press, p.117.

53 Holmes, P. 2019 *Aromatica Vol. 2: Principles and Profiles.* London: Singing Dragon, p.418.

54 Mojay, G. 1997 *Aromatherapy for Healing the Spirit.* Rochester, VT: Healing Arts Press.

55 Keim Loughram, J. and Bull, R. 2001 *Aromatherapy Anointing Oils.* Berkeley, CA: Frog.

56 Davis, P. 1991 *Subtle Aromatherapy.* Saffron Walden: C.W. Daniel, p.217; Warner, F. 2018 *Sacred Oils.* London: Hay House, p.175.

57 Warner, F. 2018 *Sacred Oils.* London: Hay House.

58 Holmes, P. 2019 *Aromatica Vol. 2: Principles and Profiles.* London: Singing Dragon, p.444.

59 Warner, F. 2018 *Sacred Oils.* London: Hay House.

Conclusion

1 Jackson, A. 2024 "People need this 'essential' cognitive ability—and fewer have it than ever before, says psychologist: 'It's a major concern.'" CNBC. www.cnbc.com/2024/06/26/technology-reliance-causes-loss-of-cognitive-ability-psychologist.html.

2 Guba, R. n.d. *The Aromatic Hologram Project.* www.aromatichologram.com.

3 Hari, J. 2018 *Lost Connections.* London: Bloomsbury Publishing, p.318.

Appendix

1 Cited in Harman, A. 2015 *Harvest to Hydrosol.* Fruitland, WA: IAG Botanics, p.7.
2 Mehmet Oz MD, cardiothoracic surgeon, cited in Buckle, J. 2015 *Clinical Aromatherapy: Essential Oils in Healthcare.* New York: Elsevier, pp.v–vi.
3 Harman, A. 2015 *Harvest to Hydrosol.* Fruitland, WA: IAG Botanics, p.7.
4 Holmes, P. 2016 *Aromatica: A Clinical Guide to Essential Oil Therapeutics*, vol. 1. London: Singing Dragon, p.26.
5 Buckle, J. 2015 *Clinical Aromatherapy: Essential Oils in Healthcare.* New York: Elsevier, p.145; Rai, M. and Kon, K. (eds) 2013 *Fighting Multidrug Resistance with Herbal Extracts, Essential Oils and Their Components.* New York: Elsevier.
6 Buckle, J. 2015 *Clinical Aromatherapy: Essential Oils in Healthcare.* New York: Elsevier, p.145; Kerkhof-Knapp Hayes, M. 2015 *Complementary Nursing in End of Life Care.* Netherlands: Kicozo; Tavares, M. 2011 *Integrating Clinical Aromatherapy in Specialist Palliative Care.* Marianne Tavares; Rose, C. 2023 *Integrating Clinical Aromatherapy in Palliative Care.* London: Singing Dragon; Schnaubelt, K. 2011 *The Healing Intelligence of Essential Oils.* Rochester, VT: Healing Arts Press.
7 Tisserand, R., Valussi, M., Cont, A. and Bowles, E.J. 2019 "Debunking functional group theory: not supported by current evidence and not a useful educational tool." Hons Tisserand Institute. https://tisserandinstitute.org/wp-content/uploads/2019/12/FGT_FINAL.pdf.
8 Bowles, E.J. 2003 *The Chemistry of Aromatherapeutic Oils*, 3rd edition. Crows Nest, NSW: Allen & Unwin.
9 Bowles, E.J. 2003 *The Chemistry of Aromatherapeutic Oils*, 3rd edition. Crows Nest, NSW: Allen & Unwin, p.65.
10 Bowles, E.J. 2003 *The Chemistry of Aromatherapeutic Oils*, 3rd edition. Crows Nest, NSW: Allen & Unwin; Holmes, P. 2016 *Aromatica Vol. 1: Principles and Profiles.* London: Singing Dragon; Holmes, P. 2019 *Aromatica Vol. 2: Principles and Profiles.* London: Singing Dragon; Pénoël, D. and Franchomme, P. 2001 *L'Aromatherapie exactement.* Paris: Roger Jollois; Battaglia, S. 2018 *The Complete Guide to Aromatherapy*, 3rd edition, vol. 1. Brisbane: Black Pepper Creative; Tisserand, R. and Young, R. 2014 *Essential Oil Safety*, 2nd edition. London: Churchill Livingstone; Harris, R. Advanced Clinical Aromatherapy Level One Residential Intensive. Provence. 26 June to 4 July 2014.
11 Harris, R. Advanced Clinical Aromatherapy Level One Residential Intensive. Provence. 26 June to 4 July 2014.
12 Pénoël, D. and Franchomme, P. 2001 *L'Aromatherapie exactement.* Paris: Roger Jollois.
13 Harris, R. Advanced Clinical Aromatherapy Level One Residential Intensive. Provence. 26 June to 4 July 2014.
14 -OH refers to a hydroxyl group which is a functional group containing one hydrogen and one oxygen atom.
15 Harris, R. Advanced Clinical Aromatherapy Level One Residential Intensive. Provence. 26 June to 4 July 2014.
16 Bowles, E.J. 2003 *The Chemistry of Aromatherapeutic Oils*, 3rd edition. Crows Nest, NSW: Allen & Unwin, p.75.
17 Bowles, E.J. 2003 *The Chemistry of Aromatherapeutic Oils*, 3rd edition. Crows Nest, NSW: Allen & Unwin, p.75.
18 GRAS is an acronym for the phrase "Generally Regarded As Safe" for substances under sections 201[s] and 409 of the Federal Food Drug and Cosmetic Act.
19 Bowles, E.J. 2003 *The Chemistry of Aromatherapeutic Oils*, 3rd edition. Crows Nest, NSW: Allen & Unwin, p.84.

20 Pénoël, D. and Franchomme, P. 2001 *L'Aromatherapie exactement.* Paris: Roger Jollois.

21 Bowles, E.J. 2003 *The Chemistry of Aromatherapeutic Oils*, 3rd edition. Crows Nest, NSW: Allen & Unwin, p.108.

22 Floracopeia 2024 "The absorption and effects of essential oils." www.floracopeia.com/the-absorption-and-effects-of-essential-oils.

23 Cited in Buckle, J. 2015 *Clinical Aromatherapy: Essential Oils in Healthcare.* New York: Elsevier, p.10.

24 Yücel, Ş.Ç., Arslan, G.G. and Bagci, H. 2020 "Effects of hand massage and therapeutic touch on comfort and anxiety living in a nursing home in Turkey: a randomized controlled trial." *Journal of Religion and Health*, 59(1), 351–64.

25 Zhihong, L. *et al.* 2021 "Benefits of hand massage on anxiety in preoperative outpatient: a quasi-experimental study with pre- and post-tests." *Explore (NY)*, 17(5), 410–16.

26 Erzincanli, S. and Kasar, K.S. 2021 "Effect of hand massage on pain, anxiety, and vital signs in patients before venipuncture procedure: a randomized controlled trial." *Pain Management Nursing*, 22(3), 356–60.

27 Chang, S.Y. 2008 "Effects of aroma hand massage on pain, state anxiety and depression in hospice patients with terminal cancer." *Taehan Kanho Hakhoe Chi*, 38(4), 493–502. Article in Korean.

28 Wang, H.L. and Keck, J.F. 2004 "Foot and hand massage as an intervention for postoperative pain." *Pain Management Nursing*, 5(2), 59–65.

29 Harvard Health Publishing 2014 "Regular massage improves circulation, stimulates muscles, reduces tension, often eases pain." www.health.harvard.edu/mind-and-mood/foot-massage-the-pause-that-refreshes-and-it-good-for-you.

30 Cheng, Y., Zhou, X. and Wang, G. 2023 "The efficacy of foot massage for pain relief of laparoscopic cholecystectomy: a meta-analysis study." *Surgical Laparoscopy, Endoscopy & Percutaneous Techniques*, 33(3), 286–90.

31 Chandrababu, R. *et al.* 2020 "Effects of foot massage and patient education in patients undergoing coronary artery bypass graft surgery: a randomized controlled trial." *Complementary Therapy Clinical Practice*, 40: 101215.

32 Sung, E.J. and Tochihara, Y. 2000 "Effects of bathing and hot footbath on sleep in winter." *Journal of Physiological Anthropology and Applied Human Science*, 19, 21–7.

33 Kim, B.S. and Chae, S.H. 2021 "The effects of aroma foot baths on stress and sleep in terminal cancer patients." *Journal of Hospice and Palliative Care*, 24(2), 109–15; Lee, J.H. *et al.* 2017 "The effects of aroma massage and foot bath on psychophysiological response in stroke patients." *Journal of Physical Therapy Science*, 29(8), 1292–6.

34 Pénoël, D. and Pénoël, R.M. 1998 *Natural Home Health Care Using Essential Oils.* La Drome, France: Editions Osmobiose, p.90.

35 Department of Health and Aged Care 2021 "Kunzea pain relief cream (360331)." www.tga.gov.au/resources/artg/360331.

36 Ming, H.T. 2017 "ALCHEMY a seemingly magical process of transformation, creation, or combination." (Unpublished document submitted in partial fulfilment of the requirements for the degree of Master of Architecture (Professional)). Unitec Institute of Technology, Auckland, New Zealand. Retrieved from https://hdl.handle.net/10652/4671

37 Harman, A. 2015 *Harvest to Hydrosol.* Fruitland, WA: IAG Botanics, p.14.

38 Catty, S. 2001 *Hydrosols: The Next Aromatherapy.* Vermont: Healing Arts Press, pp.10, 49.

39 Harman, A. 2015 *Harvest to Hydrosol.* Fruitland, WA: IAG Botanics, p.7.

40 Harman, A. 2015 *Harvest to Hydrosol.* Fruitland, WA: IAG Botanics, p.36.

Recommended Reading and Reputable Websites/Suppliers

This is by no means an exhaustive list; it is taken from my own library and experience. It is a starting point.

Recommended reading

Ashley, E. *Cannabis, CBD Rich Hemp Oil, Hemp Essential Oil and Hemp Seed Oil.* Elizabeth Ashley; 2017

Atterby, D. *Australian Essential Oil Profiles.* Australia: AAT Publishing; 2021

Battaglia, S. *The Complete Guide to Aromatherapy*, 3rd edition, vol. 1. Brisbane, Australia: Black Pepper Creative; 2018

Battaglia, S. *Aromatherapy & Chakras.* Queensland, Australia: Black Pepper Creative; 2020

Battaglia, S. *The Complete Guide to Aromatherapy*, 3rd edition, vol III *Psyche and Subtle.* Queensland, Australia: Black Pepper Creative; 2021

Baudoux, D. *Contemporary French Aromatherapy.* London: Singing Dragon; 2020

Bauermeister, E. *The Scent Keeper: A Novel.* New York: Saint Martin's Griffin; 2020

Bellebuono, H. *Women Healers of the World.* New York: Helios Press; 2014

Benavides, J. *Rest on Me, Breathe. Emotional Palliative Care.* Portugal: Edicoes Para a Alma; 2023

Bensouila, J. and Buck, P. *Aromadermatology.* Abingdon, Oxon: Radcliffe Publishing; 2006

Bowles, E.J. *The Chemistry of Aromatherapeutic Oils*, 3rd edition. NSW Australia: Allen and Unwin; 2003

Broom, B. *MEANing-full Disease.* Abingdon: Routledge; 2018

Brown, B. *Daring Greatly: How the Courage to Be Vulnerable Transforms the Way We Live, Parent, and Lead.* New York: Gotham Books; 2012

Brown, B. *Atlas of the Heart: Mapping Meaningful Connection and the Language of Human Experience.* New York: Random House; 2021

Buckle, J. *Clinical Aromatherapy: Essential Oils in Healthcare*, 3rd edition. St Louis, MO: Elsevier; 2015

Buhner, S.H. *The Lost Language of Plants.* New York: Chelsea Green Publishing; 2002

Buhner, S.H. *The Secret Teachings of Plants.* Rochester, VT: Bear and Company Books; 2004

Buhner, S.H. *Herbal Antivirals.* North Adams, MA: Storey Publishing; 2013

Buhner, S.H. *Plant Intelligence and the Imaginal Realm.* Rochester, VT: Bear and Company Books; 2014

Butje, A. *The Heart of Aromatherapy.* Carlsbad, CA: Hay House, Inc.; 2017

Cacioppo, J. *Loneliness: Human Nature and the Need for Social Connection.* New York: W.W. Norton; 2009

Catty, S. *Hydrosols: The Next Aromatherapy.* Vermont: Healing Arts Press; 2001

Chang, S.Y. "Effects of aroma hand massage on pain state, anxiety and depression in hospice patients with terminal cancer." *Taehan Kanho Hakhoe Chi,* 38(4), 493–502; 2008

Chapman, G. *The Five Love Languages.* Chicago: Northfield Publishing; 1992

Chopra, D. and Tanzi, R.E. *The Healing Self.* London: Rider; 2017

Conrad, P. *Women's Health Aromatherapy: A Clinical Evidence Based Guide for Nurses, Midwives, Doulas and Therapists.* London: Singing Dragon; 2019

Conrad, P. *Aromatherapy and Women's Mental Health: An Evidence Based Guide to Support Emotional Wellbeing.* London: Singing Dragon; 2023

Cooksley, V.G. *Aromatherapy: Soothing Remedies to Restore, Rejuvenate and Heal.* New York: Prentice Hall Press; 2002

Cope, S. *Deep Human Connection.* Carlsbad, CA: Hay House, Inc.; 2017

Davis, P. *Subtle Aromatherapy.* Saffron Walden: C.W. Daniel; 1991

De La Foret, R. *Alchemy of Herbs.* Carlsbad, CA: Hay House, Inc.; 2017

Fukuoka, M. *The One-Straw Revolution.* New York: New York Review of Books; 1978

Gattefossé, R.M. *Gattefossé's Aromatherapy,* ed. Robert Tisserand. London: Ebury Press; 1993

Goldberg, M. *Personality Types: The Enneagram for Success at Work.* London: Thorsons; 1997

Graves, J. *The Language of Plants: A Guide to the Doctrine of Signatures.* Great Barrington, MA: Lindisfarne Books; 2012

Green, J. *The Herbal Medicine Maker's Handbook.* New York: Crossing Press; 2000

Grosjean, N. *Aromatherapy from Provence.* Saffron Walden: C.W. Daniel; 1993

Guyett, C. *Sacred Plant Initiations.* Rochester, VT: Bear and Company Books; 2015

Hari, J. *Lost Connections.* London: Bloomsbury Publishing; 2018

Harman, A. *Harvest to Hydrosol,* 2nd edition. Fruitland, WA: IAG Botanics; 2023

Heckels, F. and Lawton, K. (The Seed Sistas) *The Sensory Herbal Handbook.* London: Watkins Media; 2019

Hobbs, C. *Medicinal Mushrooms: The Essential Guide.* North Adams, MA: Storey Publishing; 2020

Holmes, P. *Aromatica* Vol. 1. London: Singing Dragon; 2016

Holmes, P. *Aromatica* Vol. 2. London: Singing Dragon; 2019

Ilardi, S.S. *The Depression Cure: The 6 Step Programme to Beat Depression without Drugs.* Da Capo Press; 2009

Isted, M. *The Herball's Guide to Botanical Drinks.* London: Jacqui Small; 2018

Jones, E.A. *Awaken to Healing Fragrance: The Power of Essential Oil Therapy.* Berkeley, CA: North Atlantic Books; 2010

Kannis-Dymand, L. and Carter, J.D. *How to Deal with Anxiety.* London: John Murray Learning; 2015

Keller, J. *Healing with Water.* Bombay, India: Parker Publishing Company, Inc.; 1979

Kelly, R. *Healing Ways, A Doctor's Guide to Healing.* Auckland, NZ: Penguin Books; 2000

Kennedy, D.O. *Plants and the Human Brain.* New York: Oxford University Press; 2014

Kerkhof, M. *CO2 Extracts in Aromatherapy, 50+ Extracts for Clinical Applications.* Netherlands: Kicozo; 2018

Kerkhof, M. *Clinical AromaCare, Aromatherapy for Healthcare and Practice.* Netherlands: Kicozo; 2023

Kerkhof-Knapp Hayes, M. *Complementary Nursing in End of Life Care.* Netherlands: Kicozo-Knowledge Institute for Complementary Nursing; 2015

King, P. *Your Life Matters: The Power of Living Now.* Milson's Point, NSW: Random House Australia; 2003

Lama, D. and Tutu, D. *The Book of Joy.* London: Hutchinson; 2016

Lavabre, M. *Aromatherapy Workbook.* Vermont: Healing Arts Press; 1997

Levine, P. *In an Unspoken Voice.* California: North Atlantic Books; 2010

Low Dog, T. *Healthy at Home: Get Well and Stay Well without Prescriptions.* Washington DC: National Geographic Society; 2014

Lown, B. *The Lost Art of Healing.* New York: Ballantine Books; 1996

MacDonald, G. *Medicine Hands: Massage Therapy for People with Cancer*, 3rd edition. Findhorn: Findhorn Press; 2004

Mackereth, P. and Carter, A. (eds) *Massage and Bodywork: Adapting Therapies for Cancer Care.* Philadelphia: Churchill Livingstone; 2006

Mailhebiau, P. *Portraits in Oils.* Saffron Walden: C.W. Daniel; 1995

Mannix, K. *Listen. How to Find the Words for Tender Conversations.* Dublin: Harper-Collins; 2021

Martin, I. *Aromatherapy for Massage Practitioners.* Baltimore: Lippincott Williams & Wilkins; 2007

Mate, G. *When the Body Says No. Exploring the Stress-Disease Connection.* Nashville: Turner Publishing; 2003

Maury, M. *The Secret of Life and Youth*, trans. D. Ryman. Saffron Walden: C.W. Daniel; 1995

McGarey, W. *The Oil that Heals: A Physician's Successes with Castor Oil Treatments.* A.R.E. Press; 2002

McPherson, M. *et al.* "Social isolation in America: changes in core discussion networks over two decades." *American Sociological Review*, 71, 353–75; 2006

McTaggart, L. *The Intention Experiment: Using Your Thoughts to Change Your Life and the World.* New York: Free Press; 2007

Miflin, H. *The Green Fuse: Our Deep Connection with the Power of Plants.* Leicestershire: Matador; 2021

Mojay, G. *Aromatherapy for Healing the Spirit.* Singapore: Healing Arts Press; 1999

Montgomery, P. *Plant Spirit Healing.* Rochester, VT: Bear and Company Books; 2008

Murtagh, J. *General Practice.* Sydney: McGraw-Hill; 1998

Murthy, V. *Together: The Healing Power of Human Connection in a Sometimes Lonely World.* New York: HarperCollins; 2020

O'Donohue, J. *Anam Cara: Spiritual Wisdom from the Celtic World.* London: Bantam Press; 1997

O'Donohue, J. *Eternal Echoes: Exploring Our Hunger to Belong.* London: Bantam Press; 1998

O'Donohue, J. *To Bless the Space between Us.* New York: Doubleday; 2008

Parker, S.M. *Power of the Seed.* Port Townsend, WA: Process Media; 2014

Peace Rhind, J. *Essential Oils: A Handbook for Aromatherapy Practice.* London: Singing Dragon; 2012

Peace Rhind, J. *Essential Oils*, fully revised and updated 3rd edition: *A Comprehensive Handbook for Aromatic Therapy.* London: Singing Dragon; 2019

Pénoël, D. and Franchomme, P. (ed. Jollois, R.) *L'Aromatherapie exactement.* France: Roger Jollois; 2001

Pénoël, D. and Pénoël, R.M. *Natural Home Health Care Using Essential Oils.* La Drome, France: Osmobiose; 1998

Pert, C. *Molecules of Emotion.* New York: Scribner; 1997

Price, L. *Understanding Hydrolats: The Specific Hydrosols for Aromatherapy: A Guide for Health Professionals.* Edinburgh: Churchill Livingstone; 2004

Price, S. and Price, L. *Aromatherapy for Health Professionals*, 4th edition. Edinburgh: Churchill Livingstone; 2012

Purchon, N. and Cantele, L. *The Complete Aromatherapy and Essential Oils Handbook for Everyday Wellness.* Toronto: Robert Rose; 2014

Putnam, R. *Bowling Alone: The Collapse and Revival of American Community.* New York: Simon and Schuster; 2001

Rankin, L. *Mind over Medicine*, revised edition. Alexandria, NSW: Hay House Australia; 2020

Raven, S. *Nature Spirits: The Remembrance.* East Sussex: Clairview Books; 2012

Reynolds, M. *The Garden Awakening.* Cambridge: Green Books; 2016

Rose, C. *Integrating Clinical Aromatherapy in Palliative Care.* London: Jessica Kingsley Publishers; 2023

Rose, J. *The Aromatherapy Book.* Berkeley, CA: North Atlantic Books; 1992

Rose, J. *375 Essential Oils and Hydrosols.* Berkeley, CA: North Atlantic Books; 1999

Sade, D. *The Aromatherapy Beauty Guide.* Toronto: Robert Rose; 2017

Schnaubelt, K. *Advanced Aromatherapy: The Science of Essential Oil Therapy.* Rochester, NY: Healing Arts Press; 1995

Schnaubelt, K. Wholistic Aromatherapy: A Scientific Conference on Therapeutic Uses of Essential Oils. San Francisco, 4, 5 and 6 November 1995: Terra Linda Scent and Image; 1995

Schnaubelt, K. Science & Emotion: Proceedings of the 3rd Aromatherapy Conference on Therapeutic Uses of Essential Oils, 30, 31 October and 1 November 1998: Terra Linda Scent and Image; 1998

Schnaubelt, K. *Medical Aromatherapy.* Berkeley, CA: Frog; 1999

Schnaubelt, K. Essential Oils and Cancer: Proceedings of the 4th Scientific Wholistic Aromatherapy Conference. San Francisco, 10, 11 and 12 November 2000: Terra Linda Scent and Image; 2000

Schnaubelt, K. Essential Oils, Cancer, Degenerative and Autoimmune Disease: Proceedings of the 7th Wholistic Aromatherapy Conference, San Francisco, February 20, 21 and 22, 2009: Terra Linda Scent and Image; 2009

Schaubelt, K. *The Healing Intelligence of Essential Oils.* Vermont: Healing Arts Press; 2011

Schnaubelt, K. Unlimited Possibilities: Proceedings of the 8th International Aromatherapy Conference. San Francisco, 6, 7 and 8 November 2015: Terra Linda Scent and Image; 2015

Stringer, J. "Infection in the clinical environment: challenges and benefits of using essential oils – a therapist's perspective." *International Journal of Clinical Aromatherapy*, 4(2), 32–4; 2010

Tavares, M. *Integrating Clinical Aromatherapy in Specialist Palliative Care.* Canada: Marianne Tavares; 2011.

Tisserand, R. *The Art of Aromatherapy.* Saffron Walden: C.W. Daniel; 1997

Tisserand, R. and Young, R. *Essential Oil Safety*, 2nd edition. Churchill Livingstone; 2014

Tomkins, P. and Bird, C. *The Secret Life of Plants.* London: Allen Lane; 1974

Tree, I. *Wilding.* London: Picador; 2018

Turkle, S. *Reclaiming Conversation: The Power of Talk in a Digital Age.* New York: Penguin Random House; 2015

Valnet, J. *The Practice of Aromatherapy*, ed. R. Tisserand. Rochester, VT: Healing Arts Press; 1990

Van der Kolk, B. *The Body Keeps the Score.* New York: Viking Penguin; 2014

Waldinger, R. and Schulz, M. *The Good Life and How to Live It. Lessons from the World's Longest Study on Happiness.* London: Rider; 2023

Walker, M. *Why We Sleep.* Harmondsworth: Penguin Books; 2018

Warner, F. *The Soul Midwives' Handbook.* London: Hay House; 2013

Warner, F. *Sacred Oils.* London: Hay House; 2018

Wilson, E.O. *Biophilia*, revised edition. Cambridge, MA: Harvard University Press; 1984

Worwood, V. *The Fragrant Mind.* New World Library; 1996

Worwood, V. *Aromatherapy for the Soul.* New World Library; 1999
Young, R. *The Secret Life of Cows.* London: Faber & Faber; 2017
Youngson, R.A. *Time to Care.* Raglan, NZ: Rebelheart Publishers; 2012
Zeck, R. *The Blossoming Heart.* Invermay, Australia: Aroma Tours; 2014

Websites

https://clinicalaromatherapynetwork.com (ICAN)

www.florihana.com

www.aromaticsinternational.com

www.absoluteessential.co.nz

www.essentiallyaustralia.com.au

www.floracopeia.com

www.kicozo.com

www.oshadhi.co.uk

www.naturesgift.com

www.originalswissaromatics.com

https://circlehinstitute.com

www.alembics.co.nz

www.heartmath.org

www.lifeextension.com: The Science of a Healthier Life

www.dropsmart.io

www.labaroma.com

Courses/Classes/Lectures

Tisserand Institute

www.tisserandinstitute.org

Aromahead Institute

www.aromahead.com

Essence of Thyme College of Holistic Studies

www.essenceofthyme.com

The School of Aromatic Studies

www.aromaticstudies.com

École Internationale de Sante Bien-Etre

www.eibe-formation.com

Naturopathic CE

www.naturopathicce.com

The Herbal Hub

www.theherbalhub.com

Airmid Institute

https://airmidinstitute.org

International Clinical Aromatherapy Network (ICAN)

https://clinicalaromatherapynetwork.com

Journals

International Journal of Clinical Aromatherapy (now incorporated into the ICAN platform)

https://ijca.net

International Journal of Holistic Aromatherapy

www.ijpha.com

Aromatherapy Today

www.aromatherapytoday.com

Aromatika

www.aromatikamagazine.com

Printed in Great Britain
by Amazon

59946104R00092